METHOTREXATE

PHARMACOLOGY, CLINICAL USES AND ADVERSE EFFECTS

PHARMACOLOGY - RESEARCH, SAFETY TESTING AND REGULATION

Additional books in this series can be found on Nova's website
under the Series tab.

Additional E-books in this series can be found on Nova's website
under the E-book tab.

METHOTREXATE

PHARMACOLOGY, CLINICAL USES AND ADVERSE EFFECTS

VALENTINA S. CASTILLO
AND
LAURA A. MOYANO
EDITORS

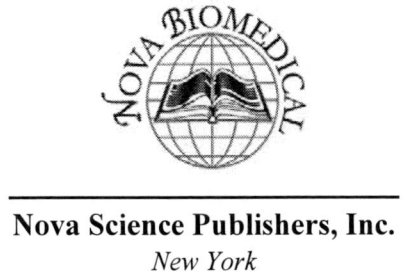

Nova Science Publishers, Inc.
New York

Library of Congress Cataloging-in-Publication Data

Methotrexate : pharmacology, clinical uses, and adverse effects / editors, Valentina S. Castillo and Laura A. Moyano.
     p. ; cm.
  Includes bibliographical references and index.
  ISBN 978-1-62100-596-4 (hardcover)
  I. Castillo, Valentina S. II. Moyano, Laura A.
  [DNLM: 1. Methotrexate. 2. Neoplasms--drug therapy. QU 188]

  615.7'39--dc23
                        2011035679

Published by Nova Science Publishers, Inc. ✛ *New York*

Contents

Preface

Methotrexate (MTX) is an important component of therapy in several immune diseases (rheumatoid arthritis, psoriasis, and cancers such as acute lymphoblastic leukemia, osteosarcoma, ovarian cancer and others). Despite its clinical success, treatment with MTX often causes toxicity, dose reduction or treatment cessation. In this book, the authors present topical research in the study of the pharmacology, clinical uses and adverse effects of methotrexate. Topics discussed include lipid alterations instigated by methotrexate; acute toxicity of high doses of methotrexate in the treatment of lymphoblastic leukemia in children; pharmacogenetics update on MTHFR and methotrexate toxicity; animal models of cognitive impairment induced by methotrexate and damage, as well as the recovery of the bone and bone marrow following methotrexate chemotherapy.

Chapter I – This chapter examines the effect of antineoplastic agent, methotrexate, on lipid composition of female reproductive tract in rats. It is well recognized that methotrexate (MTX) causes abnormal development of female reproductive tract in young women treated for non-neoplastic diseases, for whom preservation of gonadal function is important. The advent of combination therapy has made it difficult to evaluate the toxic effects of individual drugs, therefore animal models to study each drug separately becomes a necessity to understand the mechanisms of gonadal toxicity. Leucovorin (LCN), a folinic acid is an antidote to MTX, therefore, emphasis has been laid on its supplementation and withdrawal of MTX treatment to evaluate whether the effects are either rescued or reversed once the exposure ceases. Previous studies on rats distinctly revealed MTX's deleterious effects on the histopathology, hormones and steroid markers of female reproductive tract. Lipids are essential for the reproductive events and serves as an energy source. Consequently, the importance of lipids in maintenance of normal function of female reproductive tract is unequivocal. Female reproductive cells accumulate lipids for their metabolism, but there have been few attempts to carefully correlate alterations in lipid levels with the metabolic changes occurring after MTX treatment. This chapter is the first of its kind to delineate the effect of methotrexate on total lipids, cholesterol, glyceride glycerol, phospholipids and their fractions in ovary, oviduct, uterus, cervix and vagina of albino rats. MTX inhibition of total lipids was dose and tissue dependent. This was chiefly due to the reduction of phospholipids content in the organs. Total cholesterol levels increased dose dependently in all the organs except cervix. A differential tissue specific effect of the drug was observed on total glyceride glycerol levels. LCN supplementation and withdrawal of MTX treatment, did not recover these concentrations to levels observed in controls. Further exploration of the fractions of cholesterol, *viz;* free and esterified cholesterol; glyceride glycerol fractions *viz;* mono, di and triacyl glycerol and phospholipid fractions *viz;* inositol, choline, ethanolamine, serine, sphingomyelin, phosphatidic acid and cardiolipin revealed variations in their levels, which was MTX dose and tissue dependent. Some fractions recouped to normalcy or near normalcy by LCN supplementation or withdrawal of treatment, while others did not retrieve. Such changes were tissue dependent. These results unambiguously illustrate that MTX has multiple mechanisms of actions, and that lipid genes are target to the deleterious effects of the drug on female reproductive tract of rats.

Chapter II – various malignancies. With leucovorin rescue and standard supportive care, HD-MTX carries a low risk for severe treatment-related toxicity. However, some patients experience a delay in methotrexate (MTX) elimination and develop a HD-MTX induced renal failure which may be life threatening. Glucarpidase cleaves glutamate from MTX resulting in the formation of a non-toxic metabolite and in a rapid reduction in MTX serum concentration. We describe a case of HD-MTX induced renal failure in a 12 year old boy successfully treated with glucarpidase. *Design.* Case report. *Main outcome measures.* To evaluate the efficacy of glucarpidase, MTX serum concentration (MTXs) before and after glucarpidase administration were registered. Data related to renal function was also registered. *Results.* A 12 year old patient with an acute lymphoblastic leukemia started his first consolidation chemotherapy cycle with HD-MTX (5g/m2=7.2g) but during the infusion the patient developed fever and MTX administration was stopped after only 1,1g. Twenty-four hours later, MTXs was 5.50 µM. Leucovorin rescue was started, but MTXs at 36h was 4.75 µM. Serum creatinine was also increased from initial 53.04 µmol/L to 238.68 µmol/L. The calculated creatinine clearance (18 ml/min/1.73m2) demonstrated a renal failure. The patient was admitted to the pediatric intensive care unit and treated with rasburicase, hyperhidratation and furosemide, but MTXs and serum creatinine were still high: 38 h post-infusion concentration was 3.91 µM and creatinine was 256.36 µmol/L. Glucarpidase was then administered at a dose of 2000UI (50 UI/kg). A pronounced and rapid reduction in circulating MTX was observed: 0.53 µM (56h), 0.26 µM (68h), 0.13 µM (80h), 0.09 µM (92h) and renal function was normalised. *Conclusions.* In this case, glucarpidase was effective in reducing serum MTX levels and in normalizing renal function after intoxication with HD-MTX.

Chapter III - Methotrexate (MTX) is an important component of therapy in several immune diseases (rheumatoid arthritis, psoriasis...) and cancers (acute lymphoblastic leukaemia, osteosarcoma, ovarian cancer...). Despite its clinical success, treatment with MTX often causes toxicity, dose reduction or treatment cessation being necessary. Several toxicities have been reported, including nodulosis, hypersensitive pneumonitis, central nervous system toxicity, postdosing reactions, gastrointestinal symptoms such as nausea, vomiting, abdominal pain, and diarrhoea, hepatitis with elevated transaminase levels, hematologic abnormalities, rash, alopecia and osteopathy.

For drugs such as MTX, with a very narrow therapeutic index, every effort should be made to minimize interpatient variability in drug exposure in order to maximize the benefit while keeping the risk of serious adverse effects at an acceptable level. Therefore, for appropriate use of MTX, it would be useful to identify predictors of the MTX adverse effects.

In this context, pharmacogenetics is gaining relevance. Pharmacogenetics studies the inherited genetic variations involved in drug response, with the aim to prospectively individualize the selection of medications and their doses to enhance efficacy and safety.

MTHFR is a key enzyme for intracellular folate homeostasis and metabolism. The non-synonymous C677T and A1298C variants in the 5,10-methylenetetrahydrofolate reductase (MTHFR) gene are among the most studied genetic polymorphisms for identifying predictors of response to methotrexate. An alteration in reduced folate pools, derived from inherited changes in MTHFR activity, may have a significant effect on the response to methotrexate, whose activity depends on cellular composition of folate.

The MTHFR 677T allele encodes proteins with decreased enzymatic activity, so people with the CT genotype exhibit only 60% of the MTHFR activity and those with the TT genotype demonstrate 30% bioactivity. MTHFR 1298C allele is responsible for a milder decrease in MTHFR activity, CC individuals having 60% of the normal activity.

In this chapter, we perform an extensive review of the studies that analyze the association of these two MTHFR polymorphisms with MTX toxicity in different diseases. We find that there is a great heterogeneity among studies but, after a deep analysis of the literature data, we conclude that MTHFR C677T and A1298C polymorphisms do not appear to be good MTX toxicity markers in most of the cases.

Chapter IV - Methotrexate formerly known as amethopterin is an antimetabolite drug. It is a 4-amino substituted folic acid analogue. The mechanism of action of methotrexate is by competitive inhibition of dihydrofolate reductase (DHFR), an enzyme required for the synthesis of tetrahydrofolate. Tetrahydrofolate is essential for the de novo synthesis of DNA and methotrexate inhibits folate-dependent thymidylate production in cells. Thus, methotrexate inhibits DNA synthesis, which is essential for cell replication and repair in cancer and normal cells.

Methotrexate acts specifically during the S phase of the cell cycle when the cell is undergoing synthesis of DNA. Methotrexate is therefore effective in cancers involving rapidly proliferating cells. Although initially used only in cancer, methotrexate is now widely used for several nonmalignant conditions also. The latter has been possible in part with extensive research and understanding of the pharmacotherapeutics of the drug, and effective monitoring of methotrexate therapy in patients. Methotrexate for example is also used as an immunosuppresant and in small doses as an antinflammatory agent in autoimmune and other non-cancerous diseases. Since Methotrexate acts on rapidly dividing cells, the adverse effects of this medication target those tissues, which rapidly replicate with a fast turn over. We review pharmacology, clinical applications and adverse effects of methotrexate in this chapter.

Chapter V - In the late 1940's methotrexate was developed for use primarily in haematological malignancies. Used at much lower doses, it has subsequently become an established treatment for a range of autoimmune conditions including: rheumatoid arthritis, psoriasis and psoriatic arthropathy, Crohn's disease, connective tissue disease and Felty's syndrome.

Methotrexate is a structural analogue of folic acid. It competitively inhibits binding of dihydrofolic acid to the enzyme dihydrofolate reductase. The amount of intracellular folinic acid (the active metabolite of dihydrofolic acid) is thereby decreased, and intracellular metabolic pathways dependent on folinic acid affected. Purine and pyrimidine metabolism are two such pathways. Whilst these pathways are considered important, the exact mechanism of action by which methotrexate exerts clinical effect remains elusive.

Low dose methotrexate has been shown to cause aplastic marrow failure, pulmonary fibrosis and liver toxicity, including cirrhosis. Hence strict monitoring and review becomes necessary. In 1982, the dermatology community released guidelines recommending regular liver biopsy once a critical cumulative dose (1.5g) was reached. These guidelines were initially applied to patients with rheumatoid arthritis treated with low dose methotrexate. Subsequent research revealed a good correlation between liver enzymes and histological changes on liver biopsy, and regular blood test monitoring has since been widely practiced as a screening tool for early liver disease. Low dose methotrexate can also cause nausea and vomiting and a significant minority of patients become intolerant due to these troublesome adverse effects.

Methotrexate is contraindicated in certain situations namely pregnancy, localised or systemic infection, renal impairment and unexplained cytopenia associated with marrow failure. Several drug interactions are also associated with its use.

Despite these problems, methotrexate has remained the first line agent in many diseases for many years. It is generally well tolerated and displays good efficacy.

We provide an overview of the use of low dose methotrexate in autoimmune conditions with respect to pharmacology, clinical uses, adverse effects and monitoring schedules.

Chapter VI - Methotrexate (MTX) is an antimetabolic agent that affects the metabolism of folic acid. The drug entered clinical medicine as an innovative antineoplastic drug in 1948, after the detection of its indirect effects on DNA synthesis. Although by a different mechanism, it resembled corticosteroid drugs by acting on the proliferation of connective tissue. The drug has thus been used in the treatment of psoriasis, psoriatic arthritis and rheumatoid arthritis (RA). Since then, studies have been carried out on the effectiveness, toxicity, doses and other features of methotrexate. It has also been compared more recently with different rheumatic drugs, such as corticosteroids and new immunosuppressive drugs, such as inhibitors of specific molecular components of inflammation.

Increases in the number of patients treated with methotrexate and increases in doses are universal. It is now commonly administered in combination with either biological agents or other small-molecule antirheumatic drugs. Combination therapies have been more effective than either monotherapy, without increasing toxicity.

Chapter VII - Sustained elevation of serum methotrexate (MTX) concentrations (>1.0 µM) for 48 h (48-h value) has been found to have predictive significance for the development of toxicity. However, severe adverse events are sometimes encountered during high-dose (HD)-MTX therapy even if serum MTX concentrations comply with recommended values. We designed and conducted a retrospective study to identify predictors for the occurrence of adverse events, and examined whether the 48-h value alone offers a significant predictor of clinical adverse events during HD-MTX therapy. The results showed that 48-h value is not the only predictive value for clinical adverse events during HD-MTX therapy, identifying long infusion time as a significant predictor of general fatigue and neutropenia and higher doses and combination chemotherapy as predictors for stomatitis. This chapter discusses predictors for clinical adverse events during HD-MTX therapy based on our study (retrospective study, n=58 episodes) and further review of recent findings, including genetic factors.

Chapter VIII - Methotrexate is an antimetabolite commonly used in adjuvant combination chemotherapy treatments. Patients treated with methotrexate have frequently complained of cognitive impairment. This phenomenon encompasses problems with memory and concentration and is reported to occur in many cancer survivors for several years after treatment.

Attempts to quantify these effects by psychometric testing of patients has been confounded by factors, including multi drug treatments, patient stress and fatigue and the effect of the cancer itself.

This has led to the use of rodent models to study chemotherapy-induced cognitive impairment. These studies have allowed the investigation of single chemotherapy agents and are not compromised by the confounding factors associated with patient testing. Animal investigations have used a range of behavioural tests including the Morris water maze, novel object/location recognition tasks and conditioning to investigate the effects of methotrexate on behaviour.

These tests have shown that methotrexate can significantly impair a range of memory paradigms. Furthermore research in rodents has allowed the investigation of potential underlying mechanisms including the effects of methotrexate on the proliferation, survival and apoptosis of cells involved in adult hippocampal neurogenesis and the demyelination of white matter tracts. Herein, we review this research and discuss potential approaches for intervention.

Chapter IX - The bone marrow microenvironment is home to mesenchymal and haematopoietic stem cells, and the interaction between these cell types and their respective progeny allows the maintenance of a steady-state functioning marrow, bone formation and turnover throughout life. Unfortunately, cancer chemotherapy, which commonly includes the anti-metabolite methotrexate (MTX), is a serious risk factor that disrupts homeostasis of the bone marrow and compromises bone formation, leading to myelosuppression and bone loss. MTX has been shown to cause significant damage to the bone marrow and reduce bone volume in both clinical and animal studies. Although the severity of damage to the bone marrow and the degree of ensuing recovery of marrow cell populations are dependent on the MTX dose and length of treatment, in order to re-establish the depleted marrow cavity, haematopoietic stem cells maintained at endosteal niche sites are induced to enter the cell cycle and differentiate down the appropriate lineage. Associated with damaged bone marrow stromal cells and a differentiation switch to adipogenesis at the expense of osteogenesis, are bone loss, increased marrow fat and fracture risk. This chapter will discuss mechanisms of how MTX chemotherapy causes myelosuppression, bone loss and marrow adiposity as reported in both clinical and animal studies, and will summarise changes in the relationship between cells of the mesenchymal and haematopoietic lineages in relation to MTX-induced damage and recovery of the bone and bone marrow.

Chapter X - *Objective*. The purpose of this study was to evaluate the effect of Imunoglukan ® , β-(1,3/1,6)-D-glucan isolated from *Pleurotus ostreatus* (β-glucan-PO) on prophylactic treatment of adjuvant arthritis (AA) with methotrexate (MTX) in rats. *Methods*. Groups of rats with AA were treated with methotrexate (1 mg/kg/week), β-glucan-PO (1 mg/kg every second day) or their combination for the period of 28 days from adjuvant application. Body mass, hind paw swelling, arthrogram scores and a level of serum albumin were measured as markers of inflammation and arthritis. *Results*. Treatment with low dose of MTX significantly inhibited the markers of both inflammation and arthritis. MTX and its combination with β-glucan-PO significantly increased body mass of arthritic rats. β-glucan-PO administered alone significantly decreased both the hind paw swelling and arthritic score. In combination with MTX, β-glucan-PO markedly potentiated the beneficial effects of MTX, which resulted in a more significant reduction of hind paw swelling and arthritic scores. The concentration of albumin in the serum of arthritic controls was significantly lower than in healthy controls. Both MTX alone and the combination treatment with MTX + β-glucan-PO significantly inhibited the decrease in serum albumin. *Conclusion.* β-glucan-PO increased the treatment efficacy of basal treatment of AA with MTX.

Chapter XI - Methotrexate (MTX) ($C_{20}H_{22}N_8O_5$) is an antimetabolite analogue of folic acid (4-amino-10-methylfolic acid) and is derived from N_{10} methylation of its precursor amethopterin. MTX is used as anti-inflammatory, antiproliferative and immunosuppressant agents for systemic treatments of plaque psoriasis, psoriatic erythroderma, generalized pustular psoriasis, nail psoriasis, palmoplantar psoriasis, and psoriatic arthritis. MTX is also used in combination with other medicine to increase the efficacy or reduce adverse effects. Contraindications and special precautions are supposed to be considered with care during MTX administration. MTX is absorbed and intracellularly accumulated as MTX-poly glutamates. It may induce liver toxicity with high doses in a long period. During MTX administration, liver enzymes increase, but only a few patients develop liver diseases. Hematologic toxicity and serious cytopenias were reported in patients with renal insufficiency or depleted folate storages without folic acid supplements. Different from the liver and the blood whose injury and toxicity are reversible, lung toxicosis may be fatal. Following MTX application, lung injury could happen at any time, even within a few weeks. Malignancies of MTX are considered co-carcinogenic, and malignant changes are elicited by synergistical effects with compounds. In addition, other side effects of MTX include carcinogenesis teratogenicity, direct potential mutagenic action, etc. MTX toxicities are numerous and involve almost any organ system.

Chapter XII - Methotrexate (MTX) is a purine analog antimetabolite that is widely used in the treatment of neoplastic disease, rheumatoid arthritis, and severe psoriasis. Uptake of MTX into cells is dependent upon the reduced folate carriers (RFCs), while the cellular level of MTX is maintained by its polyglutamylation. The development of MTX resistance, which reduces MTX efficacy in a variety of disease treatments, has been discussed in many studies. Resistance factors include defective or slow uptake of MTX with RFCs or increased efflux via ATP-binding cassette (ABC) multidrug transporters, certain alterations in targeted enzymes, genetic polymorphisms, impaired MTX polyglutamylation, increased salvage and increased metabolism of MTX. However, the pharmacokinetic and cellular resistance mechanisms of MTX are still not completely understood. This chapter discusses current knowledge of the molecular basis of MTX resistance based on data obtained from both pre-clinical and clinical studies. In addition, emerging mechanisms for MTX treatment are also discussed. An in-depth understanding of the molecular mechanisms behind the MTX resistance could help facilitate the optimal use of antifolate therapy as well as new drug development.

In: Methotrexate
Editors: V. S. Castillo and L. A. Moyano

ISBN: 978-1-62100-596-4
© 2012 Nova Science Publishers, Inc.

Chapter I

Lipid Alterations Instigated by Methotrexate and Leucovorin in Female Reproductive Tract of Albino Rats

Karri Sritulasi[1],*, G. Vanithakumari[1]
and Coimbatore Gopalakrishnan[2]

[1]Department of Zoology, School of Life Sciences, Bharathiar University,
Coimbatore, Tamilnadu, India
[2]The Institute of Environmental and Human Health,
Texas Tech University, Lubbock, TX, US

Abstract

This chapter examines the effect of antineoplastic agent, methotrexate, on lipid composition of female reproductive tract in rats. It is well recognized that methotrexate (MTX) causes abnormal development of female reproductive tract in young women treated for non-neoplastic diseases, for whom preservation of gonadal function is important. The advent of combination therapy has made it difficult to evaluate the toxic effects of individual drugs, therefore animal models to study each drug separately becomes a necessity to understand the mechanisms of gonadal toxicity. Leucovorin (LCN), a folinic acid is an antidote to MTX, therefore, emphasis has been laid on its supplementation and withdrawal of MTX treatment to evaluate whether the effects are either rescued or reversed once the exposure ceases. Previous studies on rats distinctly revealed MTX's deleterious effects on the histopathology, hormones and steroid markers of female reproductive tract. Lipids are essential for the reproductive events and serves as an energy source. Consequently, the importance of lipids in maintenance of normal function of female reproductive tract is unequivocal. Female reproductive cells

---

* Corresponding author: Karri Sritulasi. E-mail: sritulasi@gmail.com.

accumulate lipids for their metabolism, but there have been few attempts to carefully correlate alterations in lipid levels with the metabolic changes occurring after MTX treatment. This chapter is the first of its kind to delineate the effect of methotrexate on total lipids, cholesterol, glyceride glycerol, phospholipids and their fractions in ovary, oviduct, uterus, cervix and vagina of albino rats. MTX inhibition of total lipids was dose and tissue dependent. This was chiefly due to the reduction of phospholipids content in the organs. Total cholesterol levels increased dose dependently in all the organs except cervix. A differential tissue specific effect of the drug was observed on total glyceride glycerol levels. LCN supplementation and withdrawal of MTX treatment, did not recover these concentrations to levels observed in controls. Further exploration of the fractions of cholesterol, *viz;* free and esterified cholesterol; glyceride glycerol fractions *viz;* mono, di and triacyl glycerol and phospholipid fractions *viz;* inositol, choline, ethanolamine, serine, sphingomyelin, phosphatidic acid and cardiolipin revealed variations in their levels, which was MTX dose and tissue dependent. Some fractions recouped to normalcy or near normalcy by LCN supplementation or withdrawal of treatment, while others did not retrieve. Such changes were tissue dependent. These results unambiguously illustrate that MTX has multiple mechanisms of actions, and that lipid genes are target to the deleterious effects of the drug on female reproductive tract of rats.

Keywords: Cervix, Cholesterol, Glyceride glycerol, Leucovorin, Lipids, Methotrexate, Ovary, Oviduct, Phospholipids, Uterus, Vagina

Introduction

Methotrexate (MTX), known as amethopterin was the first chemotherapeutic drug introduced in late 1940s capable of inducing complete remissions in children with acute lymphoblast leukemia [1]. MTX is extensively used as a component of combination therapy for neoplastic diseases [2,3]. MTX inhibits the synthesis of nucleic acids, thymidylates and proteins [4] by inhibiting dihydrofolate reductase (DHFR) an enzyme that participates in the tetrahydrofolate synthesis [5]. In the presence of NADPH, MTX binds to DHFR [6] and inhibits *de novo* synthesis of the nucleoside thymidine a prerequisite for DNA synthesis, thereby acts as a folic acid antagonist [4]. MTX subdues folate, an essential participant in purine base synthesis causing toxic effect on rapidly dividing cells, suppressing the growth and proliferation in malignant and some non-cancerous cells [7]. MTX is used in combination therapy to treat several non-neoplastic diseases like arthritis [8], spondylitis [9], psoriasis [10], ectopic pregnancy [11], gestational trophoblastic neoplasia [12], interstitial twin pregnancy [13], and as an abortifacient [14]. Toxicity of MTX on skeletal growth [15], hepatic [16], pulmonary [17], neuro [18], nephro [19], and reproductive systems is extensively reported [20,21,22,23]. MTX usage for non-neoplastic and non-malignant diseases across the globe and the risk factors in reproductive health of young women [24,25,26] is soaring, which is an undesirable side effect. Thus, there is a critical need to understand the mechanism(s) of MTX toxicity and prevention of its side effects in non-neoplastic conditions.

Reduction of folic acid, a pro-vitamin, in the body is by dihydrofolate reductase (DHFR) to form dihydrofolate (DHF) and tetrahydrofolate (THF) [27]. Disruption of the folate metabolism causes deficiency in either DHF or THF metabolites essential for the biosynthetic pathway of nucleic acids, lipids and proteins [28,29]. Leucovorin (LCN), a folinic acid is often expended as an antidote in MTX therapy, where it acts as a 'rescue agent' to MTX's side effects [22,30]. Folinic acid is a 5-formyl derivative of tetrahydrofolic acid [31] readily converted to THF, and thus has folic acid like vitamin activity [32]. However, since it does not require the action of DHFR for its conversion, its function as a vitamin is unaffected by MTX [30,33]. Thus, LCN given after MTX administration induced synchronous recovery of DNA synthesis and RNA transcription [34], and protects from MTX induced toxicity. Our recent reports establish the effects of MTX and LCN on the histopatholgy, carbohydrate metabolism markers, steroidogenic genes in female reproductive tissues and serum steroids and gonadotropins [35,36,37]. Studies also revealed the antiprogestational, antiestrogenic and antiimplantation activities of MTX in rats [38,39]. The current chapter explores the effect of MTX, LCN supplementation and withdrawal of MTX influence on the lipid profiles (cholesterol, glyceride glycerol and phospholipids) in female reproductive tract of rats.

Lipids play a vital role not only in providing a source of nutrient to the cell, but also in modifying the physical properties and functions of biological membranes [40]. In addition, lipids have potent effects on cell-cell interactions, cell proliferation and transport [40]. Furthermore, the activities of membrane proteins depend on their immediate lipid environment, and the ability of hormone receptor complexes to bind to effector molecules may be modulated by the head group and fatty acid composition of membrane lipids [41,42]. Cholesterol is an indispensable component of cell membranes, involved in the clearance and digestion of fats, and is the precursor of all steroid hormones [43]. Extensive modification of cholesterol dynamics in a population may lead to surprising consequences. There is evidence that a minimum amount of body fat (26 to 28%) is required for reproductive function in women [43]. Also, cholesterol concentration is related to increased fertility, number of transferable embryos [44,45] and inversely related to days to conception [46]. Cholesterol is an essential structural component of mammalian cell membranes [47,48] and is the major regulator of numerous cellular processes including signal transduction, receptor function, gene expression, cell growth, and lipoprotein synthesis [49,50]. A change in cholesterol levels is reported upon MTX treatment in arthritis patients [51]. Gonadal steroids regulate circulating concentrations of cholesterol [52]. Estradiol can increase cholesterol concentrations (*via* endogenous biosynthesis), and the highest circulating cholesterol concentrations are found during estrus [53,54]. Treatment with testosterone decreases cholesterol synthesis [53] and progesterone inhibits the synthesis *via* stimulation of sterol suppressors [55]. Gonadotropins increase available free cholesterol by increasing lipoprotein receptor number and by increasing hydrolysis of stored cholesterol ester. In the absence of available lipoprotein, gonadotropins stimulate cholesterol synthesis *de novo* from acetate in the cell [56]. StAR protein mediates the rate-limiting step in steroidogenesis, the transfer of cholesterol from the outer to the inner mitochondrial membrane, where it is cleaved to pregnenolone by the inner membrane-bound $P450_{SCC}$ enzyme [57]. Also, the expression of StAR protein is stimulated *via* a cyclic AMP signalling pathway and is correlated with an acute steroidogenic response to tropic hormone stimulation [58,59].

Glycerides, known as acylglycerols, are esters formed from glycerol and fatty acids, whose primary function is energy storage. Although glucose is the major precursor of glyceride glycerol, pyruvate and certain gluconeogenic amino acids can also be converted to glyceride-glycerol at appreciable rates [60,61,62]. For the supply of structural components for membrane production and the storage of excess calories in animal cells, the production of glycerolipids, glycerophospholipids and triacylglycerol's is important [63,64]. The dividing cells require a constant supply of glycerophospholipids for membrane production, whereas diets rich in carbohydrates result in increased production of fatty acids, which are stored as triglycerides [63]. Dysregulation of glycerolipid biosynthesis results in a number of pathologies [64].

Phospholipids are diglycerides, which are a major component of all cell membranes forming the lipid bilayer [65]. Phosphatidic acid is the precursor for the anionic phospholipids, phosphatidylinositol, phosphatidylglycerol, and cardiolipin, whereas diacylglycerol is the precursor for the quantitatively most prominent phospholipids, choline, ethanolamine, and serine, as well as for triacylglycerol [65]. Choline is the precursor for the biosynthesis of membrane phospholipids and sphingomyelin. It is well known that choline, methionine and folate metabolism are interrelated [66] and any disturbance in the folate metabolism would perturb methionine and choline synthesis. Choline is the only single nutrient for which dietary deficiency is associated with the development of cancer [67,68]. Phosphatidyl serine is an essential phospholipid for the growth of mammalian cells, localized in the inner (cytoplasmic) side of the bilayer and is a minor component of the plasma membrane [69]. The synthesis of phosphatidyl serine occurs primarily in the endoplasmic reticulum, but significant amounts are found in Golgi and nuclear membrane. Phosphatidyl serine in mitochondrial membrane is decarboxylated to form phosphatidyl ethanolamine [70]. Though sphingolipids are vital for normal function of an organism, aberrant sphingolipid metabolism participates in various pathophysiology including diabetes and ulcers [71,72]. Cardiolipin (CL) is a complex mitochondrial-specific phospholipid that regulates numerous enzyme activities especially those related to oxidative phosphorylation and coupled respiration. CL is found exclusively in the inner mitochondrial membrane where it constitutes about 20% of the total lipid composition and is essential for the optimal function of numerous enzymes that are involved in mitochondrial energy metabolism. It is suggested that abnormalities in CL can impair mitochondrial function and bioenergetics [73]. In addition to inherited mutations, somatic mutations in tumor suppressor/oncogenes or aneuploidy could also produce mitochondrial defects, thus causing CL abnormalities [74,75,76]. CL abnormalities might also arise from a variety of epigenetic causes involving abnormalities in cellular proliferation, metabolic flux, and calcium homeostasis [77,78]. A variety of environmental insults, including necrosis, hypoxia/ischemia, dietary imbalances, and reactive oxygen species, could also alter CL content and/or composition, thus contributing to tumor initiation or progression [79,80,81]. CL abnormalities through numerous genetic, epigenetic, and environmental factors is linked to tumor cells [73].

Significant differences in lipid homeostasis in female reproductive tract organs lead to various clinical complications [74,82] and lipid signaling plays a vital role in the function and pathology of reproductive system [83]. Alterations in membrane lipid levels can also influence cell proliferation and viability [84]. Control of ovary, oviduct, uterus, cervix and vagina functions represents a very complex and intriguing regulatory pattern of cell growth and steroid production. The nature of granulosa cells changes from the chief protein-synthesizing cells in follicles to the lipid synthesizing cells in the corpora lutea [85]. Lipid granules in ovaries are confined to the interstitial tissue and comprise cholesteryl esters, triacylglycerol and phospholipids. Free cholesterol and the cholesterol ester triacylglycerol ratio fall during follicular growth [86]. Total lipids increase progressively and significantly with the growth of the follicles in the rat ovary [87]. Glycerides are the main fraction of total lipids in regressing corpora lutea [88]. The low phospholipid content in the ovary is attributed to the decreased intracellular membranes of the follicle cells. The luteal cells show abundant diffuse lipoproteins and lipid droplets consisting of triglycerides, phospholipids and some triglycerides, which are indicative of steroidogenesis [87]. Sphingomyelin although synthesized in the intracellular region is transported to the plasma membranes of ovarian cells [89]. An increase in phosphatidic acid synthesis is observed when phosphatidyl inositol hydrolysis increases [90]. Terminally differentiated gamete cells, various sterols, sphingolipids, glycolipids, and glycosyl phosphatidyl inositol (GPI) anchored proteins are localized on cell membrane microdomains that are called lipid rafts [91,92]. Since lipid rafts in gametes contain signaling proteins that regulate intracellular functions and cell signaling, these domains are important for sperm maturation, fertilization, and early embryogenesis [93,94].

Various lipids influence events that normally take place within the oviduct, such as sperm capacitation, the acrosome reaction, and early embryo development [95,96]. Lipid droplets have been detected in epithelial cells of the oviduct and their numbers are reported to fluctuate with endocrine status. Cellular lipids increase in oviduct epithelial monolayers in response to estradiol treatment [97]. Regional differences in the relative ability of oviducal explants to synthesize lipids were also apparent. The predominant lipid synthesized and detected in culture supernatants was cholesterol. Lipid content in oviduct cells varied in composition with the ovarian cycle and oviducal region [98]. Oviduct epithelium exhibits regional differences in phospholipid and neutral lipid distribution [99]. Oviduct is capable of significant de novo synthesis of a variety of lipids in vitro, and that this synthesis is affected by the stage of the ovarian cycle and the increase in total lipid present in oviducal fluid around oestrous [100]. Fatty acids apparently are essential for the survival of rabbit [101] and mouse embryos [102], which are taken up by zygotes [103], and are incorporated into neutral glycerides by embryos developing in vitro [104]. Oviducal lipids also serve as a source of substrates for embryos to synthesize phospholipids [105] and sterols [106]. The role of the oviducal epithelium may be to regulate cholesterol availability within the lumen. Loss of membrane cholesterol results in a decreased cholesterol: phospholipid ratio and increased membrane fluidity associated with capacitation and the acrosome reaction [107]. Regional differences exist in localization of oviducal neutral lipid droplets and phospholipid containing choline. Concentrations of neutral lipid droplets, free cholesterol, and glycerides were highest in the preampulla and ampulla and least in the isthmus. These differences in epithelial lipids may reflect changes in the luminal environment and may affect the membranes of sperm and early embryos. In the isthmus, phospholipid-containing choline in mucosal crypts and high amounts of epithelial esterified cholesterol may play a role in sperm storage [99,108].

Many factors are known to influence uterine contractility *via* interaction with the myometrial cell membrane, e.g., receptors and ion channels. Estrogen increases total lipid content in rat uterus, while progesterone and LH decrease activity and lipid accumulation in cells [97,109,110]. The presence of lipid in epithelium and stroma seems mainly a degenerative phenomenon associated with cell break down and convergent tissue disruption [111]. The influence of hormones on lipids and their role in uterine signaling and contractility, cholesterol levels are well established [112,113]. Bulk phospholipids do not change in the myometrium with pregnancy [114], but changes in membrane fluidity and increased cholesterol occur [115]. With the use of thin-layer chromatography [116], it has also been reported that there are higher cholesterol levels compared with total phospholipid content in pregnant myometrium. Many changes in lipid metabolism occur in pregnant women, including significant increases in cholesterol and triglycerides [117,118]. These changes in lipid metabolism have been suggested to help maintain an adequate supply of nutrients to the growing fetus [119]. Women with low cholesterol levels might be at risk for increased uterine activity and possibly premature labor [120]. The synthesis of triacylglycerol (TAG) is an important metabolic pathway for the control of lipid metabolism and maintenance of energy homeostasis in all mammals [121].

Lipid content, and the fatty acid composition are related to the three phases of the menstrual cycle and correlate with the hormonal variation [122]. The amount of total lipids decrease during mid cycle and variations in lipid components persists in menstrual cycle. Cyclic changes in human cervical mucus glycerides, free fatty acids and sterol ester fatty acids were reported. Triglycerides differ from mono, diglycerides, and free fatty acids, containing the most saturated fatty acids in cervix [122]. The lipid content of cervical and vaginal cells is related to the stage of differentiation of their epithelium in the estrogenic and progesteronic phases and in atrophy. Four main fractions of lipids: triglycerides, phospholipids, cholesterol and cholesterol esters are major components of cervix and vaginal cells [123]. Lipid globules in vaginal epithelium vary with cyclic variations in volume and quantity as a function of the phase of the cycle [124]. Enhanced phosphatidylinositol lipid turnover in immature rats demonstrates involvement in the early events of oestradiol-induced rat vaginal cell differentiation [125]. Lipid metabolism undergoes an alteration as pregnancy advances in the placenta. The nature of the lipid changes suggests an increase in physiological activity beginning as early as the 20th day and this increase in physiological activity is concerned with the transfer of lipids from mother to fetus through the mediation of placental tissues. Such an increase in placental physiological activity may be related to the production of sex hormones [126,127].

The reproductive health effects of cancer treatments specifically affect younger women as adjuvant chemotherapy often causes ovarian failure and amenorrhea leading to early menopause [128,129]. Ovarian failure after chemotherapy has an unfavorable effect on serum lipids in premenopausal cancer patients [130]. Menopause causes changes in serum lipids that are explained by the deficiency of estrogens [131,132]. The defect in lipid rafts may result in failed tolerance induction at the maternal-fetal interface, which would lead to the occurrence of recurrent spontaneous abortion [133]. Patients with cervical cancer show low mean values of all lipid fractions [134]. Phosphatidylcholine and sphingomyelin are shown to be the major phospholipids in cancerous and normal cervical tissues respectively with a significant elevation in all the phospholipid levels of cancerous ones in comparison with the normal [135]. The above-mentioned literature evidently indicates the importance of lipids and its fractions in maintenance of normal reproductive cell function. In addition, lipids serve as the biomarkers in clinical complications hence this study to address the lipid alterations by methotrexate in female reproductive tract of albino rats is therefore unequivocal.

Protection of MTX toxicity is a serious concern in combination therapy in non-neoplastic diseases. Studies involving alterations in lipid markers occurring in female reproductive tract due to MTX treatment may help detect metabolism alterations occurring in reproductive tissues. Reproductive failure is a common trend in young women subjected to MTX treatment for non-neoplastic diseases. Like cancer cells reproductive cells are fast proliferating and MTX treatment causes reproductive failure. Our recent reports unravel the effects of MTX and LCN on the histopatholgy of ovary, oviduct, uterus, cervix and vagina, carbohydrate metabolism markers, steroidogenic genes, progesterone, estradiol, FSH and LH [35,36,37].

Studies also reveal the antiprogestational, antiestrogenic and antiimplantation activity of MTX in rats [38,39]. Therefore, the current study aims to evaluate the effect of MTX and LCN on lipid profiles in female reproductive tract of albino rats.

Although several clinical studies address the discrepancies brought about in lipid profiles in neoplastic diseases, very few studies are available on the effects of individual anticancer drugs on lipid profiles in female reproductive tract in non-neoplastic condition. We hypothesize that lipids being vital for cell differentiation, growth and hormone synthesis may also be a target to MTX in non-neoplastic condition. Hence, it is vital to establish studies pertaining to the effect of methotrexate on lipid profiles in female rat model. The purpose of the present study was therefore, to enquire into the possible alterations in the lipid fractions in the female reproductive tract of rats. Consequently, the aim was to study (a) the effects of MTX on lipids and its fractions in female reproductive system (b) if the use of leucovorin (LCN) acts as a rescue agent and (c) if withdrawal of treatment brings back the MTX-caused effects to normalcy. The focus was to investigate the following parameters (a) total lipids (b) total cholesterol and its fractions free and esterified cholesterol (c) total glyceride glycerol and its fractions mono, di and triacyl glycerol (d) total phospholipids, phosphatidyl inositol, choline, ethanolamine, serine, sphingomyelin, phosphatidic acid and cardiolipin in ovary, oviduct, uterus, cervix and vagina of rats.

Materials and Methods

Animals

Procedures for treatment and harvesting tissues were adapted from recently published work [37]. Briefly, healthy adult female albino rats of Wistar strain, showing normal 4-5 days oestrous cycle, were used in this study. They were housed with 12h alternate light-dark cycle. Food and water were provided ad libitum. All animal experiments were carried out in accordance with the guidelines of the Institutional Animals Ethics Committee.

Study Design

Methotrexate (MTX) sodium salt and leucovorin (LCN) calcium salt were obtained from M/S Cynamide India Ltd., (Lederle division), India. Two different doses of MTX, 0.05mg and 0.15mg/kg body weight were chosen to study the long-term effects. The doses were used based on our previous studies for inhibition of various markers in female reproductive tract [37]. The period for complete follicle maturation has been calculated to be 19 days [136] and such matured follicles were disrupted by MTX in 20 days [37]. As LCN supplementation is an antidote to MTX, we included LCN and withdrawal of MTX treatment in the present chapter.

Rats with regular oestrous cycle were randomly divided into five groups (n=6) as follows:

- Group 1: Control: Vehicle saline
- Group 2: MTX LD (low dose): 0.05mg/kg body weight
- Group 3: MTX HD (high dose): 0.15mg/kg body weight
- Group 4: MTXHD + LCN (leucovorin): 0.015mg/kg body weight (LCN)
- Group 5: MTXHD+WD (withdrawal): 20 days withdrawal

Animals were treated once per day intramuscularly (im) for 20 days to study the effects for 4 consecutive oestrous cycles. LCN was injected after 4h of MTXHD treatment. Rats were sacrificed on day 21. High dose MTX treated rats with respective control group were separated and the treatment was withdrawn for additional 20 days and animals sacrificed on day 41 [37]. The ovary, oviduct, uterus, cervix and vagina were dissected and used for lipid analysis.

Analytical Methods

Extraction of Lipids

Ovarian, oviduct, uterine, cervix and vagina lipids were extracted as by the method of Folch [137]. Briefly, tissue was homogenized in chloroform: methanol (2:1 v/v) containing butylated hydroxy toluene (BHT) and centrifuged at 3000xg for 10min. The process was repeated thrice, the supernatants were pooled and concentrated at 40-45°C in a flask rotator vacuum evaporator. Evaporated sample was resuspended in 20ml chloroform: methanol (2:1v/v) containing 4% water and evaporated at 40°C in vacuo. This process was repeated thrice and residue was quantitatively taken up in 100ml chloroform: methanol (2:1 v/v) containing 0.1% BHT in a separating funnel. After the addition of 20ml of 0.1M NaCl, the funnel was swirled for few minutes and allowed to stand without disturbance. The lower phase which contains the lipid component was collected and evaporated at 40°C in vacuo. The residue of total lipid extract was taken up quantitatively in 5ml of $CHCl_3$ and stored at -20°C for further analysis of lipid classes.

Total Lipid Analysis

Total lipids were estimated by the method of Frings et al [138]. Briefly, 200 µl of concentrated H_2SO_4 was added to 200µl lipid extract and vortexed rigorously and incubated at 100°C for 10 min in an oven and cooled for 5 min. The phospho-vanillin reagent was prepared by adding 800 ml of 85% phosphoric acid to 200 ml of 0.6% (w/v) vanillin in water. After adding 10ml of phosphovanillin reagent, the contents were vortexed and incubated at 37°C in a water bath for 15 min. Following cooling the color developed was measured at 540nm. A reagent blank and set of standards using olive oil 10mg/dl diluted in absolute ethanol were run simultaneously. The total lipid concentration of the sample was calculated from the standard graphs and expressed as mg/g tissue.

Total Cholesterol Analysis

Cholesterol was analyzed by the method of Hanel and Dam [139]. In brief, 100 µl of lipid extract was evaporated to dryness, the residue was dissolved in 2ml of chloroform, 26.14% ZnCl2 in glacial acetic acid (w/v) and 98% of acetyl chloride and mixed well. The tubes were incubated in a water bath at 65°C for 15 min. The tubes were chilled on an ice bath and then allowed to come to room temperature. The intensity of eosin red color was read at 528 nm against a reagent blank. Standards were run parallel to the samples using cholesterol (Sigma) and values expressed as mg/g tissue.

Total Glyceride Glycerol Analysis

A method described by Van Handel and Silver smith [140] was used to analyze glyceride glycerol. 50µl of lipid extract was evaporated to dryness. 500µl of 0.1N alcoholic KOH was added to the tubes and kept at 60-70°C in oven for 15min. After cooling to room temperature 500µl of 0.4N H_2SO_4 was added, tubes were placed in a boiling water bath for 15 min. Subsequent to cooling 100µl of 0.05M sodium metaperiodate was added. After 10 mins 100µl of 20% $NaSO_4$ (w/v) was added. Then 5ml of 1.92% of chromotrophic acid reagent (w/v) was added, mixed and incubated for 30 min in boiling water bath. After cooling, the color was measured at 570nm. A reagent blank and standard of tripalmitin were run simultaneously and the glyceride concentration was calculated from the standard value and expressed as mg/g tissue.

Total Phospholipids Analysis

The method of Fiske and Subbarow [141], as per Marinetti [142] was employed for phospholipid analysis. 100 µl of lipid extract was evaporated to dryness. 1ml of 60% perchloric acid was added and the contents were digested on a hot sand bath (150-200°C) for 15min. After cooling 7ml of distilled water, 2.5% ammonium molybdate (w/v) and 0.2ml of 1-amino-2-naphthol-4-sulfonic acid (ANSA) reagent were added in that order. After each addition the tubes were vortexed and placed in boiling water bath for 7 min. Tubes were brought to room temperature for 20 min and the blue color formed was measured at 830nm. A reagent blank and a set of standards of sodium dihydrogenphosphate were also run simultaneously with the samples. The amount of phosphorous obtained was multiplied by 25 [143] and the phospholipid concentration expressed as mg/g tissue.

Separation of Neutral Lipids

Separation of neutral lipids; free cholesterol, esterified cholesterol, mono, di and triacyl glycerol was achieved by thin layer chromatography coated with Silica Gel G using three solvent systems of n hexane: diethyl ether: glacial acetic acid (60:40:1; 90:10:1; 30:70:1, respectively) [144]. 50 µg of lipid extract was applied, the spots were identified in an iodine chamber, scraped into tubes, and individual fractions were eluted with 5ml chloroform. Individual neutral lipids were quantified by the methods of total cholesterol and total glyceride glycerol as described earlier [139,140].

Separation of Phospholipid Fractions

Individual phosphatides were also separated by thin-layer chromatography on Silica Gel G by using a solvent system of chloroform: methanol: ammonia (7N) (115:45:7.5 v/v) as described by Abramson and Bleecher [145]. 15 µg of lipid extract was applied in each lane and the Phosphatides were identified as blue spots by spraying molybdenum blue spray as proposed by Dittmer and Wells [146]. The identified spots were scraped out into test tubes and eluted with a mixture of chloroform: methanol: formic acid: water (97:97:4:2 v/v). The phosphorous in individual fractions was quantified as described earlier [142,143].

Statistical Analysis

Prism software (version 4.02, Graph Pad Inc., San Diego, CA, USA) was used for graphical presentation and statistical analysis. Data are presented as standard error mean (SEM) values of 'n' independent experiments with variability given as mean ± SE. Analyses of variance (ANOVA) performed included one-way ANOVA for matched samples followed by Newman–Keuls post-hoc test of differences between all group means. P < 0.05 was considered statistically significant.

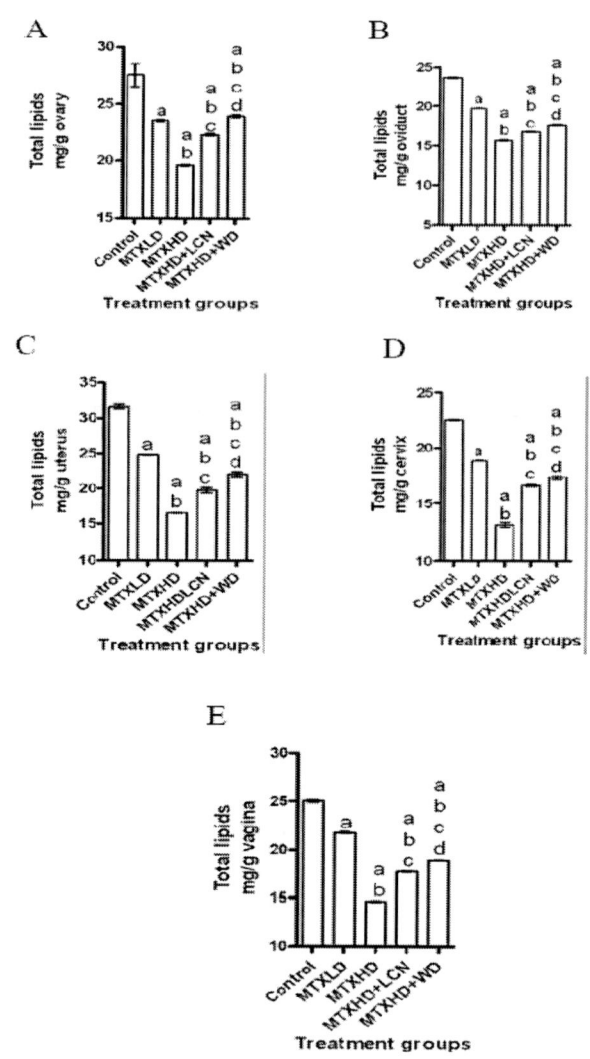

Figure 1 (A–E). Effect of MTX on total lipids in ovary (A), oviduct (B), uterus (C), cervix (D) and vagina (E) of rats. MTX = methotrexate, LD = low dose, HD =high dose, LCN = leucovorin, WD = withdrawal. P < 0.05, 'a' vs. Control, 'b' vs. MTX LD, 'c' vs. MTX HD, 'd' vs. MTX+LCN. Note marked reduction in total lipids in the tissues dose dependently by MTX treatment. Total lipid levels remained low after LCN supplementation and withdrawal of MTX treatment compared to control groups.

Results

Effect of MTX on Total Lipids (Figures 1A-E)

Ovary (Figure 1A): Total lipid concentrations in the ovary decreased perceptibly by MTX and such levels were dose dependent. Compared to the control group, total lipids significantly (P<0.001) decreased in MTXLD, MTXHD, MTXHD+LCN and MTXHD+WD groups. The levels further decreased significantly (P<0.001) in MTXHD and MTXHD+LCN groups compared to MTXLD. While, in MTXHD+WD the levels increased significantly (P<0.001) compared to the rest of the groups, although such levels were lower than the control group.

Oviduct (Figure 1B): A marked decrease in total lipid concentrations in the oviduct by MTX was dose dependent. The total lipids concentrations in MTXLD, MTXHD, MTXHD+LCN and MTXHD+WD significantly (P<0.001) decreased compared to the control group. These levels further decreased significantly (P<0.001) in MTXHD, MTXHD+LCN and MTXHD+WD groups compared to MTXLD. The levels increased significantly (P<0.001) in MTXHD+LCN and MTXHD+WD compared to MTXHD. In MTXHD+WD group such levels were further increased significantly (P<0.001) compared to MTXHD+LCN group.

Uterus (Figure 1C): Total lipid levels significantly (P<0.001) decreased in uterus of MTX treated rats dose dependently. Compared to the control group, total lipid concentrations in MTXLD, MTXHD, MTXHD+LCN and MTXHD+WD decreased significantly (P<0.001). In MTXHD, MTXHD+LCN and MTXHD+WD groups total lipid levels further decreased significantly (P<0.001) compared to MTXLD. Although, the levels increased significantly (P<0.001) in MTXHD+LCN and MTXHD+WD groups compared to MTXHD. In MTXHD+WD group further significant (P<0.001) increase was observed compared to MTXHD+LCN group.

Cervix (Figure 1D): Significant (P<0.001) levels of total lipid decreased by MTX dose dependently in the cervix of rats. Compared to the control group, the total lipids in MTXLD, MTXHD, MTXHD+LCN and MTXHD+WD decreased significantly (P<0.001). In MTXHD, MTXHD+LCN and MTXHD+WD groups the levels further decreased significantly (P<0.001) compared to MTXLD. In MTXHD+LCN and MTXHD+WD groups the levels increased significantly (P<0.001) compared to MTXHD. Levels in MTXHD+WD group further increased significantly (P<0.001) compared to MTXHD+LCN group.

Vagina (Figure 1E): MTX treatment significantly (P<0.001) decreased vaginal total lipid, which was dose dependent. Compared to the control group, the total lipid concentrations in MTXLD, MTXHD, MTXHD+LCN and MTXHD+WD decreased significantly (P<0.001). In MTXHD, MTXHD+LCN and MTXHD+WD groups the levels further decreased significantly (P<0.001) compared to MTXLD. Although, in MTXHD+LCN and MTXHD+WD groups the levels increased significantly (P<0.001) compared to MTXHD. Levels in MTXHD+WD group further increased significantly (P<0.001) compared to MTXHD+LCN group.

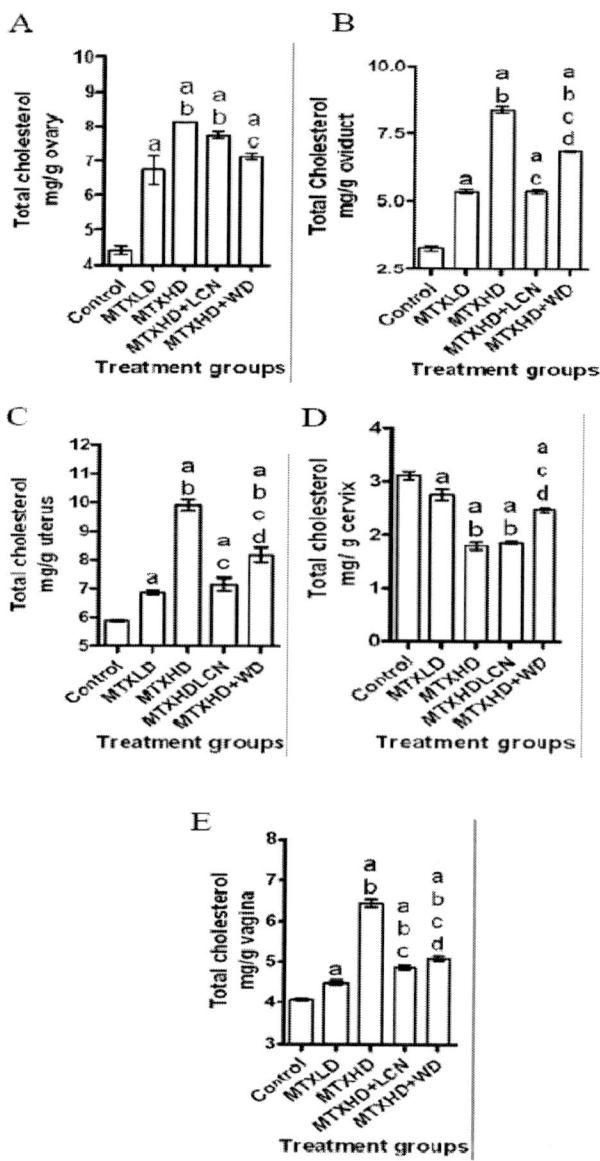

Figure 2 (A–E). Effect of MTX on total cholesterol in ovary (A), oviduct (B), uterus (C), cervix (D) and vagina (E) of rats. MTX = methotrexate, LD = low dose, HD =high dose, LCN = leucovorin, WD = withdrawal. P < 0.05, 'a' vs. Control, 'b' vs. MTX LD, 'c' vs. MTX HD, 'd' vs. MTX+LCN. Note marked increase in total cholesterol in ovary, oviduct, uterus and vagina and a decrease in the levels in cervix dose dependently. Also note the reduction in the levels after LCN supplementation and withdrawal of MTX treatment and a reverse effect in cervix.

Effect of MTX on Total Cholesterol (Figures 2A-E)

Ovary (Figure 2A): MTX caused a dose dependent shift in the total cholesterol concentrations in the ovary. Compared to the control group, total cholesterol concentrations in MTXLD, MTXHD, MTXHD+LCN and MTXHD+WD increased significantly (P<0.001). In

MTXHD, MTXHD+LCN groups the levels further increased significantly (P<0.001) compared to MTXLD. Although, in MTXHD+WD group the levels decreased significantly (P<0.001) compared to MTXHD.

Oviduct (Figure 2B): MTX caused a dose dependent change in the total cholesterol concentrations in the oviduct. Compared to the control group, total cholesterol concentrations in MTXLD, MTXHD, MTXHD+LCN and MTXHD+WD increased significantly (P<0.001). Cholesterol concentrations in MTXHD group increased significantly (P<0.001) compared to MTXLD. In MTXHD+LCN and MTXHD+WD groups the cholesterol levels decreased significantly (P<0.001) compared to MTXHD. Nevertheless, MTXHD+WD group cholesterol levels were significantly higher than MTXLD and MTXHD+LCN groups.

Uterus (Figure 2C): MTX caused a dose dependent change in the total cholesterol concentrations in the uterus. Compared to the control group, total cholesterol concentrations in MTXLD, MTXHD, MTXHD+LCN and MTXHD+WD increased significantly (P<0.001). Cholesterol concentrations increased significantly (P<0.001) in MTXHD group compared to MTXLD. While in MTXHD+LCN and MTXHD+WD groups the cholesterol levels decreased significantly (P<0.001) compared to MTXHD. On the other hand, MTXHD+WD group cholesterol levels were significantly higher than MTXLD and MTXHD+LCN groups.

Cervix (Figure 2D): Compared to other organs, MTX had a dose dependent reverse effect in total cholesterol concentrations in cervix. Compared to the control group, total cholesterol concentrations in MTXLD, MTXHD, MTXHD+LCN and MTXHD+WD decreased significantly (P<0.001). Additional decrease in cholesterol concentrations was significant (P<0.001) in MTXHD group compared to MTXLD, while the levels remained unchanged in MTXHD+LCN group compared to MTXHD group. MTXHD+WD group cholesterol levels increased significantly (P<0.001) compared to MTXHD and MTXHD+LCN groups. In MTXHD+WD group cholesterol levels significantly (P<0.001) increased compared to MTXHD and MTXHD+LCN groups.

Vagina (Figure 2E): MTX caused dose dependent alterations in the vaginal total cholesterol. Compared to the control group, total cholesterol concentrations in MTXLD, MTXHD, MTXHD+LCN and MTXHD+WD increased significantly (P<0.001). Further, total cholesterol concentration increased significantly (P<0.001) in MTXHD group compared to MTXLD. While in MTXHD+LCN and MTXHD+WD groups the cholesterol levels decreased significantly (P<0.001) compared to MTXHD. On the other hand, cholesterol levels in MTXHD+LCN and MTXHD+WD groups were significantly (P<0.001) higher than MTXLD and MTXHD+LCN groups.

Effect of MTX on Free Cholesterol (Figures 3A-E)

Ovary (Figure 3A): MTX caused a significant decrease in free cholesterol levels in ovary dose dependently. Compared to the control group, free cholesterol concentrations in MTXLD, MTXHD, MTXHD+LCN and MTXHD+WD decreased significantly (P<0.001) in the ovary. Further, free cholesterol concentration decreased significantly (P<0.001) in MTXHD group compared to MTXLD. While in MTXHD+LCN group the free cholesterol levels increased significantly (P<0.001) compared to MTXHD. Cholesterol levels in MTXHD+WD groups remained significantly (P<0.001) lower than MTXLD, MTXHD and MTXHD+LCN groups.

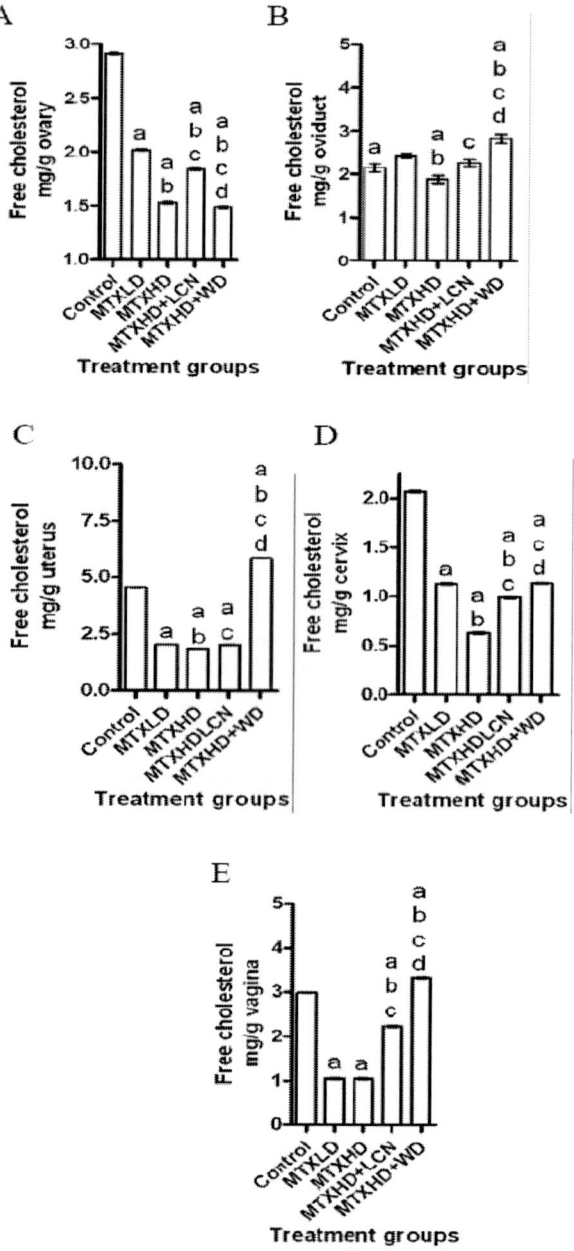

Figure 3 (A–E). Effect of MTX on free cholesterol in ovary (A), oviduct (B), uterus (C), cervix (D) and vagina (E) of rats. MTX = methotrexate, LD = low dose, HD =high dose, LCN = leucovorin, WD = withdrawal. P < 0.05, 'a' vs. Control, 'b' vs. MTX LD, 'c' vs. MTX HD, 'd' vs. MTX+LCN. Note marked reduction in free cholesterol in the organs dose dependently by MTX treatment. LCN supplementation brought about a partial restoration and withdrawal of MTX treatment brought about a complete reversal in oviduct, uterus and vagina.

Oviduct (Figure 3B): MTX caused a significant (P<0.001) decrease in free cholesterol levels in oviduct in MTXHD group and an increase (P<0.001) in MTXHD+WD group, no significant change in MTXLD and MTXHD+LCN groups were observed compared to the control group. Free cholesterol concentration decreased significantly (P<0.001) in MTXHD group compared to MTXLD. In MTXHD+LCN group free cholesterol levels increased significantly (P<0.001) compared to MTXHD. Cholesterol levels in MTXHD+WD groups significantly (P<0.001) increased compared to the control, MTXLD, MTXHD and MTXHD+LCN groups.

Uterus (Figure 3C): MTX caused a significant (P<0.001) decrease in free cholesterol levels in the uterus. Compared to the control group free cholesterol levels decreased significantly in MTXLD, MTXHD and MTXHD+LCN groups, while an increase (P<0.001) was observed in MTXHD+WD group. Further, free cholesterol concentration decreased significantly (P<0.001) in MTXHD group compared to MTXLD. While in MTXHD+LCN group the free cholesterol levels increased significantly (P<0.001) compared to MTXHD. In MTXHD+WD group significant (P<0.001) increase in free cholesterol levels was observed compared to the control, MTXLD, MTXHD and MTXHD+LCN groups.

Cervix (Figure 3D): MTX caused a dose dependent decrease in free cholesterol levels in the cervix. Compared to the control group free cholesterol levels decreased significantly (P<0.001) in MTXLD, MTXHD and MTXHD+LCN and MTXHD+WD groups. Further, significant (P<0.001) decrease was observed in MTXHD group compared to MTXLD. In MTXHD+LCN group the levels increased significantly (P<0.001) compared to MTXHD. In MTXHD+WD group significant (P<0.001) increase in levels was observed compared to MTXHD and MTXHD+LCN groups.

Vagina (Figure 3E): MTX caused a decrease in free cholesterol levels in the vagina. Compared to the control group the levels decreased significantly (P<0.001) in MTXLD, MTXHD and MTXHD+LCN groups. No significant differences were observed between MTXLD and MTXHD groups. In MTXHD+LCN and MTXHD+WD groups levels increased significantly (P<0.001) compared to MTXLD and MTXHD. Such levels were further increased significantly (P<0.001) in MTXHD+WD group compared to MTXHD+LCN group.

Effect of MTX on Esterified Cholesterol (Figures 4A-E)

Ovary (Figure 4A): MTX caused a significant increase in esterified cholesterol levels in ovary dose dependently. Compared to the control group, esterified cholesterol concentrations in MTXLD, MTXHD, MTXHD+LCN and MTXHD+WD increased significantly (P<0.001) in the ovary. Further, esterified cholesterol concentration increased significantly (P<0.001) in MTXHD group compared to MTXLD. While in MTXHD+LCN group the esterified cholesterol levels decreased significantly (P<0.001) compared to MTXHD. On the other hand, although esterified cholesterol levels in MTXHD+WD were significantly (P<0.001) higher than MTXLD group, such levels remained considerably (P<0.001) lower than MTXHD group.

Oviduct (Figure 4B): MTX caused a significant increase in esterified cholesterol levels in oviduct dose dependently. Compared to the control group, esterified cholesterol concentrations in MTXLD, MTXHD, MTXHD+LCN and MTXHD+WD increased significantly (P<0.001). Further, esterified cholesterol concentration increased significantly (P<0.001) in MTXHD group compared to MTXLD. In MTXHD+LCN group the esterified cholesterol levels decreased significantly (P<0.001) compared to MTXHD. On the other hand, although esterified cholesterol levels in MTXHD+WD were significantly (P<0.001) higher than MTXLD group, such levels remained considerably (P<0.001) lower than MTXHD group.

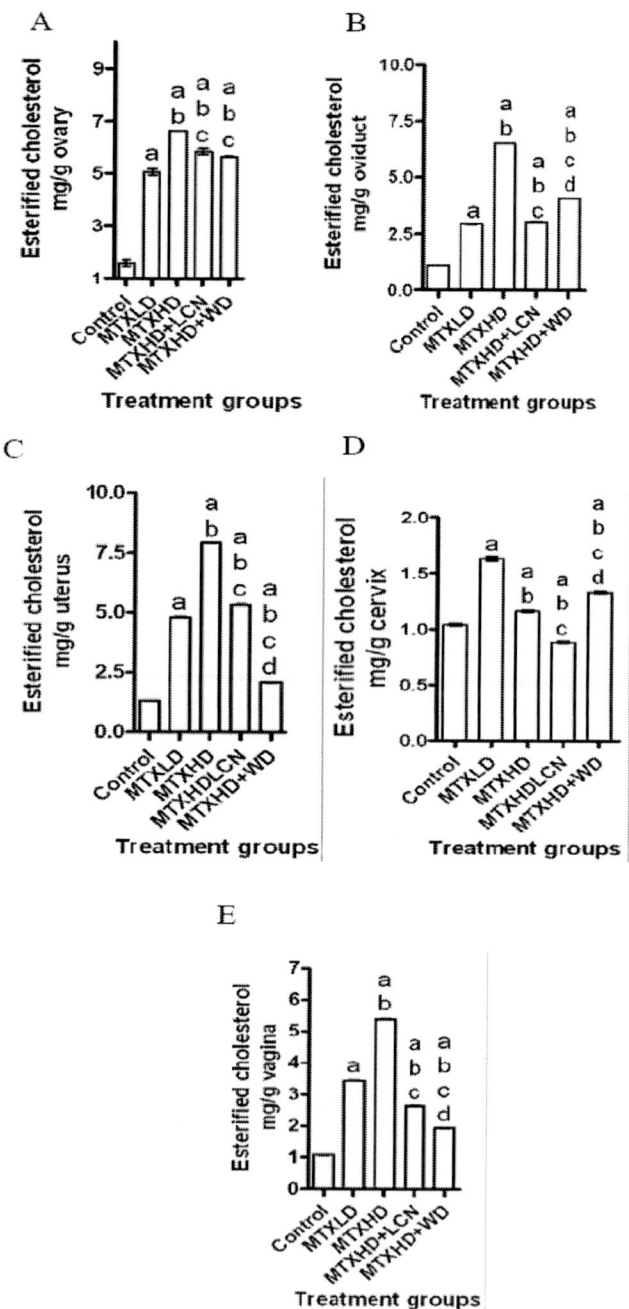

Figure 4 (A–E). Effect of MTX on esterified cholesterol in ovary (A), oviduct (B), uterus (C), cervix (D) and vagina (E) of rats. MTX = methotrexate, LD = low dose, HD =high dose, LCN = leucovorin, WD = withdrawal. P < 0.05, 'a' vs. Control, 'b' vs. MTX LD, 'c' vs. MTX HD, 'd' vs. MTX+LCN. Note marked increase in esterified cholesterol levels dose dependently by MTX treatment in the tissues. Neither LCN supplementation nor withdrawal of MTX treatment brought back the levels to normalcy.

Uterus (Figure 4C): MTX caused a significant increase in esterified cholesterol levels in uterus dose dependently. Compared to the control group, esterified cholesterol concentrations in MTXLD, MTXHD, MTXHD+LCN and MTXHD+WD increased significantly (P<0.001) in the uterus. Further, esterified cholesterol levels increased significantly (P<0.001) in MTXHD group compared to MTXLD. In MTXHD+LCN group the esterified cholesterol levels decreased significantly (P<0.001) compared to MTXHD, however such levels remained higher than MTXLD group. On the other hand, esterified cholesterol levels in MTXHD+WD were significantly (P<0.001) lower than MTXLD, MTXHD and MTXHD+LCN groups.

Cervix (Figure 4D): MTX caused a significant increase in esterified cholesterol levels in cervix. Compared to the control group, esterified cholesterol concentrations increased in MTXLD, MTXHD and MTXHD+WD increased significantly (P<0.001) in the cervix. Further, esterified cholesterol levels decreased significantly (P<0.001) in MTXHD group compared to MTXLD. In addition the esterified cholesterol levels decreased significantly (P<0.001) in MTXHD+LCN group compared to the control, MTXLD MTXHD and MTXHD+WD groups. On the other hand, esterified cholesterol levels in MTXHD+WD were significantly (P<0.001) decreased compared to MTXLD and increased compared to MTXHD and MTXHD+LCN groups.

Vagina (Figure 4E): MTX caused an increase in esterified cholesterol levels in the vagina. Compared to the control group, esterified cholesterol concentrations increased significantly (P<0.001) in MTXLD, MTXHD, MTXHD+LCN and MTXHD+WD groups. Further, esterified cholesterol levels decreased significantly (P<0.001) in MTXHD compared to MTXLD. In addition the esterified cholesterol levels decreased significantly (P<0.001) in MTXHD+LCN group compared to MTXLD and MTXHD groups. Further, esterified cholesterol levels in MTXHD+WD were significantly (P<0.001) decreased compared to MTXLD, MTXHD and MTXHD+LCN groups.

Effect of MTX on Total Glyceride Glycerol (TGG) (Figures 5A-E)

Ovary (Figure 5A): TGG levels in ovary increased dose dependently after MTX treatment. Compared to the control group, TGG levels increased significantly (P<0.001) in MTXLD, MTXHD, MTXHD+LCN and MTXHD+WD groups. Further, TGG levels increased significantly (P<0.001) in MTXHD compared to MTXLD. In addition the TGG levels elevated significantly (P<0.001) in MTXHD+LCN group compared to MTXLD and MTXHD groups. Although TGG levels in MTXHD+WD were significantly (P<0.001) higher compared to MTXLD and MTXHD groups, however the levels were significantly lower compared to MTXHD+LCN group.

Oviduct (Figure 5B): TGG levels in oviduct decreased dose dependently after MTX treatment. Compared to the control group, TGG levels decreased significantly (P<0.001) in MTXLD, MTXHD, MTXHD+LCN and MTXHD+WD groups. Further, TGG levels decreased significantly (P<0.001) in MTXHD compared to MTXLD. Although, TGG levels were significantly (P<0.001) high in MTXHD+LCN group compared to MTXLD and MTXHD groups, the levels in MTXHD+WD were significantly (P<0.001) lower compared to MTXLD, MTXHD and MTXHD+LCN groups.

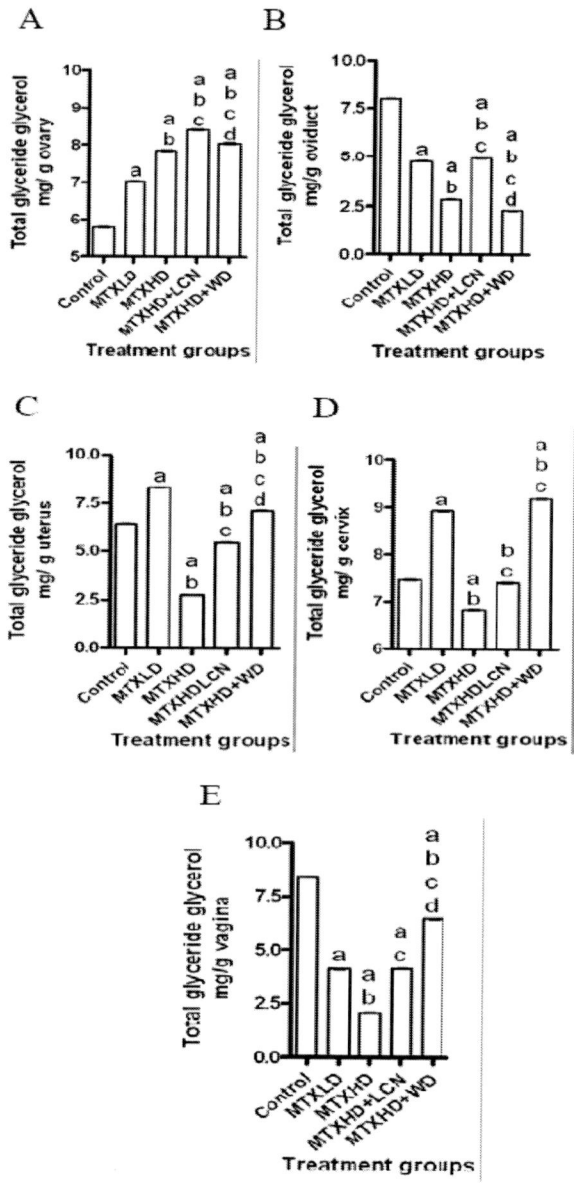

Figure 5 (A–E). Effect of MTX on total glyceride glycerol in ovary (A), oviduct (B), uterus (C), cervix (D) and vagina (E) of rats. MTX = methotrexate, LD = low dose, HD =high dose, LCN = leucovorin, WD = withdrawal. P < 0.05, 'a' vs. Control, 'b' vs. MTX LD, 'c' vs. MTX HD, 'd' vs. MTX+LCN. Note marked increase in the total glyceride glycerol levels in ovary and a reduction in oviduct dose dependently. Note the mixed effect in uterus, cervix and vagina. LCN supplementation restored the levels in ovary alone while withdrawal of MTX treatment restored the levels not only in ovary but also in uterus and cervix.

Uterus (Figure 5C): Compared to the control group TGG levels in uterus increased significantly (P<0.001) in MTXLD, MTXHD+LCN and MTXHD+WD groups, while a decrease was observed in MTXHD group. Further, TGG levels decreased significantly (P<0.001) in MTXHD compared to MTXLD, although, the levels were significantly (P<0.001) high in MTXHD+LCN and MTXHD+WD groups compared to MTXHD groups.

However, such levels in MTXHD+WD were significantly (P<0.001) low compared to MTXLD.

Cervix (Figure 5D): Compared to the control group TGG levels in cervix increased significantly (P<0.001) in MTXLD and MTXHD+WD groups, while a decrease was observed in MTXHD group. Further, TGG levels decreased significantly (P<0.001) in MTXHD compared to MTXLD, although, the levels were significantly (P<0.001) high in MTXHD+LCN and MTXHD+WD groups compared to MTXHD groups. TGG levels were also significantly (P<0.001) higher in MTXHD+WD compared to MTXLD group.

Vagina (Figure 5E): Compared to the control group TGG levels in vagina decreased significantly (P<0.001) in MTXLD, MTXHD, MTXHD+LCN and MTXHD+WD groups. Further, TGG levels decreased significantly (P<0.001) in MTXHD and MTXHD+LCN groups compared to MTXLD. However, in MTXHD+WD the levels were significantly (P<0.001) high compared to MTXLD, MTXHD and MTXHD+LCN.

Effect of MTX on Monoacyl Glycerol (MAG) (Figures 6A-E)

Ovary (Figure 6A): MTX treatment caused an increase in MAG levels in the ovary. Compared to the control group MAG levels in ovary increased significantly (P<0.001) in MTXLD, MTXHD, MTXHD+LCN and MTXHD+WD groups. Further, MAG levels increased significantly (P<0.001) in MTXHD and MTXHD+LCN groups compared to MTXLD. However, in MTXHD+WD the levels were significantly (P<0.001) low compared to MTXLD, MTXHD and MTXHD+LCN.

Oviduct (Figure 6B): MTX treatment caused a decrease in MAG levels in the oviduct. Compared to the control group MAG levels in ovary decreased significantly (P<0.001) in MTXLD, MTXHD, MTXHD+LCN and MTXHD+WD groups. Further, MAG levels decreased significantly (P<0.001) in MTXHD and MTXHD+LCN groups compared to MTXLD. However, in MTXHD and MTXHD+WD the levels were significantly (P<0.001) high compared to MTXHD. The levels in MTXHD+WD further increased significantly compared to MTXHD+LCN.

Uterus (Figure 6C): MTX treatment caused a significant (P<0.001) increase in MAG levels in the MTXLD group compared to the control group in the uterus. While the MAG levels decreased significantly (P<0.001) in MTXHD, MTXHD+LCN and MTXHD+WD groups compared to the control and MTXLD groups. However, in MTXHD+LCN and MTXHD+WD the levels were significantly (P<0.001) high compared to MTXHD. Further significant (P<0.001) increase in the levels was observed in MTXHD+WD group compared to MTXHD+LCN.

Cervix (Figure 6D): MTX treatment caused a significant (P<0.001) increase in MAG levels in the MTXLD group compared to the control group in the cervix. While the MAG levels decreased significantly (P<0.001) in MTXHD and MTXHD+LCN groups compared to control and MTXLD groups. However, in MTXHD+LCN and MTXHD+WD the levels were significantly (P<0.001) high compared to MTXHD. Further significant (P<0.001) increase in the levels was observed in MTXHD+WD group compared to MTXHD+LCN.

Vagina (Figure 6E): MTX treatment caused a significant (P<0.001) decrease in MAG levels in the MTXLD, MTXHD, MTXHD+LCN and MTXHD+WD groups compared to the control group. Such levels further decreased in MTXHD compared to MTXLD group.

However, in MTXHD+LCN and MTXHD+WD the levels were significantly (P<0.001) high compared to MTXHD. Further significant (P<0.001) increase in the levels was observed in MTXHD+WD group compared to MTXHD+LCN.

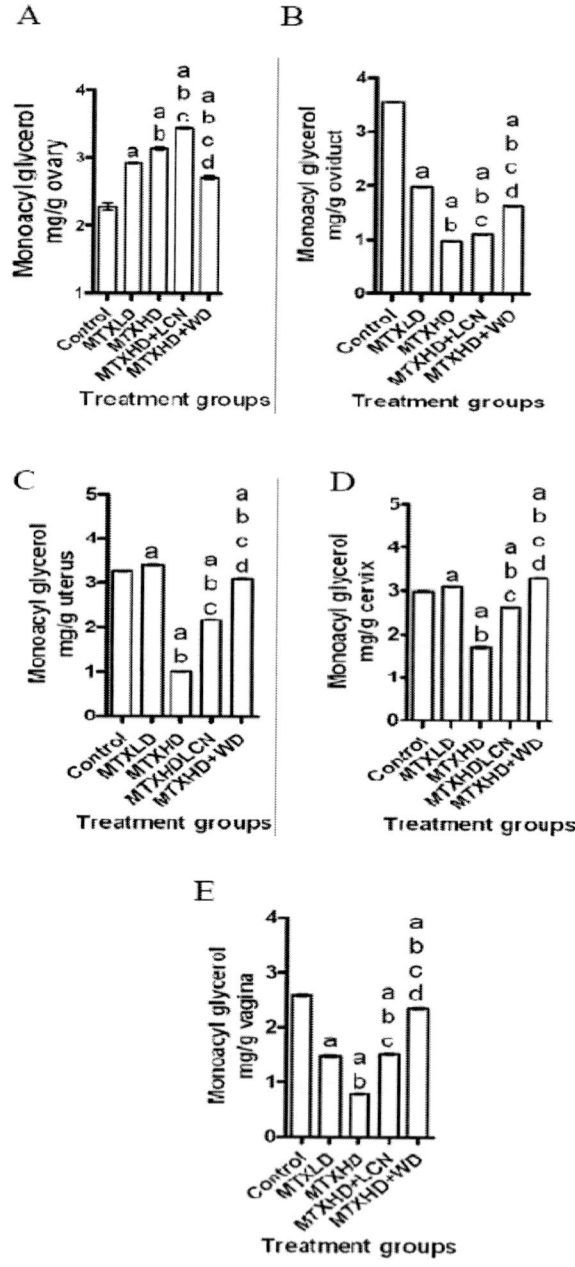

Figure 6 (A–E). Effect of MTX on monoacyl glycerol (MAG) in ovary (A), oviduct (B), uterus (C), cervix (D) and vagina (E) of rats. MTX = methotrexate, LD = low dose, HD =high dose, LCN = leucovorin, WD = withdrawal. P < 0.05, 'a' vs. Control, 'b' vs. MTX LD, 'c' vs. MTX HD, 'd' vs. MTX+LCN. Note marked increase in MAG levels in ovary and a decrease in other tissues dose dependently by MTX treatment. LCN supplementation restored the levels in ovary and remained low in other tissues. While withdrawal effect restored the levels in ovary, uterus, cervix and vagina.

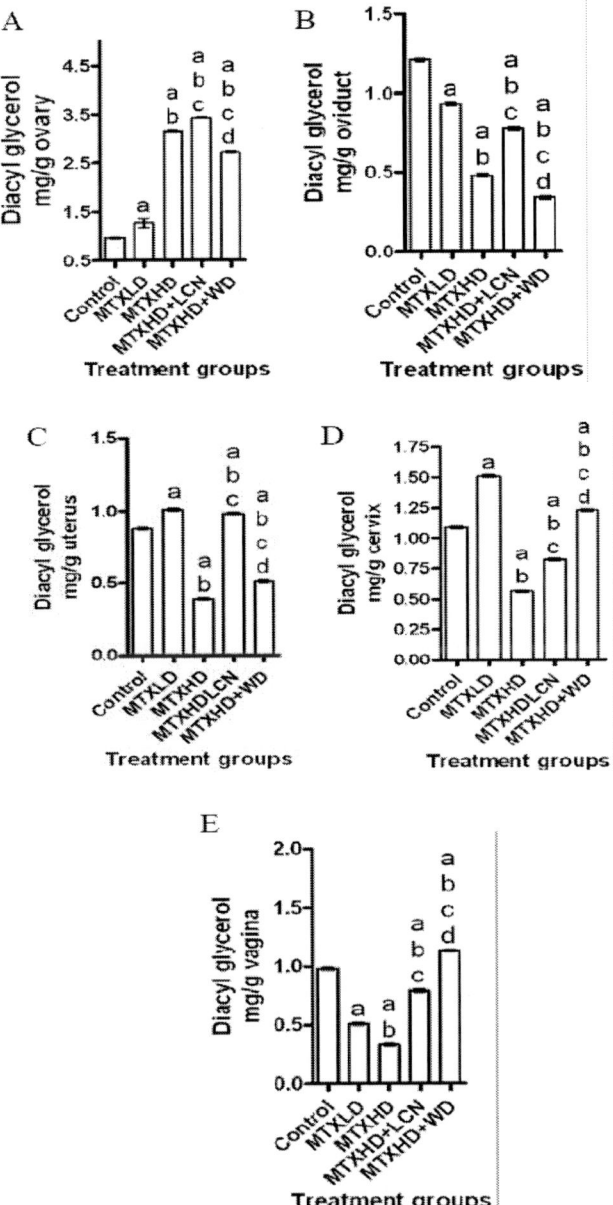

Figure 7 (A–E). Effect of MTX on diacyl glycerol (DAG) in ovary (A), oviduct (B), uterus (C), cervix (D) and vagina (E) of rats. MTX = methotrexate, LD = low dose, HD =high dose, LCN = leucovorin, WD = withdrawal. P < 0.05, 'a' vs. Control, 'b' vs. MTX LD, 'c' vs. MTX HD, 'd' vs. MTX+LCN. Note the differential effect of MTX, LCN and withdrawal treatment on DAG levels depending on the dose and tissue.

Effect of MTX on Diacyl Glycerol (DAG) (Figures 7A-E)

Ovary (Figure 7A): MTX treatment caused a significant (P<0.001) increase in DAG levels in the MTXLD, MTXHD, MTXHD+LCN and MTXHD+WD groups compared to the control group in ovary. DAG levels also increased significantly (P<0.001) in MTXHD,

MTXHD+LCN and MTXHD+WD groups compared to MTXLD group. Further, increase in the MTXHD+LCN levels were significant (P<0.001) compared to MTXHD. However, significant (P<0.001) decrease in the levels was observed in MTXHD+WD group compared to MTXHD and MTXHD+LCN groups.

Oviduct (Figure 7B): MTX treatment caused a significant (P<0.001) decrease in DAG levels in the MTXLD, MTXHD, MTXHD+LCN and MTXHD+WD groups compared to the control group. DAG levels decreased significantly (P<0.001) in MTXHD, MTXHD+LCN and MTXHD+WD groups compared to MTXLD group. An increase in the MTXHD+LCN levels was significant (P<0.001) compared to MTXHD. However, significant (P<0.001) decrease in the levels was observed in MTXHD+WD group compared to control, MTXLD, MTXHD and MTXHD+LCN groups.

Uterus (Figure 7C): MTX treatment caused a significant (P<0.001) increase in DAG levels in the MTXLD and MTXHD+LCN groups compared to the control group in uterus. DAG levels decreased significantly (P<0.001) in MTXHD, MTXHD+LCN and MTXHD+WD groups compared to MTXLD group. An increase in the MTXHD+LCN levels was significant (P<0.001) compared to MTXHD. However, significant (P<0.001) decrease in the levels was observed in MTXHD+WD group compared to the control, MTXLD and MTXHD+LCN groups, although such levels were higher than MTXHD group.

Cervix (Figure 7D): MTX treatment caused a significant (P<0.001) increase in DAG levels in the MTXLD and MTXHD+WD groups compared to the control group in cervix. DAG levels decreased significantly (P<0.001) in MTXHD and MTXHD+LCN groups compared to both control and MTXLD groups. An increase in the MTXHD+LCN levels was significant (P<0.001) compared to MTXHD. Further significant (P<0.001) increase in the levels was observed in MTXHD+WD group compared to control, MTXHD and MTXHD+LCN groups.

Vagina (Figure 7E): MTX treatment caused a significant (P<0.001) decrease in DAG levels in the MTXLD, MTXHD and MTXHD+LCN groups compared to the control group in vagina. DAG levels decreased significantly (P<0.001) in MTXHD group compared to MTXLD group. An increase in the MTXHD+LCN levels was significant (P<0.001) compared to MTXLD and MTXHD groups. Further significant (P<0.001) increase in the levels was observed in MTXHD+WD group compared to the control, MTXLD, MTXHD and MTXHD+LCN groups.

Effect of MTX on Triacyl Glycerol (TAG) (Figures 8A-E)

Ovary (Figure 8A): MTX treatment caused a significant (P<0.001) increase in TAG levels in MTXLD, MTXHD, MTXHD+LCN and MTXHD+WD groups compared to the control group in ovary. TAG levels increased significantly (P<0.001) in MTXHD group compared to MTXLD group. An increase in the MTXHD+LCN levels was significant (P<0.001) compared to MTXLD and MTXHD groups. Further significant (P<0.001) increase in the levels was observed in MTXHD+WD group compared to MTXLD, MTXHD and MTXHD+LCN groups.

Oviduct (Figure 8B): MTX treatment caused a significant (P<0.001) decrease in TAG levels in MTXLD, MTXHD, MTXHD+LCN and MTXHD+WD groups compared to the control group in oviduct. TAG levels increased significantly (P<0.001) in MTXHD group compared to MTXLD group. An increase in the MTXHD+LCN levels was significant (P<0.001) compared to MTXHD group. Further significant (P<0.001) decrease in the levels was observed in MTXHD+WD group compared to MTXLD, MTXHD and MTXHD+LCN groups.

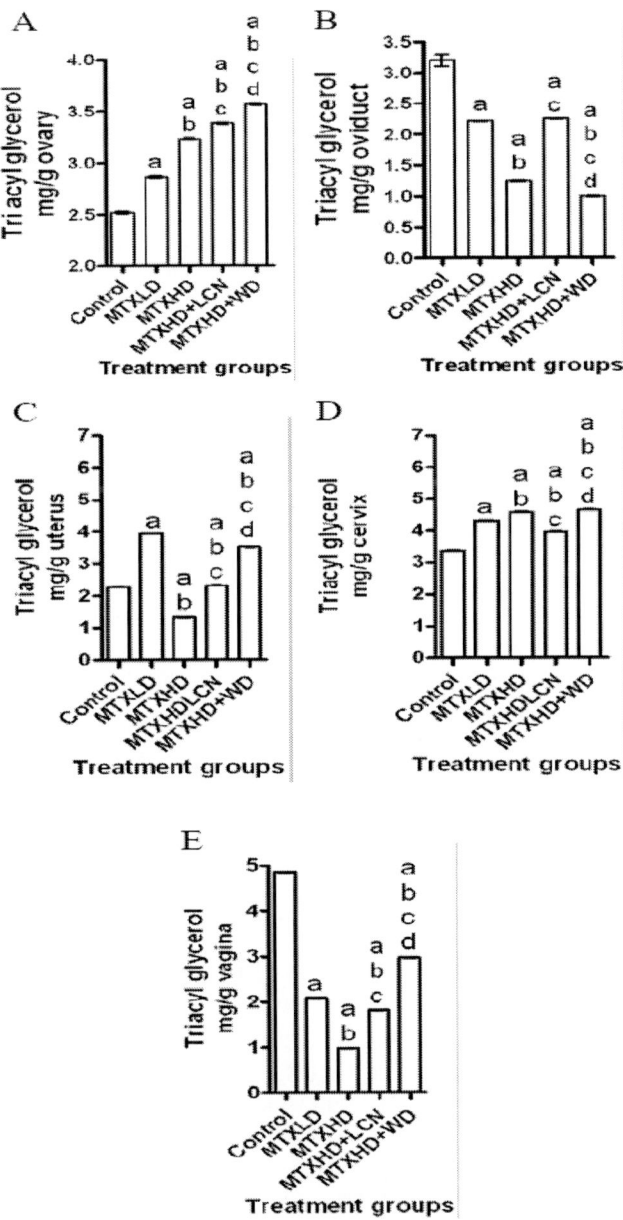

Figure 8 (A–E). Effect of MTX on triacyl glycerol (TAG) in ovary (A), oviduct (B), uterus (C), cervix (D) and vagina (E) of rats. MTX = methotrexate, LD = low dose, HD =high dose, LCN = leucovorin, WD = withdrawal. P < 0.05, 'a' vs. Control, 'b' vs. MTX LD, 'c' vs. MTX HD, 'd' vs. MTX+LCN. Note marked increase in TAG levels in ovary, cervix and a decrease in oviduct and vagina in all treatment groups. Uterus showed a mixed effect. LCN and withdrawal groups brought back the levels to normalcy in ovary, uterus and cervix.

Uterus (Figure 8C): MTX treatment caused a significant (P<0.001) increase in TAG levels in MTXLD, MTXHD+LCN and MTXHD+WD groups compared to the control group in uterus. TAG levels decreased significantly (P<0.001) in MTXHD group compared to MTXLD group. An increase in the MTXHD+LCN levels was significant (P<0.001) compared to MTXHD group. Further significant (P<0.001) increase in the levels was observed in MTXHD+WD group compared to MTXHD and MTXHD+LCN groups. However such levels were significantly (P<0.001) lower than MTXLD group.

Cervix (Figure 8D): MTX treatment caused a significant (P<0.001) increase in TAG levels in MTXLD, MTXHD, MTXHD+LCN and MTXHD+WD groups compared to the control group in cervix. TAG levels increased significantly (P<0.001) in MTXHD group compared to MTXLD group. A decrease in the MTXHD+LCN levels was significant (P<0.001) compared to MTXLD and MTXHD group. Further, significant (P<0.001) increase in the levels was observed in MTXHD+WD group compared to MTXHD+LCN group.

Vagina (Figure 8E): MTX treatment caused a significant (P<0.001) decrease in TAG levels in MTXLD, MTXHD, MTXHD+LCN and MTXHD+WD groups compared to the control group in vagina. TAG levels decreased significantly (P<0.001) in MTXHD group compared to MTXLD group. An increase in the MTXHD+LCN levels was significant (P<0.001) compared to MTXHD group. However, such levels were lower than MTXLD group. Further, significant (P<0.001) increase in the levels was observed in MTXHD+WD group compared to MTXLD, MTXHD and MTXHD+LCN group.

Effect of MTX on Total Phospholipids (TPL) (Figures 9A-E)

Ovary (Figure 9A): Total phospholipids decreased in ovary in all the MTX treated groups. MTX treatment caused a significant (P<0.001) decrease in TPL levels in MTXLD, MTXHD, MTXHD+LCN and MTXHD+WD groups compared to the control group in ovary. TPL levels decreased significantly (P<0.001) in MTXHD group compared to MTXLD group. An increase in the MTXHD+LCN levels was significant (P<0.001) compared to MTXHD group. However, such levels were lower than MTXLD group. Further, significant (P<0.001) increase in the TPL level was observed in MTXHD+WD group compared to MTXHD and MTXHD+LCN groups.

Oviduct (Figure 9B): Total phospholipids decreased in oviduct in all the MTX treated groups. MTX treatment caused a significant (P<0.001) decrease in TPL levels in MTXLD, MTXHD, MTXHD+LCN and MTXHD+WD groups compared to the control group in oviduct. TPL levels decreased significantly (P<0.001) in MTXHD group compared to MTXLD group. An increase in the MTXHD+LCN levels was significant (P<0.001) compared to MTXHD group. However, such levels were lower than MTXLD group. Further, significant (P<0.001) increase in the TPL level was observed in MTXHD+WD group compared to MTXHD and MTXHD+LCN groups.

Uterus (Figure 9C): Total phospholipids decreased in uterus in all the MTX treated groups. MTX treatment caused a significant (P<0.001) decrease in TPL levels in MTXLD, MTXHD, MTXHD+LCN and MTXHD+WD groups compared to the control group in uterus. TPL levels decreased significantly (P<0.001) in MTXHD group compared to MTXLD group. An increase in the MTXHD+LCN levels was significant (P<0.001) compared to MTXHD group. However, such levels were lower than MTXLD group. Further, significant (P<0.001) increase in the TPL level was observed in MTXHD+WD group compared to MTXHD. However, such levels were significantly lower than MTXLD and MTXHD+LCN groups.

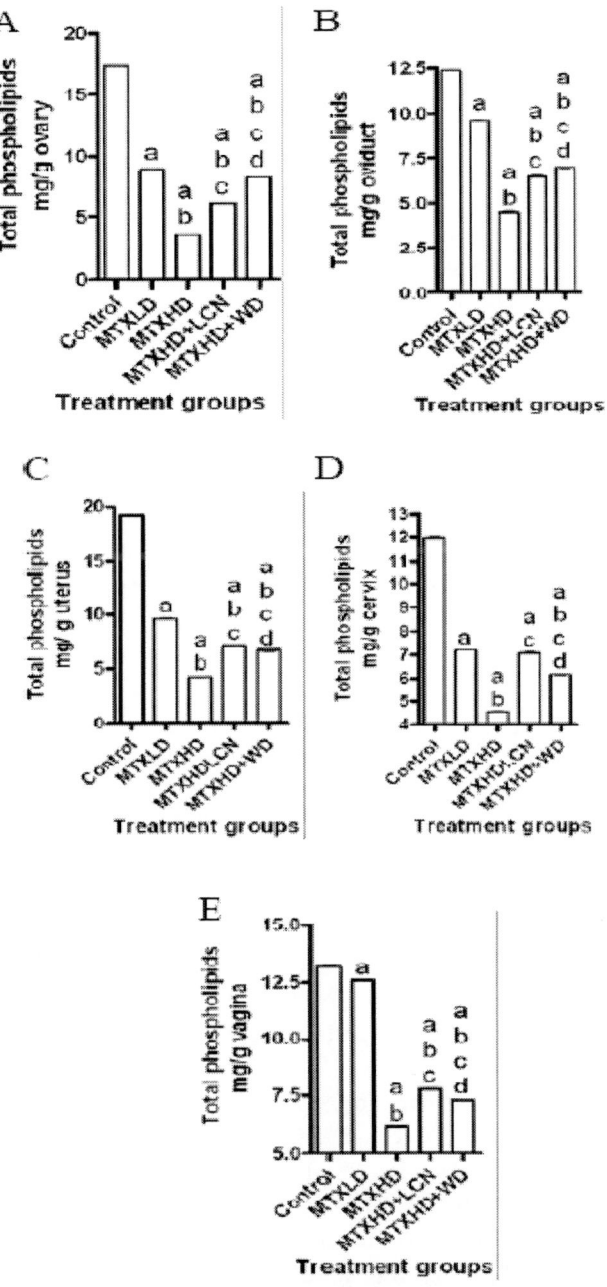

Figure 9 (A–E). Effect of MTX on total phospholipids in ovary (A), oviduct (B), uterus (C), cervix (D) and vagina (E) of rats. MTX = methotrexate, LD = low dose, HD =high dose, LCN = leucovorin, WD = withdrawal. P < 0.05, 'a' vs. Control, 'b' vs. MTX LD, 'c' vs. MTX HD, 'd' vs. MTX+LCN. Note marked reduction in total phospholipids in the tissues dose dependently by MTX treatment. Neither LCN nor withdrawal of MTX treatment brought back the levels to normalcy.

Cervix (Figure 9D): Total phospholipids decreased in cervix in all the MTX treated groups. MTX treatment caused a significant ($P<0.001$) decrease in TPL levels in MTXLD, MTXHD, MTXHD+LCN and MTXHD+WD groups compared to the control group in cervix. TPL levels decreased significantly ($P<0.001$) in MTXHD group compared to MTXLD group. An increase in the MTXHD+LCN levels was significant ($P<0.001$) compared to MTXHD group. Further, significant ($P<0.001$) increase in the TPL level was observed in MTXHD+WD group compared to MTXHD. However, such levels were significantly lower than MTXLD and MTXHD+LCN groups.

Vagina (Figure 9E): Total phospholipids decreased in vagina in all the MTX treated groups. MTX treatment caused a significant ($P<0.001$) decrease in TPL levels in MTXLD, MTXHD, MTXHD+LCN and MTXHD+WD groups compared to the control group in ovary. TPL levels decreased significantly ($P<0.001$) in MTXHD group compared to MTXLD group. An increase in the MTXHD+LCN levels was significant ($P<0.001$) compared to MTXHD group. However, such levels were lower than MTXLD group. Further, significant ($P<0.001$) increase in the TPL level was observed in MTXHD+WD group compared to MTXHD. However, such levels were significantly lower than MTXLD and MTXHD+LCN groups.

Effect of MTX on Phosphatidyl Inositol (PI) (Figures 10A-E)

Ovary (Figure 10A): MTX treatment caused a significant ($P<0.001$) decrease in PI levels in MTXLD, MTXHD, MTXHD+LCN and MTXHD+WD groups compared to the control group in ovary. PI levels decreased significantly ($P<0.001$) in MTXHD group compared to MTXLD group. An increase in the MTXHD+LCN levels was significant ($P<0.001$) compared to MTXHD group. However, such levels were lower than MTXLD group. Further, significant ($P<0.001$) increase in the PI level was observed in MTXHD+WD group compared to MTXHD.

Oviduct (Figure 10B): MTX treatment caused a significant ($P<0.001$) decrease in PI levels in MTXLD, MTXHD, MTXHD+LCN and MTXHD+WD groups compared to the control group in oviduct. PI levels decreased significantly ($P<0.001$) in MTXHD group compared to MTXLD group. An increase in the MTXHD+LCN levels was significant ($P<0.001$) compared to MTXHD group. However, such levels were lower than MTXLD group. Further, significant ($P<0.001$) increase in the PI level was observed in MTXHD+WD group compared to MTXHD.

Uterus (Figure 10C): MTX treatment caused a significant ($P<0.001$) decrease in PI levels in MTXLD, MTXHD, MTXHD+LCN and MTXHD+WD groups compared to the control group in uterus. PI levels decreased significantly ($P<0.001$) in MTXHD group compared to MTXLD group. An increase in the MTXHD+LCN levels was significant ($P<0.001$) compared to MTXHD group. However, such levels were lower than MTXLD group. Further, significant ($P<0.001$) increase in the PI level was observed in MTXHD+WD group compared to MTXHD.

Cervix (Figure 10D): MTX treatment caused a significant ($P<0.001$) decrease in PI levels in MTXLD, MTXHD, MTXHD+LCN and MTXHD+WD groups compared to the control group in cervix. PI levels decreased significantly ($P<0.001$) in MTXHD group compared to MTXLD group. An increase in the MTXHD+LCN levels was significant ($P<0.001$) compared to MTXHD group. Further, significant ($P<0.001$) increase in the PI level was observed in

MTXHD+WD group compared to MTXHD. However, such levels were significantly lower than MTXLD and MTXHD+LCN.

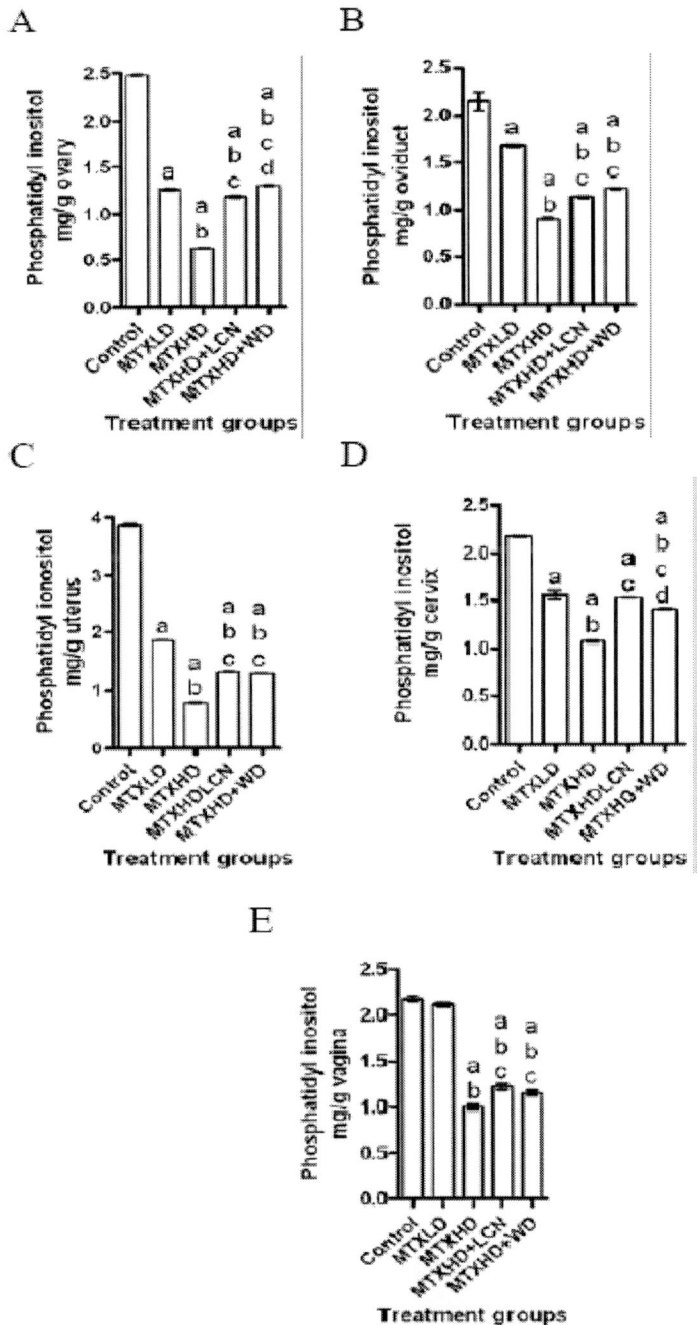

Figure 10 (A–E). Effect of MTX on phosphatidyl inositol in ovary (A), oviduct (B), uterus (C), cervix (D) and vagina (E) of rats. MTX = methotrexate, LD = low dose, HD =high dose, LCN = leucovorin, WD = withdrawal. $P < 0.05$, 'a' vs. Control, 'b' vs. MTX LD, 'c' vs. MTX HD, 'd' vs. MTX+LCN. Note marked reduction in phosphatidyl inositol in the tissues dose dependently by MTX treatment. Neither LCN nor withdrawal of MTX treatment brought back the levels to normalcy.

Vagina (Figure 10E): MTX treatment caused a significant (P<0.001) decrease in PI levels in MTXHD, MTXHD+LCN and MTXHD+WD groups compared to the control and MTXLD groups in vagina. An increase in the MTXHD+LCN and MTXHD+WD levels was significant (P<0.001) compared to MTXHD group. Further, significant (P<0.001) increase in the PI level was observed in MTXHD+WD group compared to MTXHD. However, such levels were lower than MTXHD+LCN group.

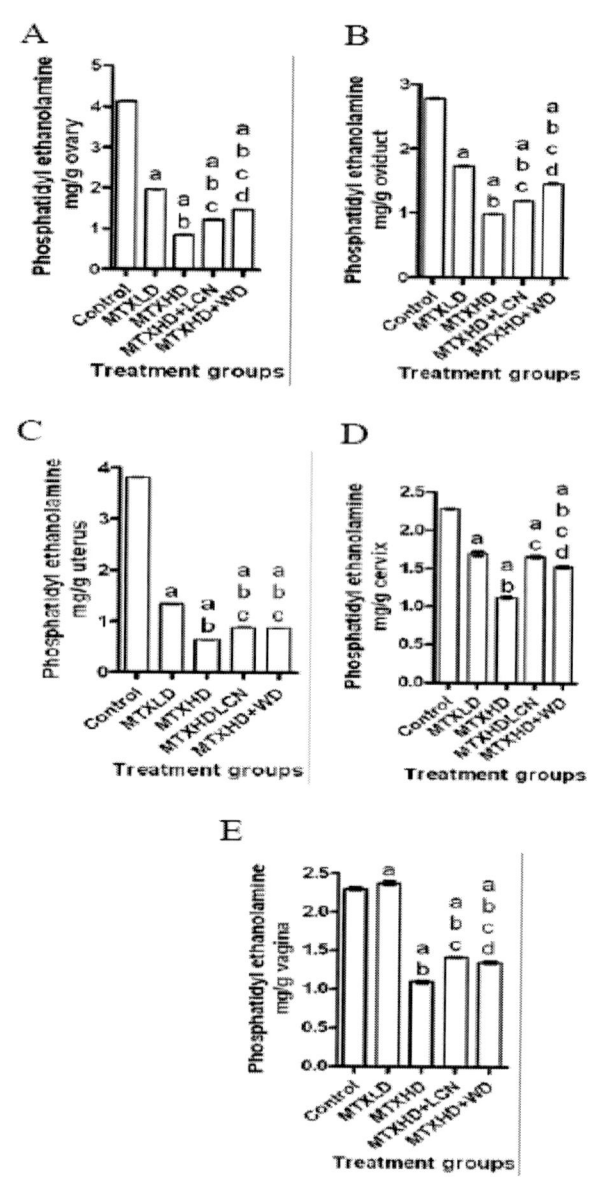

Figure 11 (A–E). Effect of MTX on phosphatidyl ethanolamine in ovary (A), oviduct (B), uterus (C), cervix (D) and vagina (E) of rats. MTX = methotrexate, LD = low dose, HD =high dose, LCN = leucovorin, WD = withdrawal. P < 0.05, 'a' vs. Control, 'b' vs. MTX LD, 'c' vs. MTX HD, 'd' vs. MTX+LCN. Note marked reduction in phosphatidyl ethanolamine in the tissues dose dependently by MTX treatment. Neither LCN nor withdrawal of MTX treatment brought back the levels to normalcy.

Effect of MTX on Phosphatidyl Ethanolamine (PE)(Figures 11A-E)

Ovary (Figure 11A): MTX treatment caused a significant (P<0.001) decrease in PE levels in MTXHD, MTXHD+LCN and MTXHD+WD groups compared to the control and MTXLD groups in ovary. An increase in MTXHD+LCN and MTXHD+WD was significant (P<0.001) compared to MTXHD group. Further, significant (P<0.001) increase in the PE level was observed in MTXHD+WD group compared to MTXHD+LCN groups.

Oviduct (Figure 11B): MTX treatment caused a significant (P<0.001) decrease in PE levels in MTXHD, MTXHD+LCN and MTXHD+WD groups compared to the control and MTXLD groups in oviduct. An increase in the MTXHD+LCN and MTXHD+WD levels was significant (P<0.001) compared to MTXHD group. Further, significant (P<0.001) increase in the PE level was observed in MTXHD+WD group compared to MTXHD+LCN groups.

Uterus (Figure 11C): MTX treatment caused a significant (P<0.001) decrease in PE levels in MTXHD, MTXHD+LCN and MTXHD+WD groups compared to the control and MTXLD groups. An increase in the MTXHD+LCN and MTXHD+WD levels was significant (P<0.001) compared to MTXHD group. Further, significant (P<0.001) increase in the PE level was observed in MTXHD+WD group compared to MTXHD+LCN groups.

Cervix (Figure 11D): MTX treatment caused a significant (P<0.001) decrease in PE levels in MTXLD, MTXHD, MTXHD+LCN and MTXHD+WD groups compared to the control group. Further a decrease in MTXHD compared to MTXLD was observed. An increase in the MTXHD+LCN and MTXHD+WD levels was significant (P<0.001) compared to MTXHD group. Further, significant (P<0.001) decrease in the PE level was observed in MTXHD+WD group compared to MTXHD+LCN groups.

Vagina (Figure 11E): MTX treatment caused a significant (P<0.001) increase in PE levels in MTXLD group and a decrease in MTXHD, MTXHD+LCN and MTXHD+WD groups compared to the control group. Further, a decrease in MTXHD compared to MTXLD was observed. An increase in the MTXHD+LCN and MTXHD+WD levels was significant (P<0.001) compared to MTXHD group. Further, significant (P<0.001) decrease in the PE level was observed in MTXHD+WD group compared to MTXHD+LCN group.

Effect of MTX on Phosphatidyl Choline (PC) (Figures 12A-E)

Ovary (Figure 12A): MTX treatment caused a significant (P<0.001) decrease in PC levels in MTXLD group and a decrease in MTXHD, MTXHD+LCN and MTXHD+WD groups compared to the control group. Further, a decrease in MTXHD compared to MTXLD was observed. An increase in the MTXHD+LCN and MTXHD+WD levels was significant (P<0.001) compared to MTXHD group. Further, significant (P<0.001) increase in the PC level was observed in MTXHD+WD group compared to MTXHD+LCN group.

Oviduct (Figure 12B): MTX treatment caused a significant (P<0.001) decrease in PC levels in MTXLD group and a decrease in MTXHD, MTXHD+LCN and MTXHD+WD groups compared to the control group. Further, a decrease in MTXHD compared to MTXLD was observed. An increase in the MTXHD+LCN and MTXHD+WD levels was significant (P<0.001) compared to MTXHD group. Further, significant (P<0.001) increase in the PC level was observed in MTXHD+WD group compared to MTXHD+LCN group.

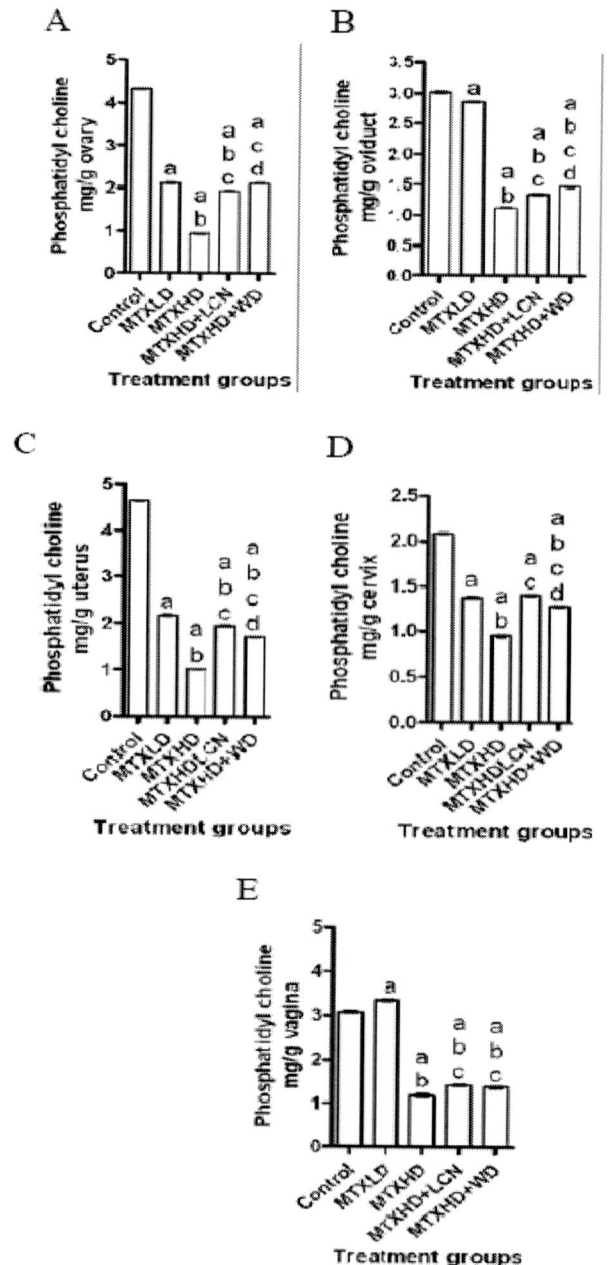

Figure 12 (A–E). Effect of MTX on phosphatidyl choline in ovary (A), oviduct (B), uterus (C), cervix (D) and vagina (E) of rats. MTX = methotrexate, LD = low dose, HD =high dose, LCN = leucovorin, WD = withdrawal. P < 0.05, 'a' vs. Control, 'b' vs. MTX LD, 'c' vs. MTX HD, 'd' vs. MTX+LCN. Note marked reduction in phosphatidyl choline in the tissues dose dependently by MTX treatment. Neither LCN nor withdrawal of MTX treatment brought back the levels to normalcy.

Uterus (Figure 12C): MTX treatment caused a significant (P<0.001) decrease in PC levels in MTXLD group and a decrease in MTXHD, MTXHD+LCN and MTXHD+WD groups compared to the control group in uterus. Further, a decrease in MTXHD compared to MTXLD was observed. An increase in the MTXHD+LCN and MTXHD+WD levels was significant (P<0.001) compared to MTXHD group. Further, significant (P<0.001) decrease in the PC level was observed in MTXHD+WD group compared to MTXHD+LCN group.

Cervix (Figure 12D): MTX treatment caused a significant (P<0.001) decrease in PC levels in MTXLD, MTXHD, MTXHD+LCN and MTXHD+WD groups compared to the control group. Further, a decrease in MTXHD compared to MTXLD was observed. An increase in the MTXHD+LCN and MTXHD+WD levels was significant (P<0.001) compared to MTXHD group. A significant (P<0.001) decrease in the PC level was observed in MTXHD+WD group compared to MTXHD+LCN group.

Vagina (Figure 12E): MTX treatment caused a significant (P<0.001) increase in PC levels in MTXLD group and a decrease in MTXHD, MTXHD+LCN and MTXHD+WD groups compared to the control group. Further, a decrease in MTXHD compared to MTXLD was observed. An increase in the MTXHD+LCN and MTXHD+WD levels was significant (P<0.001) compared to MTXHD group.

Effect of MTX on Phosphatidyl Serine (PS) (Figures 13A-E)

Ovary (Figure 13A): MTX treatment caused a significant (P<0.001) increase in PS levels in MTXLD, MTXHD, MTXHD+LCN and MTXHD+WD groups compared to the control group. Further, a decrease in MTXHD compared to MTXLD was observed. An increase in the MTXHD+LCN and MTXHD+WD levels was significant (P<0.001) compared to MTXHD group. A significant (P<0.001) increase in the PS level was observed in MTXHD+WD group compared to MTXHD+LCN group.

Oviduct (Figure 13B): MTX treatment caused a significant (P<0.001) increase in PS levels in MTXLD, MTXHD, MTXHD+LCN and MTXHD+WD groups compared to the control group. Further, a decrease in MTXHD compared to MTXLD was observed. An increase in the MTXHD+LCN and MTXHD+WD levels was significant (P<0.001) compared to MTXHD group. A significant (P<0.001) increase in the PS level was observed in MTXHD+WD group compared to MTXHD+LCN group.

Uterus (Figure 13C): MTX treatment caused a significant (P<0.001) increase in PS levels in MTXLD, MTXHD, MTXHD+LCN and MTXHD+WD groups compared to the control group in uterus. Further, a decrease in MTXHD compared to MTXLD was observed. An increase in the MTXHD+LCN and MTXHD+WD levels was significant (P<0.001) compared to MTXHD group.

Cervix (Figure 13D): MTX treatment caused a significant (P<0.001) increase in PS levels in MTXLD, MTXHD, MTXHD+LCN and MTXHD+WD groups compared to the control group in cervix. Further, a decrease in MTXHD compared to MTXLD was observed. An increase in the MTXHD+LCN and MTXHD+WD levels was significant (P<0.001) compared to MTXHD group. A significant (P<0.001) decrease in the PS level was observed in MTXHD+WD group compared to MTXHD+LCN group.

Vagina (Figure 13E): MTX treatment caused a significant (P<0.001) increase in PS levels in MTXLD, MTXHD, MTXHD+LCN and MTXHD+WD groups compared to the control group in vagina. Further, a decrease in MTXHD compared to MTXLD was observed. An increase in the MTXHD+LCN and MTXHD+WD levels was significant (P<0.001) compared to MTXHD group. A significant (P<0.001) decrease in the PS level was observed in MTXHD+WD group compared to MTXHD+LCN group.

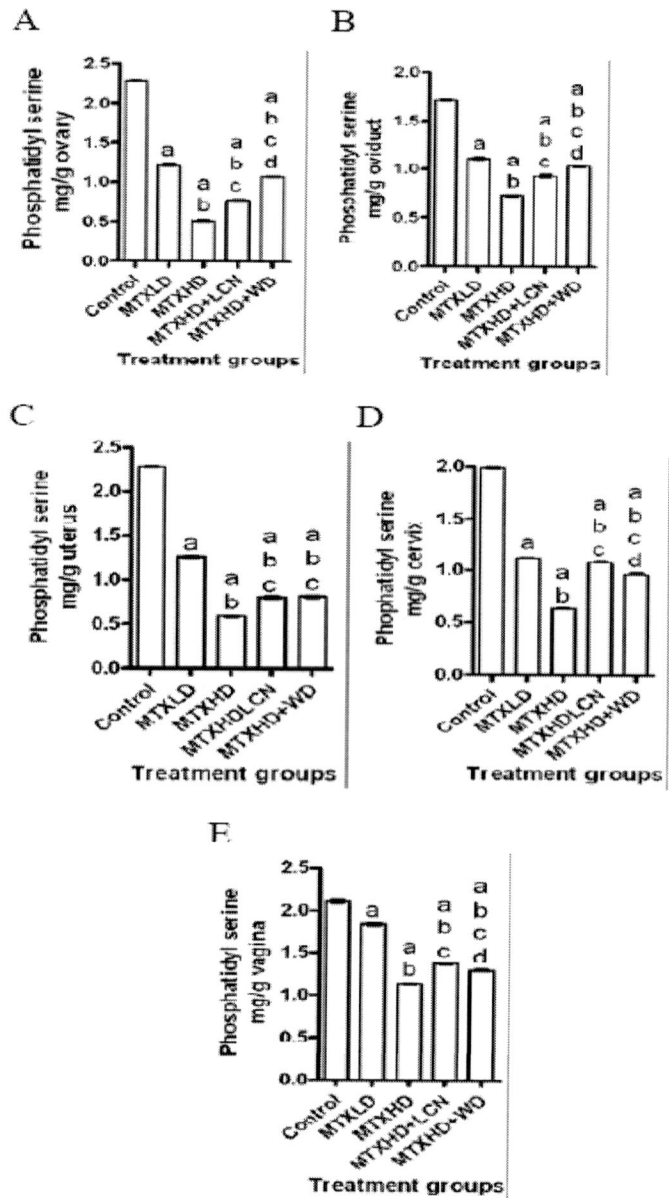

Figure 13 (A–E). Effect of MTX on phosphatidyl serine in ovary (A), oviduct (B), uterus (C), cervix (D) and vagina (E) of rats. MTX = methotrexate, LD = low dose, HD =high dose, LCN = leucovorin, WD = withdrawal. P < 0.05, 'a' vs. Control, 'b' vs. MTX LD, 'c' vs. MTX HD, 'd' vs. MTX+LCN. Note marked reduction in phosphatidyl serine in the tissues dose dependently by MTX treatment. Neither LCN nor withdrawal of MTX treatment brought back the levels to normalcy.

Effect of MTX on Sphingomyelin (Figures 14A-E)

Ovary (Figure 14A): MTX treatment caused a significant (P<0.001) decrease in sphingomyelin levels in MTXLD, MTXHD, MTXHD+LCN and MTXHD+WD groups compared to the control group. Further, a decrease in MTXHD compared to MTXLD was observed. An increase in the MTXHD+LCN and MTXHD+WD levels was significant (P<0.001) compared to MTXHD group. A significant (P<0.001) decrease in the PS level was observed in MTXHD+WD group compared to MTXHD+LCN group.

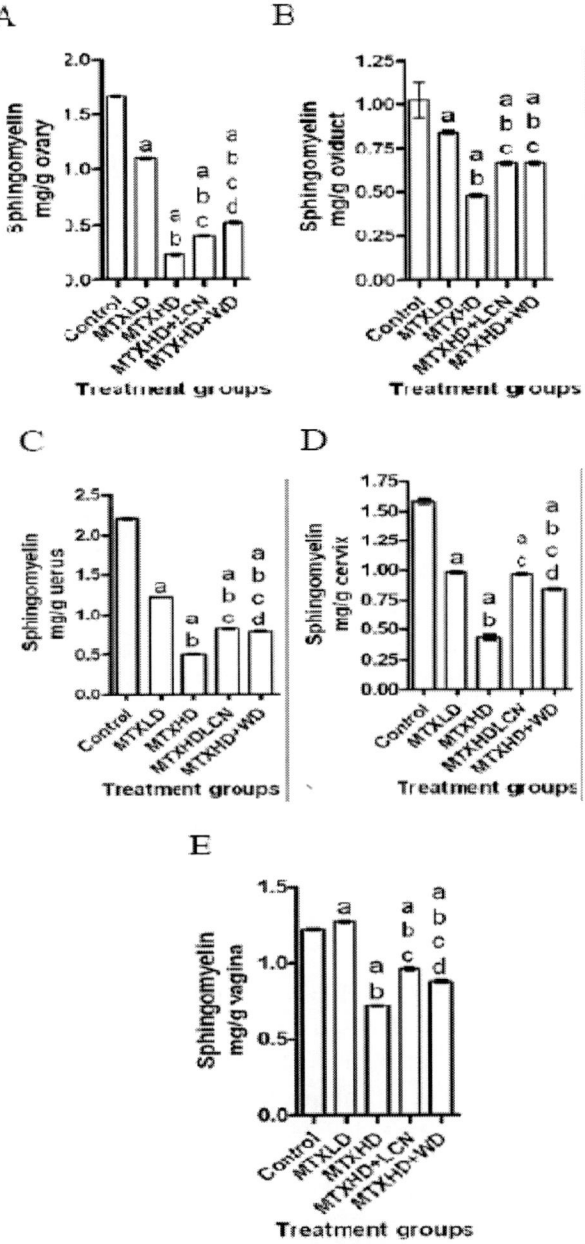

Figure 14 (A–E). Effect of MTX on sphingomyelin in ovary (A), oviduct (B), uterus (C), cervix (D) and vagina (E) of rats. MTX = methotrexate, LD = low dose, HD =high dose, LCN = leucovorin, WD = withdrawal. P < 0.05, 'a' vs. Control, 'b' vs. MTX LD, 'c' vs. MTX HD, 'd' vs. MTX+LCN. Note marked reduction in the levels is tissues and dose dependent. Neither LCN nor withdrawal of MTX treatment brought back the levels to normalcy.

Oviduct (Figure 14B): MTX treatment caused a significant (P<0.001) decrease in sphingomyelin levels in MTXLD, MTXHD, MTXHD+LCN and MTXHD+WD groups compared to the control group in oviduct. Further, a decrease in MTXHD compared to MTXLD was observed. An increase in the MTXHD+LCN and MTXHD+WD levels was significant (P<0.001) compared to MTXHD group. A significant (P<0.001) increase in the PS level was observed in MTXHD+WD group compared to MTXHD+LCN group.

Uterus (Figure 14C): MTX treatment caused a significant (P<0.001) decrease in sphingomyelin levels in MTXLD, MTXHD, MTXHD+LCN and MTXHD+WD groups compared to the control group. Further, a decrease in MTXHD compared to MTXLD was observed. An increase in the MTXHD+LCN and MTXHD+WD levels was significant (P<0.001) compared to MTXHD group. A significant (P<0.001) decrease in the PS level was observed in MTXHD+WD group compared to MTXHD+LCN group.

Cervix (Figure 14D): MTX treatment caused a significant (P<0.001) decrease in sphingomyelin levels in MTXLD, MTXHD, MTXHD+LCN and MTXHD+WD groups compared to the control group. Further, a decrease in MTXHD compared to MTXLD was observed. An increase in the MTXHD+LCN and MTXHD+WD levels was significant (P<0.001) compared to MTXHD group. A significant (P<0.001) decrease in the PS level was observed in MTXHD+WD group compared to MTXHD+LCN group.

Vagina (Figure 14E): MTX treatment caused a significant (P<0.001) an increase in sphingomyelin levels in MTXLD and a decrease in the levels in MTXHD, MTXHD+LCN and MTXHD+WD groups compared to the control group. Further, a decrease in MTXHD compared to MTXLD was observed. An increase in the MTXHD+LCN and MTXHD+WD levels was significant (P<0.001) compared to MTXHD group. A significant (P<0.001) decrease in the PS level was observed in MTXHD+WD group compared to MTXHD+LCN group.

Effect of MTX on Phosphatidic Acid (PA) (Figures 15A-E)

Ovary (Figure 15A): MTX treatment caused a significant (P<0.001) decrease in PA levels in MTXLD, MTXHD, MTXHD+LCN and MTXHD+WD groups compared to the control group. Further, a decrease in MTXHD compared to MTXLD was observed. An increase in the MTXHD+LCN and MTXHD+WD levels was significant (P<0.001) compared to MTXHD group. A significant (P<0.001) increase in the PA level was observed in MTXHD+WD group compared to MTXHD+LCN group.

Oviduct (Figure 15A): MTX treatment caused a significant (P<0.001) an increase in PA levels in MTXLD and a decrease in the levels in MTXHD, MTXHD+LCN and MTXHD+WD groups compared to the control group. Further, a decrease in MTXHD compared to MTXLD was observed. An increase in the MTXHD+LCN and MTXHD+WD levels was significant (P<0.001) compared to MTXHD group. A significant (P<0.001) increase in the PA level was observed in MTXHD+WD group compared to MTXHD+LCN group.

Uterus (Figure 15A): MTX treatment caused a significant (P<0.001) decrease in PA levels in MTXLD, MTXHD, MTXHD+LCN and MTXHD+WD groups compared to the control group. Further, a decrease in MTXHD compared to MTXLD was observed. An increase in the levels in MTXHD+LCN was significant (P<0.001) compared to MTXHD group. A significant (P<0.001) decrease in the PA level was observed in MTXHD+WD group compared to MTXHD+LCN group.

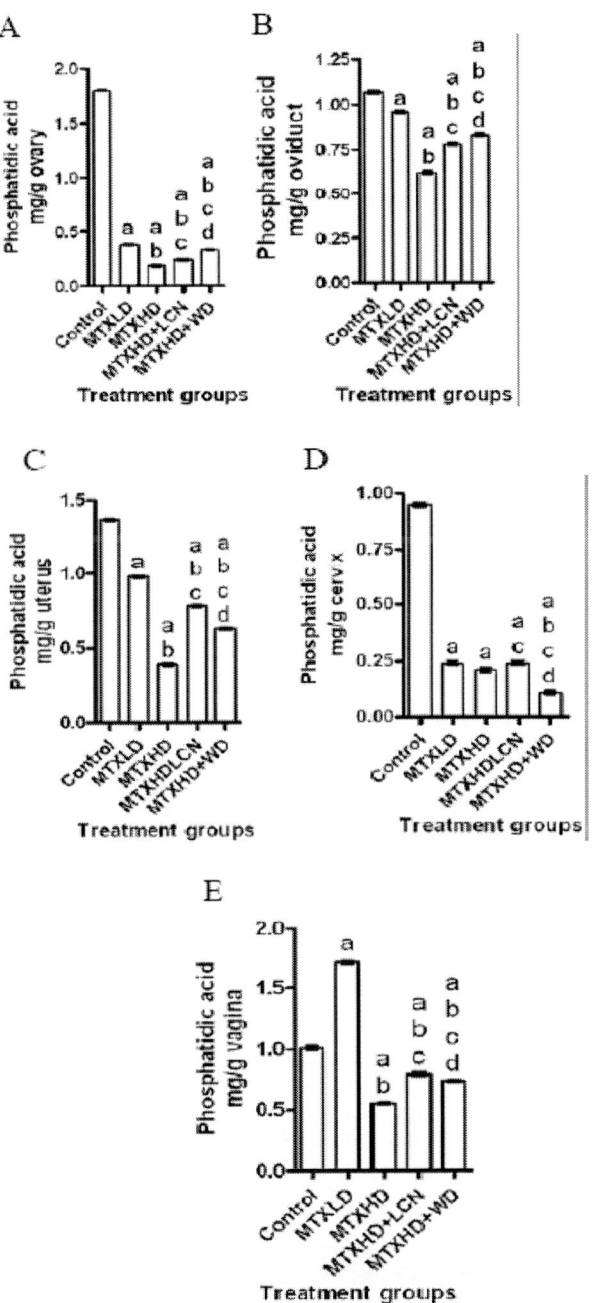

Figure 15 (A–E). Effect of MTX on phosphatidic acid in ovary (A), oviduct (B), uterus (C), cervix (D) and vagina (E) of rats. MTX = methotrexate, LD = low dose, HD =high dose, LCN = leucovorin, WD = withdrawal. P < 0.05, 'a' vs. Control, 'b' vs. MTX LD, 'c' vs. MTX HD, 'd' vs. MTX+LCN. Note marked reduction in phosphatidic acid is tissue and dose dependent. Neither LCN nor withdrawal of MTX treatment brought back the levels to normalcy.

Cervix (Figure 15A): MTX treatment caused a significant (P<0.001) decrease in PA levels in MTXLD, MTXHD, MTXHD+LCN and MTXHD+WD groups compared to the control group. Further, a decrease in MTXHD compared to MTXLD was observed. An increase in the levels in MTXHD+LCN was significant (P<0.001) compared to MTXHD group. A significant (P<0.001) decrease in the PA level was observed in MTXHD+WD group compared to all other treated groups.

Vagina (Figure 15A): MTX treatment caused a significant (P<0.001) increase in PA levels in MTXLD and a decrease in MTXHD, MTXHD+LCN and MTXHD+WD groups compared to the control group. Further, a decrease in MTXHD compared to MTXLD was observed. An increase in the levels in MTXHD+LCN was significant (P<0.001) compared to MTXHD group. A significant (P<0.001) decrease in the PA level was observed in MTXHD+WD group compared to MTXLD and MTXHD+LCN groups.

Effect of MTX on Cardiolipin (Figures 16A-E)

Ovary (Figure 16A): MTX treatment caused a significant (P<0.001) increase in cardiolipin levels in MTXLD and a decrease in MTXHD, MTXHD+LCN and MTXHD+WD groups compared to the control group. Further, a decrease in MTXHD compared to MTXLD was observed. An increase in the levels in MTXHD+LCN was significant (P<0.001) compared to MTXHD group. A significant (P<0.001) decrease in the PA level was observed in MTXHD+WD group compared to MTXLD and MTXHD+LCN groups.

Oviduct (Figure 16B): MTX treatment caused a significant (P<0.001) increase in PA levels in MTXLD and a decrease in MTXHD, MTXHD+LCN and MTXHD+WD groups compared to the control group. Further, a decrease in MTXHD compared to MTXLD was observed. An increase in the levels in MTXHD+LCN was significant (P<0.001) compared to MTXHD group. A significant (P<0.001) decrease in the cardiolipin level was observed in MTXHD+WD group compared to MTXLD, MTXHD and MTXHD+LCN groups.

Uterus (Figure 16C): MTX treatment caused a significant (P<0.001) decrease in cardiolipin levels in MTXLD, MTXHD, MTXHD+LCN and MTXHD+WD groups compared to the control group. Further, a decrease in MTXHD compared to MTXLD was observed. An increase in the levels in MTXHD+LCN and MTXHD+WD was significant (P<0.001) compared to MTXHD group. A significant (P<0.001) increase in the cardiolipin level was observed in MTXHD+WD group compared to MTXLD, MTXHD and MTXHD+LCN groups.

Cervix (Figure 16D): MTX treatment caused a significant (P<0.001) decrease in cardiolipin levels in MTXLD, MTXHD, MTXHD+LCN and MTXHD+WD groups compared to the control group. Further, a decrease in MTXHD compared to MTXLD was observed. An increase in the levels in MTXHD+LCN was significant (P<0.001) compared to MTXHD group. A significant (P<0.001) decrease in the cardiolipin level was observed in MTXHD+WD group compared to MTXLD, MTXHD and MTXHD+LCN groups.

Vagina (Figure 16E): MTX treatment caused a significant (P<0.001) increase in cardiolipin levels in MTXLD and a decrease in MTXHD and MTXHD+WD groups compared to the control group. Further, a decrease in MTXHD compared to MTXLD was observed. An increase in the levels in MTXHD+LCN and MTXHD+WD was significant (P<0.001) compared to MTXHD group. A significant (P<0.001) decrease in the cardiolipin level was observed in MTXHD+WD group compared to MTXLD and MTXHD+LCN groups.

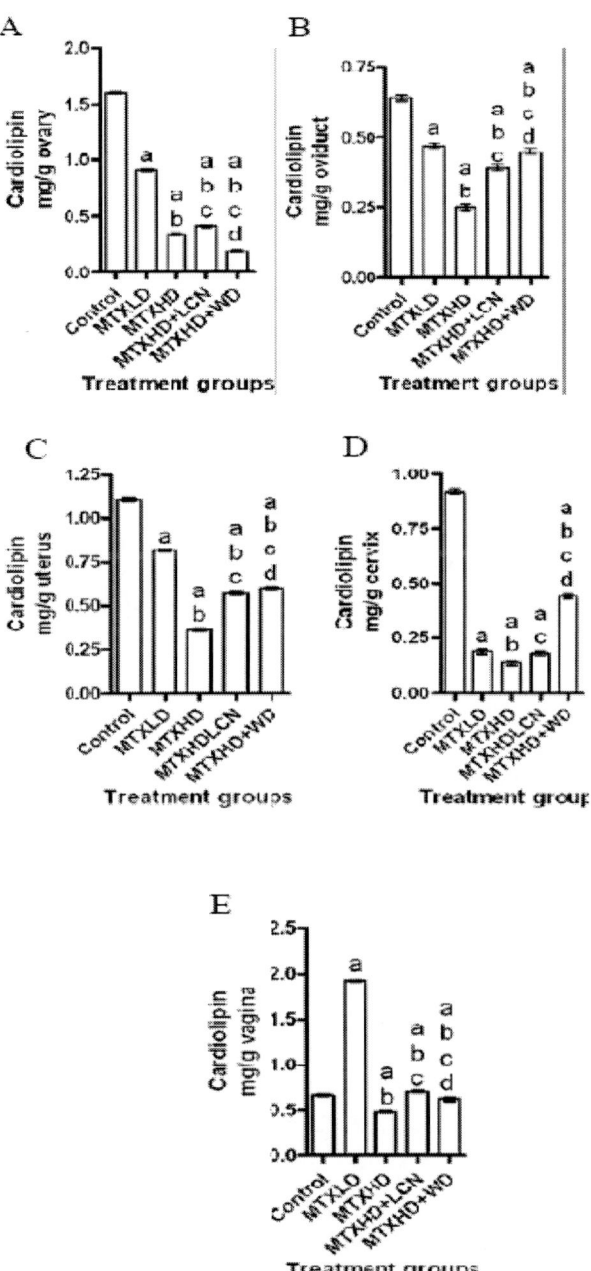

Figure 16 (A–E). Effect of MTX on cardiolipin in ovary (A), oviduct (B), uterus (C), cervix (D) and vagina (E) of rats. MTX = methotrexate, LD = low dose, HD =high dose, LCN = leucovorin, WD = withdrawal. P < 0.05, 'a' vs. Control, 'b' vs. MTX LD, 'c' vs. MTX HD, 'd' vs. MTX+LCN. Note marked reduction in the levels is tissues and dose dependent. Neither LCN nor withdrawal of MTX treatment brought back the levels to normalcy.

Discussion

Lipids like any other cellular components are considered as an active source of nutrient to the cell, cell growth, functions of biological membranes and most importantly for hormone synthesis in the female reproductive tract [40,56]. Significant differences in lipid homeostasis in female reproductive tract lead to various clinical complications [74,82]. Lipid signaling plays a vital role in the function and pathology of the reproductive system [83]. Studies show abnormalities in lipid blood levels in cancer patients as well as changes in lipid fractions in relation to cancer progression [147,148,149]. However, studies elucidating the lipid levels after treatment with individual anticancer drugs are limited. MTX is used extensively as a component of combination therapy for the treatment of neoplastic diseases [2,150]. MTX usage for non-neoplastic and non-malignant diseases across the globe and the risk factors in reproductive health of young women [24,25,26] is soaring, which is an undesirable side effect. MTX toxicity studies on the lipid levels in non-neoplastic conditions are meager in animal studies.

This chapter is the first to describe the induction of abnormalities in lipids and their fractions, in reproductive tissues of female rats exposed to two doses (50μg and 150μg/kg body weight) of MTX. The profile of changes in lipids is also mitigated by LCN supplementation and withdrawal of MTX treatment. Hence, we report the influence of LCN and withdrawal of MTX treatment as the lipid modifying factors in female reproductive tract. Lipids constitute cholesterol, glyceride glycerol and phospholipids among the broad group of naturally occurring molecules, in female reproductive tract. Consequently, the current chapter demonstrates the MTX caused lipid alterations in ovary, oviduct, uterus, cervix and vagina, thereby, establishing yet another mechanism of action of the drug. The present study adds to the growing body of literature that reports adverse effects following non-neoplastic diseases exposure to low doses of MTX in young women.

Among the abnormalities was a general incidence of decreased ovarian total lipids caused by MTX. The incidence is significantly lower than that of controls, which was dose dependent and attributes to the loss in ovary weight, low steroid levels and disruption of folliculogenesis caused by MTX [37]. Increase in total cholesterol content in ovary after MTX treatment appears to be related to the decreased synthesis and secretion of steroid hormones, which did not utilize cholesterol as substrate. Gonadal steroids regulate circulating concentrations of cholesterol [52,53,54]. MTX caused increase in gonadotropins may also be a reason for increased levels of cholesterol in ovary, as gonadotropins stimulate cholesterol synthesis in the cell [56]. The observed elevation of both total cholesterol and esterified cholesterol concentrations may also be due to the lack of corpora lutea/luteolysis and destruction of the growing follicles by MTX [37]. The nature of granulosa cells changes from the chief protein synthesizing cells in follicles to the lipid synthesizing cells in the corpora lutea [85]. Luteolysis results in concomitant increases in both cholesteryl ester and unesterified cholesterol [158]. Steroidogenic acute regulatory (StAR) protein facilitates the acute induction of steroidogenesis in endocrine organs including gonads [57,59]. Previous studies revealed that MTX treatment decreased StAR protein and P450scc gene levels in ovary [35]. Therefore, the non-availability of sufficient amounts of StAR protein may be responsible for not recruiting cholesterol and hence high levels of cholesterol in ovary.

Interestingly, an increase in total cholesterol in current chapter is similar to that reported following MTX treatment in arthritis patients [51].

MTX caused an increase in total glyceride levels in ovary. Glycerides form the main fraction of total lipids in regressing corpora lutea [88]. The effect of MTX on the histology of ovary illustrates the depletion of follicles in the ovary [37]. Therefore, it is possible that there is a decrease in the utilization of glycerides as energy source by the follicles, as a result of MTX treatment and hence, high levels of glycerides. This is supported further by an increase in the glycerides after LCN supplementation and withdrawal of MTX treatment. The elevated levels of glycerides in ovary may also be due to possible decrease in the synthesis of phospholipids [162]. Decreased total phospholipids caused by MTX in ovary can be correlated to the decreased intracellular membranes of the follicle cells [88]. LCN supplementation and withdrawal of MTX treatment increased the total phospholipid levels with an increase in small follicles and corpora lutea. These results concur with the previous reports that phospholipids form a major component of total lipids in small sized follicles and developed corpus luteum [88]. The luteal cells show abundant diffuse lipoproteins and lipid droplets composed mainly of phospholipids and some triglycerides, which are indicative of steroidogenesis [87].

Lipids influence the functions of oviduct *viz;* sperm capacitation, the acrosome reaction, and early embryo development [95,96]. Epithelial cells of the oviduct comprise lipid droplets and their numbers are reported to fluctuate with endocrine status [97]. A decrease in oviduct total lipids was observed by MTX treatment in the current chapter. Oviduct is capable of significant *de novo* synthesis of a variety of lipids, and is affected by the stage of the ovarian cycle [98, 100]. Disruption in oestrous cycle and decrease in oviduct weights [35] may be the reason for decreased total lipid levels by MTX. Oviducal epithelium regulates cholesterol availability within the lumen. Regional differences exist in localization of oviducal lipid droplets and phospholipid containing choline. Concentrations of neutral lipid droplets, free cholesterol, and glycerides were highest in the preampulla and ampulla and least in the isthmus. In the isthmus, phospholipid-containing choline in mucosal crypts and high amounts of epithelial esterified cholesterol may play a role in sperm storage [99,108]. Low levels of glyceride glycerol and phospholipids may attribute to the overall decrease in oviducal lipids. MTX caused differences in oviducal cholesterol, glyceride glycerol and phospholipids and their fractions may reflect the changes in the luminal environment and the histoarchitecture of oviduct [37].

Another abnormality induced in all MTX dose groups is low lipid levels of uterus. Uterine signaling and contractility has been described by the influence of hormones on lipids and cholesterol levels [112,113]. Hormones were shown to attenuate total lipid content in rat uterus and in cells [109,110]. MTX interference with hormone levels clearly indicates one of the reasons for the decrease in total lipid content in uterus, resulting in structural and cellular alterations [37,38]. Changes in membrane fluidity increase cholesterol in the uterus [114]. The presence of lipid in epithelium and stroma seems mainly a degenerative phenomenon associated with cell break down and tissue disruption [115]. This suggestion is supported by the observation of break down in the uterine cellular structure by MTX [37,38]. The molecular mechanism involves altered StAR protein expression in the differentiation of uterus as MTX reduced the expression this gene [38]. Subsequent studies suggest the antiestrogenic and antiprogestational activity of MTX [37,38]. Increase in total cholesterol levels in uterus by MTX involves an increase in the esterified cholesterol compared to free cholesterol. While, a decrease in total glyceride content observed in uterus may be due to increased utilization to compensate the levels of other lipid fractions. Many changes in lipid metabolism occur in progesterone-primed uterus, including significant increases in cholesterol and triglycerides [117,118]. These changes in lipid metabolism have been suggested to help maintain an adequate supply of nutrients to the growing tissue [119]. The lesions occurred in the uterus of rats treated with MTX, and the incidence was significantly different from controls. Although these lesions were histologically drastic and MTX dose dependent, the lesions were more severe and their involvement in the uterine horns was more extensive in the high-dose treated groups compared with controls reported previously [37,38].

Bulk phospholipids change in the myometrium with changes in membrane fluidity and increased cholesterol [115]. Phospholipid fractions choline, inositol and ethanolamine are estrogen dependent and their reduction in the uterus concurs with the reduction in steroid levels reported previously [37]. MTX is also known to cause choline deficiency [6,163]. Choline, methionine and folate metabolism are interrelated and any disturbance in the folate metabolism would perturb methionine and choline synthesis [66]. The consistent decrease observed in phosphatidyl choline, serine and ethanolamine in MTX treated groups suggests severe derangement in folate metabolism, resulting in low provision of precursors. An increase after LCN supplementation suggests improvement in the folate metabolism thereby increasing the levels of these fractions. Phosphatidic acid is dephosphorylated to give diacyl glycerol, the immediate precursor of both phospholipids and neutral triglycerides. Phosphatidic acid is the precursor for the anionic phospholipids (phosphatidylinositol, phosphatidylglycerol, and cardiolipin), whereas diacylglycerol is the precursor for the quantitatively most prominent phospholipids (phosphatidyl choline, phosphatidyl ethanolamine, and phosphatidyl serine) as well as for triacylglycerol [65]. Variations in the total glyceride glycerol and phospholipids fractions may be due to the fluctuation in phosphatidic acid and diacylglycerol levels. Decrease in sphingomyelin in uterus may be due to the MTX effect on the cell membranes. Although synthesized in the intra-cellular region sphingomyelin is transported to the plasma membranes [89]. Estradiol increases phospholipid content in plasma membranes [164] and modulates phosphatidyl inositol turnover through an estrogen receptor mediated mechanism. The metabolic products of lipids are important for signal transduction and cellular proliferation. Altered metabolism of lipids may play an integral role in estrogenic–induced mitogenesis [159]. Cardiolipin is a potent stimulator of luteal mitochondrial steroidogenesis [165]. Alteration in cardiolipin content by MTX in uterus may be associated with the inhibition of cellular proliferation, metabolic flux and necrosis [35,36,37,38,39]. These studies also correspond to the reports that cardiolipin content/composition or abnormalities happen due to various environmental factors contributing to tumor initiation and progression [73,77,79].

Total lipid decrease in cervix and vagina of MTX treated rats also indicates that the lipid content in these tissues is related to the stage of differentiation of the epithelium and in atrophy [35]. Partial protective effect of LCN supplementation and withdrawal of treatment also reflects on the hormonal levels and improvement in histoarchitecture of ovary, oviduct, uterus, cervix and vagina from previous studies [37]. Cholesterol and cholesterol esters, triglycerides, phospholipids, are major components of cervix and vaginal cells [123]. The triglycerides content of cervical and vaginal cells is also related to the stage of differentiation of the cervical and vaginal epithelium in the estrogenic and progesteronic phases and in atrophy [123]. Decrease in total glycerides and phospholipids also contribute to this decrease in total lipids of these tissues. Epithelium exhibits regional differences in lipid distribution in cervix and vagina [98,99]. Histopathology reveals disruption of epithelium by MTX causing a decrease in steroids [37], which may be the cause for accumulation of esterified cholesterol in the current chapter. However, decrease in cholesterol levels in cervix depicts low levels of free cholesterol. This also indicates the reduction in uptake of blood cholesterol, the cause for accumulation of cholesterol in the current study, which agrees with the previous reports [159]. The general trend in the increase of cholesterol in these tissues may be a compensation for the decreased total phospholipids.

Phospholipids and its fractions are the major lipid classes in the reproductive tissues. Therefore, the decrease in the phospholipid fractions in the MTX treated groups observed in cervix and vagina may account for the decrease in total lipids concentrations. Phospholipids are a major component of all cell membranes forming the lipid bilayer [65]. Enhanced phosphatidylinositol lipid turnover in immature rats demonstrates involvement in the early events of estradiol-induced rat vaginal cell differentiation [125]. Structural defects of cervix and vagina and the low levels of estrogen caused by MTX in rats was evident by histological and hormone analysis [37], these results also concur with the previous reports [109]. The decrease in total phospholipids in these organs may be correlated to the decrease in cell proliferation and protein synthesis from the data on nucleic acids [37]. LCN supplementation did not rescue MTX effects completely in all the tissues. It is well known that choline, methionine and folate metabolism are interrelated [66] and any disturbance in the folate metabolism would perturb methionine and choline synthesis. Choline is the only single nutrient for which dietary deficiency is associated with the development of cancer [67,68].

Thus, the present chapter clearly identifies adverse effects by MTX on the lipid markers, in ovary, oviduct, uterus, cervix and vagina. MTX high-dose has a profound action on the lipids and its fractions. Interestingly, lipid fractions in LCN supplemented and withdrawal of MTX treatment groups were also equally affected and the rescue was minimal in all the tissues. Thus, the present chapter extends the knowledge on MTX induced damage to female reproductive tract lipids in albino rats. Explicitly, previous studies [35,36,37,38,39] and the current chapter from our group show that MTX works through multiple gene pathways. Thus, molecular "misprogramming" is most likely responsible for MTX-induced female reproductive tract alterations.

Conclusion

In summary, the findings of the present study raise concerns about widespread exposure to MTX and, in particular, exposure affecting lipids and its fractions in the female reproductive tissues considered in the current chapter. Such effects confirm that MTX has disrupted endocrine function at the hypothalamic/pituitary and ovarian level through lipid genes. The effect of low and high doses of MTX, LCN supplementation and withdrawal of MTX treatment unambiguously revealed variation in (a) total lipids (b) total cholesterol and its fractions free and esterified cholesterol (c) total glyceride glycerol and its fractions mono, di and triacyl glyceride glycerol (d) total phospholipids, and its fractions phosphatidyl inositol, phosphatidyl choline, phosphatidyl ethanolamine, phosphatidyl serine, sphingomyelin, phosphatidic acid and cardiolipin in female reproductive tract of rats. Low levels of phospholipids observed in these tissues were the basis of decline in the total lipids caused by MTX treatment. Although LCN and withdrawal of MTX treatment rescued some fractions, overall their restoration was not effective. To the best of our knowledge, this is the first report to emphasize lipid markers as an additional mechanism by which MTX restrains the vital functions of the female reproductive tract in rats.

Acknowledgments

Financial support for this work by Bharathiar University, Coimbatore, India, to SK is gratefully acknowledged.

References

[1]   Bertino, JR. Methotrexate: historical aspects.In: Cronstein BN, Bertino, J.R., editor. Methotrexate.Basel/Switzerland:Birkhauser Verlag;2000. p.1-5.

[2]   Goldman, ID; Chattopadhyay, S; Zhao, R, Moran, R.(2010). The antifolates: Evolution, new agents in the clinic, and how targeting delivery via specific membrane transporters is driving the development of a next generation of folate analogs. *Curr. Opin. Investig. Drugs* 11,1409-23.

[3]   Singer, O, Gibofsky, A.(2011).Methotrexate versus leflunomide in rheumatoid arthritis: what is new in 2011? *Curr. Opin. Rheumatol.* 23,288-92.

[4]   Bertino, JR.(1963). The Mechanism of Action of the Folate Antagonists in Man. *Cancer Res.* 23,1286-306.

[5]   Goldman, ID.(1974). The mechanism of action of methotrexate. I. Interaction with a low-affinity intracellular site required for maximum inhibition of deoxyribonucleic acid synthesis in L-cell mouse fibroblasts. *Mol. Pharmacol.* 10,257-74.

[6]   Jackson, RC.(1984). Biological effects of folic acid antagonists with antineoplastic activity. *Pharmacol. Ther.* 25,61-82.

[7]   Skipper, HE;Schabel, FM, Jr., Wilcox, WS.(1967).Experimental evaluation of potential anticancer agents. XXI. Scheduling of arabinosylcytosine to take advantage of its S-phase specificity against leukemia cells. *Cancer Chemother. Rep.* 51,125-65.

[8]   Black, RL; O'Brien, WM; Vanscott, EJ; Auerbach, R; Eisen, AZ, Bunim, JJ. (1964). Methotrexate Therapy in Psoriatic Arthritis; Double-Blind Study on 21 Patients. *JAMA* 189,743-7.

[9]   Braun, J, Baraliakos, X.(2009). Treatment of ankylosing spondylitis and other spondyloarthritides. *Curr. Opin. Rheumatol.* 21,324-34.

[10]   De Moragas, JM.(1965). Psoriasis and methotrexate. *Rev. Clin. Esp.* 99,122-6.

[11]   Stovall, TG;Ling, FW;Gray, LA;Carson, SA, Buster, JE.(1991). Methotrexate treatment of unruptured ectopic pregnancy: a report of 100 cases. *Obstet. Gynecol.* 77,749-53.

[12]   Shiina, H;Oka, K;Okane, M;Tanno, W;Kawasaki, T, Nakayama, M.(2002). Coexisting true hermaphroditism and partial hydatidiform mole developing metastatic gestational trophoblastic tumors. A case report. *Virchows Arch.* 441,514-8.

[13] Karsdorp, VH;Van der Veen, F;Schats, R;Boer-Meisel, ME, Kenemans, P.(1992). Successful treatment with methotrexate of five vital interstitial pregnancies. *Hum. Reprod.* 7,1164-9.

[14] Trojano, G;Colafiglio, G;Saliani, N;Lanzillotti, G, Cicinelli, E.(2009). Successful management of a cervical twin pregnancy: neoadjuvant systemic methotrexate and prophylactic high cervical cerclage before curettage. *Fertil. Steril.* 91,935 e17-9.

[15] Iqbal, MP;Ahmed, M;Umer, M;Mehboobali, N, Qureshi, AA.(2003). Effect of methotrexate and folinic acid on skeletal growth in mice. *Acta Paediatr.* 92,1438-44.

[16] Aarsaether, N;Berge, RK;Aarsland, A;Svardal, A, Ueland, PM.(1988). Effect of methotrexate on long-chain fatty acid metabolism in liver of rats fed a standard or a defined, choline-deficient diet. *Biochim. Biophys. Acta.* 958,70-80.

[17] Costajde, S, Lima, RR.(1963). Pulmonary Metastases of Choriocarcinoma Treated with Methotrexate and Radiotherapy. *Arq. Bras. Endocrinol. Metabol.* 12,39-48.

[18] Pochedly, C.(1977). Neurotoxicity due to CNS therapy for leukemia. *Med. Pediatr. Oncol.* 3,101-15.

[19] Soga, N;Arima, K, Sugimura, Y.(2008). Adjuvant methotrexate, vinblastine, adriamycin, and cisplatin chemotherapy has potential to prevent recurrence of bladder tumors after surgical removal of upper urinary tract transitional cell carcinoma. *Int. J. Urol.* 15,800-3.

[20] Averette, HE;Boike, GM, Jarrell, MA.(1990). Effects of cancer chemotherapy on gonadal function and reproductive capacity. *CA Cancer J. Clin.*40,199-209.

[21] Badri, SN;Vanithakumari, G, Malini, T.(2000). Studies on methotrexate effects on testicular steroidogenesis in rats. *Endocr. Res.* 26,247-62.

[22] Padmanabhan, S;Tripathi, DN;Vikram, A;Ramarao, P, Jena, GB.(2009). Methotrexate-induced cytotoxicity and genotoxicity in germ cells of mice: intervention of folic and folinic acid. *Mutat. Res.* 673,43-52.

[23] Chapman, RM.(1983). Gonadal injury resulting from chemotherapy. *Am. J. Ind. Med.* 4,149-61.

[24] Aggarwal, A; Thomas, M; Spitzer, RF; Kives, S, Allen, L.(2009). Methotrexate in the management of adolescents with ectopic pregnancies: a physician survey. *J. Obstet. Gynaecol. Can.* 31,254-62.

[25] Creemers, MC; Franssen, MJ; van de Putte, LB; Gribnau, FW, van Riel, PL. (1995).Methotrexate in severe ankylosing spondylitis: an open study. *J. Rheumatol.* 22,1104-7.

[26] Beghin, D; Cournot, MP; Vauzelle, C, Elefant, E.(2011). Paternal Exposure to Methotrexate and Pregnancy Outcomes. *J. Rheumatol.* 386,28-32.

[27] Albert, A.Selective Toxicity.In: Clay R, editor.The Physico-chemical basis of therapy.Bungay, Suffolk, UK:The Chaucer Press;1981. p.309-13.

[28] Zeisel, SH.Choline deficiency. J Nutr Biochem 1990.1(issue): 332-49.

[29] Erbe, RE.Inborn errors of folate metabolism (first of two parts). N Engl J Med 1975.293(issue):753-7.

[30] Bertino, JR; Levitt, M; McCullough, JL, Chabner, B.(1971). New approaches to chemotherapy with folate antagonists: use of leucovorin "rescue" and enzymic folate depletion. *Ann. N. Y. Acad. Sci.* 186,486-95.

[31] Rosen, G;Suwansirikul, S;Kwon, C;Tan, C;Wu, SJ;Beattie, EJ, Jr., Murphy, ML.(1974). High-dose methotrexate with citrovorum factor rescue and adriamycin in childhood osteogenic sarcoma. *Cancer* 33, 1151-63.

[32] Stover, P, Schirch, V.(1993).The metabolic role of leucovorin. *Trends Biochem. Sci.* 18,102-6.

[33] Black, DJ, Livingston, RB.(1990). Antineoplastic drugs in 1990. A review (Part I). *Drugs* 39,489-501.

[34] Sirotnak, FM; Donsbach, RC; Moccio, DM, Dorick, DM. (1976). Biochemical and pharmacokinetic effects of leucovorin after high-dose methotrexate in a murine leukemia model. *Cancer Res.* 36,4679-86.

[35] Karri, S, Vanithakumari, G.(2011). Methotrexate and leucovorin exposure modulates biochemical markers in female accessory reproductive organs of albino rats. Acta endocrinologica (Buc). In press,

[36] Karri, S, Vanithakumari, G.(2011). Influence of methotrexate and leucovorin on glycogen content in female reproductive tract of albino rats. Acta Endocrinologica (Buc), In press,

[37] Karri, S, Vanithakumari, G.(2011). Effect of methotrexate and leucovorin on female reproductive tract of albino rats. *Cell Biochem. and Funct.* 29,1-21.

[38] Karri, S;Vanithakumari, G, Gopalakrishnan, CR.(2010). Antiestrogenic and Antiprogestational Activity of Methotrexate and its Effect on Uterine Histoarchitecture of Ovariectomized Albino Rats. *Bioresearch Bulletin* 4,166-75.

[39] Karri, S, Vanithakumari, G.(2011). Anti-implantation activity of methotrexate and leucovorin in albino rats. Acta Endocrinologica (Buc), In press,

[40] Stubbs, CD, Smith, AD.(1984). The modification of mammalian membrane polyunsaturated fatty acid composition in relation to membrane fluidity and function. *Biochim. Biophys. Acta* 779,89-137.

[41] Hirata, F;Strittmatter, WJ, Axelrod, J.(1979). beta-Adrenergic receptor agonists increase phospholipid methylation, membrane fluidity, and beta-adrenergic receptor-adenylate cyclase coupling. *Proc. Natl. Acad. Sci. USA* 76,368-72.

[42] Galo, MG;Unates, LE, Farias, RN.(1981). Effect of membrane fatty acid composition on the action of thyroid hormones on $(Ca^{2+} + Mg^{2+})$-adenosine triphosphatase from rat erythrocyte. *J. Biol. Chem.* 256,7113-4.

[43] Frisch, RE.(1991). Body weight, body fat, and ovulation. *Trends Endocrinol. Metab.* 2,191-7.

[44] Kweon, OK; Kanagawa, H; Takahashi, Y; Yamashina, H; Seike, N; Iwazumi, Y; Aoyagi, Y, Ono, H.(1986). Factors affecting superovulation response in cattle. Nippon Juigaku Zasshi. 48,495-503.

[45] Kweon, OK; Ono, H; Seta, T; Onda, M; Oboshi, K, Kanagawa, H.(1985). Relationship between serum total cholesterol levels before calving and occurrence rate of diseases after calving in Holstein heifers and cows. *Jpn. J. Vet. Res.* 33,11-7.

[46] Kappel, LC; Ingraham, RH; Morgan, EB; Zeringue, L; Wilson, D, Babcock, DK.(1984). Relationship between fertility and blood glucose and cholesterol concentrations in Holstein cows. *Am. J. Vet. Res.* 45,2607-12.

[47] Yeagel, PL.(1985). Cholesterol and the cell membrane. *Biochim. Biophy. Acta* 822,267-87.

[48]   Pomorski, T; Hrafnsdottir, S; Devaux, PF, van Meer, G.(2001). Lipid distribution and transport across cellular membranes. *Semin. Cell Dev. Biol.* 12,139-48.

[49]   Liscum, L, Munn, NJ.(1999). Intracellular cholesterol transport. *Biochim. Biophys. Acta* 1438,19-37.

[50]   Burger, K; Gimpl, G, Fahrenholz, F.(2000). Regulation of receptor function by cholesterol. *Cell Mol. Life Sci.* 57,1577-92.

[51]   Chih, HM; Chang, HY; Chen, DY; Lan J La, Chiang, EP.Low-dose methotrexate treatment is associated with increased total cholesterol and HDL-cholesterol in blood: a pilot study (Chinese). Nutri Sci J. in press

[52]   Gal, D; MacDonald, PC; Porter, JC, Simpson, ER.(1981).Cholesterol metabolism in cancer cells in monolayer culture. III. Low-density lipoprotein metabolism. *Int. J. Cancer* 28,315-9.

[53]   Fillios, LC; Kaplan, R; Martin, RS, Stare, FJ.(1958). Some aspects of the gonadal regulation of cholesterol metabolism. *Am. J. Physiol.* 193,47-51.

[54]   Fillios, LC.(1957).The gonadal regulation of cholesteremia in the rat. *Endocrinology* 60,22-7.

[55]   Panini, SR; Gupta, A; Sexton, RC; Parish, EJ, Rudney, H.(1987). Regulation of sterol biosynthesis and of 3-hydroxy-3-methylglutaryl-coenzyme A reductase activity in cultured cells by progesterone. *J. Biol. Chem.* 262,14435-40.

[56]   Dorfman, RI.Endocrinology.In: Greep ROaA, E.B, editor. Handbook of Physiology. Baltimore, MD:Waverly Press;1973. p.537-46.

[57]   Clark, BJ;Wells, J;King, SR, Stocco, DM.The purification, cloning, and expression of a novel luteinizing hormone-induced mitochondrial protein in MA-10 mouse Leydig tumor cells. Characterization of the steroidogenic acute regulatory protein (StAR). J Biol Chem 1994.269(issue):28314-22.

[58]   Clark, BJ, Stocco, DM.Expression of the steroidogenic acute regulatory (StAR) protein: a novel LH-induced mitochondrial protein required for the acute regulation of steroidogenesis in mouse Leydig tumor cells. Endocr Res 1995.21(issue):243-57.

[59]   Pon, LA, Orme-Johnson, NR.Acute stimulation of corpus luteum cells by gonadotrophin or adenosine 3',5'-monophosphate causes accumulation of a phosphoprotein concurrent with acceleration of steroid synthesis. Endocrinology 1988.123(issue):1942-8.

[60]   Ballard, FJ;Hanson, RW, Leveille, GA.(1967). Phosphoenolpyruvate carboxykinase and the synthesis of glyceride-glycerol from pyruvate in adipose tissue. *J. Biol. Chem.* 242,2746-50.

[61]   Reshef, L; Niv, J, Shapiro, B.(1967). Effect of propionate on pyruvate metabolism in adipose tissue. *J. Lipid Res.* 8,688-91.

[62]   Winegrad, AI, Renold, AE.(1958). Studies on rat adipose tissue in vitro. I. Effects of insulin on the metabolism of glucose, pyruvate, and acetate. *J. Biol. Chem.* 233,267-72.

[63]   Mittra, S;Bansal, VS, Bhatnagar, PK.(2008). From a glucocentric to a lipocentric approach towards metabolic syndrome. *Drug Discov. Today* 13,211-8.

[64]   Cheung, O, Sanyal, AJ.(2008). Abnormalities of lipid metabolism in nonalcoholic fatty liver disease. *Semin. Liver Dis.* 28,351-9.

[65]   Ansell, GBa, Spanner, S. The phospholipids- Chemistry, Metabolism and Function.In: Ansell GB, Hawthrone JN, editors. New Comprehensive Biochemistry. Amsterdam, The Netherlands: Elsevier Biomedical; 1964. p.1-41.

[66] Davis, RE.Clinical Chemistry of Folic Acid.In: Davis RE, editor. Advances in Clinical Chemistry. New York:Academic press; 1986. p.233-94.

[67] Newberne, PM, Rogers, AE.(1986). Labile methyl groups and the promotion of cancer. *Annu. Rev. Nutr.* 6,407-32.

[68] Zeisel, SH; Da Costa, KA; Franklin, PD; Alexander, EA; Lamont, JT; Sheard, NF, Beiser, A.(1991). Choline, an essential nutrient for humans. *FASEB J.* 5,2093-8.

[69] Connor, J, Schroit, AJ.(1991). Transbilayer movement of phosphatidylserine in erythrocytes. Inhibitors of aminophospholipid transport block the association of photolabeled lipid to its transporter. *Biochim. Biophys. Acta* 1066,37-42.

[70] Hovius, R; Faber, B; Brigot, B; Nicolay, K, de Kruijff, B.(1992).On the mechanism of the mitochondrial decarboxylation of phosphatidylserine. *J. Biol. Chem.* 267,16790-5.

[71] Summers, SA, Nelson, DH.(2005).A role for sphingolipids in producing the common features of type 2 diabetes, metabolic syndrome X, and Cushing's syndrome. *Diabetes* 54,591-602.

[72] Uehara, K; Miura, S; Takeuchi, T; Taki, T; Nakashita, M; Adachi, M; Inamura, T; Ogawa, T; Akiba, Y; Suzuki, H; Nagata, H, Ishii, H. (2003).Significant role of ceramide pathway in experimental gastric ulcer formation in rats. *J. Pharmacol. Exp. Ther.* 305,232-9.

[73] Kiebish, MA;Han, X;Cheng, H;Chuang, JH, Seyfried, TN.(2008). Cardiolipin and electron transport chain abnormalities in mouse brain tumor mitochondria: lipidomic evidence supporting the Warburg theory of cancer. *J. Lipid Res.*49,2545-56.

[74] Limoli, CL;Giedzinski, E;Morgan, WF;Swarts, SG;Jones, GD, Hyun, W.(2003).Persistent oxidative stress in chromosomally unstable cells. *Cancer Res.* 63,3107-11.

[75] Hardy, S;El-Assaad, W;Przybytkowski, E;Joly, E;Prentki, M, Langelier, Y.(2003). Saturated fatty acid-induced apoptosis in MDA-MB-231 breast cancer cells. A role for cardiolipin. *J. Biol. Chem.* 278,31861-70.

[76] Matoba, S; Kang, JG; Patino, WD; Wragg, A; Boehm, M; Gavrilova, O; Hurley, PJ; Bunz, F, Hwang, PM.(2006). p53 regulates mitochondrial respiration. *Science* 312,1650-3.

[77] Houtkooper, RH, Vaz, FM.(2008). Cardiolipin, the heart of mitochondrial metabolism. *Cell Mol. Life Sci.* 65,2493-506.

[78] Petrosillo, G; Ruggiero, FM; Pistolese, M, Paradies, G.(2004). Ca2+-induced reactive oxygen species production promotes cytochrome c release from rat liver mitochondria via mitochondrial permeability transition (MPT)-dependent and MPT-independent mechanisms: role of cardiolipin. *J. Biol. Chem.* 279,53103-8.

[79] McMillin, JB, Dowhan, W.(2002). Cardiolipin and apoptosis. *Biochim. Biophys. Acta* 1585, 97-107.

[80] Cheng, P, Hatch, GM.(1995). Inhibition of cardiolipin biosynthesis in the hypoxic rat heart. *Lipids* 30,513-9.

[81] Yamaoka, S;Urade, R, Kito, M.(1990). Cardiolipin molecular species in rat heart mitochondria are sensitive to essential fatty acid-deficient dietary lipids. *J. Nutr.* 120,415-21.

[82] Wild, RA; Rizzo, M; Clifton, S, Carmina, E. Lipid levels in polycystic ovary syndrome: systematic review and meta-analysis. *Fertil. Steril.* 95,1073-9 e1-11.

[83] Ye, X.(2008). Lysophospholipid signaling in the function and pathology of the reproductive system. *Hum. Reprod.* Update 14,519-36.

[84] Singh, GK; Miller, BA; Hankey, BF, Edwards, BK.(2004). Persistent area socioeconomic disparities in U.S. incidence of cervical cancer, mortality, stage, and survival, 1975-2000. *Cancer* 101,1051-7.

[85] Guraya, SS.Biology of the ovary. In: Motta PMaH, E.S.E, editor. Developments in obstetrics and gynecology. The Hague, Netherlands: Martinus Nijhoff; 1980. p.344.

[86] Tuckey, RC; Lee, G;Costa, ND, Stevenson, PM.(1984). The composition and distribution of lipid granules in the rat ovary. *Mol. Cell Endocrinol.* 38,187-95.

[87] Guraya, SS.Biology of Ovarian Follicles in Mammals. Berlin: Springer-Verlag; 1985.

[88] Sangha, GK, Guraya, SS.(1989). Biochemical changes in lipids during follicular growth and corpora lutea formation and regression in rat ovary. *Indian J. Exp. Biol.* 27,998-1000.

[89] Kobayashi, T, Pagano, RE.(1989). Lipid transport during mitosis. Alternative pathways for delivery of newly synthesized lipids to the cell surface. *J. Biol. Chem.* 264,5966-73.

[90] Tyson, CA;Vande Zande, H, Green, DE.(1976). Phospholipids as ionophores. *J. Biol. Chem.* 251,1326-32.

[91] Brown, DA, Rose, JK.(1992). Sorting of GPI-anchored proteins to glycolipid-enriched membrane subdomains during transport to the apical cell surface. *Cell* 68,533-44.

[92] Harder, T;Scheiffele, P;Verkade, P, Simons, K.(1998). Lipid domain structure of the plasma membrane revealed by patching of membrane components. *J. Cell Biol.* 141, 929-42.

[93] Tanphaichitr, N;Smith, J;Mongkolsirikieart, S;Gradil, C, Lingwood, CA.(1993). Role of a gamete-specific sulfoglycolipid immobilizing protein on mouse sperm-egg binding. *Dev. Biol.* 156,164-75.

[94] Maehashi, E; Sato, C; Ohta, K; Harada, Y; Matsuda, T; Hirohashi, N; Lennarz, WJ, Kitajima, K.(2003). Identification of the sea urchin 350-kDa sperm-binding protein as a new sialic acid-binding lectin that belongs to the heat shock protein 110 family: implication of its binding to gangliosides in sperm lipid rafts in fertilization. *J. Biol. Chem.* 278,42050-7.

[95] Mukherjee, AB, Lippes, J.(1972). Effect of human follicular and tubal fluids on human, mouse and rat spermatozoa in vitro. *Can. J. Genet. Cytol.* 14,167-74.

[96] Elliott, DS.Ova and embryo metabolism: functions of the oviduct. .In: Foley ADJCW, editor. The Oviduct and its Functions.New York: Academic Press; 1974. p.301-32.

[97] Witkowska, E.(1979). Reactivity of the epithelial cells of the bovine oviduct in vitro on the exogenic gonadotropic and steroid hormones. Part I: The effect of gonadotropic and steroid hormones on the amount of lipids and activity of dehydrogenases. *Folia Histochem. Cytochem.* (Krakow). 17,225-38.

[98] Wordinger, RJ; Dickey, JF, Ellicott, AR.(1977). Histochemical evaluation of the lipid droplet content of bovine oviductal and endometrial epithelial cells. *J. Reprod. Fertil.* 49,113-4.

[99] Henault, MA, Killian, GJ.(1993). Neutral lipid droplets in bovine oviductal epithelium and lipid composition of epithelial cell homogenates. *J. Dairy Sci.* 76,691-700.

[100] Killian, GJ; Chapman, DA; Kavanaugh, JF; Deaver, DR, Wiggin, HB.(1989). Changes in phospholipids, cholesterol and protein content of oviduct fluid of cows during the oestrous cycle. *J. Reprod. Fertil.* 86, 419-26.

[101] Kane, MT.(1979). Fatty acids as energy sources for culture of one-cell rabbit ova to viable morulae. *Biol. Reprod.* 20,323-32.

[102] Quinn, P, and , Whittingham, DG.(1982.). Effect of fatty acids on fertilization and development of mouse embryos in vitro. *J. Androl.* 3,440-44.

[103] Waterman, RA, Wall, RJ.(1988). Lipid interactions with in vitro development of mammalian zygotes. *Gamete Res.* 21,243-54.

[104] Hillman, N, Flynn, TJ.(1980). The metabolism of exogenous fatty acids by preimplantation mouse embryos developing in vitro. *J. Embryol. Exp. Morphol.* 56,157-68.

[105] Pratt, HP.(1980). Phospholipid synthesis in the preimplantation mouse embryo. *J. Reprod. Fertil.* 58,237-48.

[106] Pratt, HP.(1982). Preimplantation mouse embryos synthesize membrane sterols. *Dev. Biol.* 89,101-10.

[107] Langlais, Ja, Roberts., KD.(1985). A molecular membrane model of sperm capacitation and the acrosome reaction of mammalian spermatozoa. *Gamete Res.* 12,183.

[108] Henault, MA, Killian, GJ.(1993). Synthesis and secretion of lipids by bovine oviduct mucosal explants. *J. Reprod. Fertil.* 98,431-8.

[109] Sakai, Y;Kogo, H, Aizawa, Y.(1980). Effects of estrogen on fatty acid composition in rat uterine lipids (author's transl). Nippon Yakurigaku Zasshi. 76,429-34.

[110] Witkowska, E.(1979). Reactivity of the epithelial cells of the bovine oviduct in vitro on the exogenic, gonadotropic and steroid hormones. Part II: The effect of gonadotropic hormones on the amount of glycogen and of acid and alkaline phosphatases. *Folia Histochem. Cytochem.* (Krakow).17,239-50.

[111] Hall, K.(1975). Lipids in the mouse uterus during early pregnancy. *J. Endocrinol.* 65,233-43.

[112] Wray, S, Noble, K.(2008). Sex hormones and excitation-contraction coupling in the uterus: the effects of oestrous and hormones. *J. Neuroendocrinol.* 20,451-61.

[113] Wray, S.(2007). Insights into the uterus. *Exp. Physiol.* 92,621-31.

[114] Pulkkinen, MO; Hamalainen, MM; Nyman, S; Pihlaja, K, Mattinen, J.(1996). Tissue phospholipids during human pregnancy by 31P NMR: myometrium, decidua, placenta and fetal membranes. *NMR Biomed.* 9,53-8.

[115] Pulkkinen, MO; Nyman, S; Hamalainen, MM, Mattinen, J.(1998). Proton NMR spectroscopy of the phospholipids in human uterine smooth muscle and placenta. *Gynecol. Obstet. Invest.* 46,220-4.

[116] Diveky, L; Handzo, I; Krizko, M; Suska, P; Vozar, I; Bella, J; Valuch, J; Turecky, L, Pohlodek, K.(1990). Phospholipids in the human myometrium in various stages of contraction before and during labor. *Bratisl. Lek. Listy*.91,720-6.

[117] Piechota, W, Staszewski, A.(1992). Reference ranges of lipids and apolipoproteins in pregnancy. *Eur. J. Obstet. Gynecol. Reprod. Biol.* 45,27-35.

[118] Toescu, V; Nuttall, SL; Martin, U; Nightingale, P; Kendall, MJ; Brydon, P, Dunne, F.(2004). Changes in plasma lipids and markers of oxidative stress in normal pregnancy and pregnancies complicated by diabetes. *Clin. Sci.* (Lond).106,93-8.

[119] .Brizzi, P; Tonolo, G; Esposito, F; Puddu, L; Dessole, S; Maioli, M, Milia, S.(1999). Lipoprotein metabolism during normal pregnancy. *Am. J. Obstet. Gynecol.* 181,430-4.

[120] Smith, RD; Babiychuk, EB; Noble, K; Draeger, A, Wray, S.(2005). Increased cholesterol decreases uterine activity: functional effects of cholesterol alteration in pregnant rat myometrium. *Am. J. Physiol. Cell Physiol.* 288,C982-8.

[121] Martins-Santos, ME; Chaves, VE; Frasson, D; Boschini, RP;Garofalo, MA; Kettelhut Ido, C, Migliorini, RH.(2007). Glyceroneogenesis and the supply of glycerol-3-phosphate for glyceride-glycerol synthesis in liver slices of fasted and diabetic rats. *Am. J. Physiol. Endocrinol. Metab.* 293,E1352-7.

[122] Singh, EJ, Swartwout, JR.(1972). Human cervical mucus lipids. A preliminary report. *J. Reprod. Med.* 8,35-40.

[123] Bibbo, M; Camargo, AC, Valeri, V.(1969). Studies of cell lipids from the human vaginal and cervical epithelium during the menstrual cycle. *Acta Cytol.* 13,260-3.

[124] Masin, F, Masin, M.(1964). Lipid Patterns in Cervical and Vaginal Cells under Hormonal Stimulus. *Acta Cytol.* 8,263-9.

[125] Singh, S, Gupta, PD.(1997). Induction of phosphoinositide-mediated signal transduction pathway by 17 beta-oestradiol in rat vaginal epithelial cells. *J. Mol. Endocrinol.* 19,249-57.

[126] Boyd, EM.(1934). The Lipemia of Pregnancy. *J. Clin. Invest.* 13,347-63.

[127] Boyd, EM.(1935). The role of the placenta in the fat metabolism of the rabbit foetus. *Biochem. J.* 29,985-93.

[128] Bines, J; Oleske, DM, Cobleigh, MA.(1996). Ovarian function in premenopausal women treated with adjuvant chemotherapy for breast cancer. *J. Clin. Oncol.* 14,1718-29.

[129] Goodwin, PJ; Ennis, M; Pritchard, KI; Trudeau, M, Hood, N.(1999). Risk of menopause during the first year after breast cancer diagnosis. *J. Clin. Oncol.* 17,2365-70.

[130] Saarto, T; Blomqvist, C; Ehnholm, C; Taskinen, MR, Elomaa, I.(1996). Effects of chemotherapy-induced castration on serum lipids and apoproteins in premenopausal women with node-positive breast cancer. *J. Clin. Endocrinol. Metab.* 81,4453-7.

[131] Stevenson, JC; Crook, D, Godsland, IF.(1993). Influence of age and menopause on serum lipids and lipoproteins in healthy women. *Atherosclerosis* 98,83-90.

[132] Fukami, K; Koike, K; Hirota, K; Yoshikawa, H, Miyake, A.(1995). Perimenopausal changes in serum lipids and lipoproteins: a 7-year longitudinal study. *Maturitas* 22,193-7.

[133] Chen, LJ; Zhou, H, Zou, L.(2008). Defect in lipid rafts results in failed tolerance induction at the maternal-fetal interface: a possible cause for the recurrent spontaneous abortion. *Med. Hypotheses* 71,275-8.

[134] Ray, A; Sharma, BK; Bahadur, AK; Pasha, ST; Bhadola, P, Murthy, NS.(1997).Serum lipid profile and its relationship with host immunity in carcinomas of the breast and uterine cervix. *Tumori* 83,943-7.

[135] Preetha, A; Banerjee, R, Huilgol, N.(2005). Surface activity, lipid profiles and their implications in cervical cancer. *J. Cancer Res. Ther.* 1,180-6.

[136] Richards, JS, Hedin, L.(1988). Molecular aspects of hormone action in ovarian follicular development, ovulation, and luteinization. *Annu. Rev. Physiol.* 50,441-63.

[137] Folch, J; Lees, M, Sloane Stanley, GH.(1957). A simple method for the isolation and purification of total lipides from animal tissues. *J. Biol. Chem.* 226,497-509.

[138] Frings, CS; Fendley, TW; Dunn, RT, Queen, CA.(1972). Improved determination of total serum lipids by the sulfo-phospho-vanillin reaction. *Clin. Chem.*18,673-4.

[139] Hanel, HK, Dam, H.(1955). Determination of small amounts of total cholesterol by Tschugalff reaction with a note on the determination of lanosterol. *Acta Chem. Scand.* 9,677-82.

[140] Van Handel, E, Silversmit, DB.(1957). Micromethod for the direct determination of serum triglycerides. *J. Lab. Clin. Med.* 50,152-7.

[141] Fiske, CH, Subbarow, Y.(1925). The calorimetric determination of phosphorous. *J. Biol. Chem.* 66,375-400.

[142] Marinetti, GV.(1962). Chromatographic separation, identification and analysis of phosphatides. *J. Lipid Research.* 3,1-20.

[143] Bieri, JG, Prival, EL.(1965). Lipid composition of testes from various species. *Comp. Biochem. Physiol.* 15,275-82.

[144] Mangold, H.Thin layer chromatography. New York:Academic Press; 1965.

[145] Abramson, D, Blecher, M.(1964). Quantitative Two-Dimensional Thin-Layer Chromatography of Naturally Occurring Phospholipids. *J. Lipid Res.* 5,628-31.

[146] Dittmer, JC, Wells, MA. Quantitative and qualitative analysis of lipids and lipid components. In: Lowenstein JM, editor.Lipids: Methods in Enzymology.New York:Academic Press;1969. p.482-530.

[147] Alexopoulos, CG; Blatsios, B, Avgerinos, A.(1987). Serum lipids and lipoprotein disorders in cancer patients. *Cancer* 60,3065-70.

[148] Boyd, NF; Connelly, P; Lynch, H; Knaus, M; Michal, S; Fili, M; Martin, LJ; Lockwood, G, Tritchler, D.(1995). Plasma lipids, lipoproteins, and familial breast cancer. *Cancer Epidemiol. Biomarkers Prev.* 4,117-22.

[149] Kumar, K; Sachdanandam, P, Arivazhagan, R.(1991). Studies on the changes in plasma lipids and lipoproteins in patients with benign and malignant breast cancer. *Biochem. Int.* 23,581-9.

[150] Schmitt, L; Inhoff, O, Dippel, E.(2011). Oral alitretinoin for the treatment of recalcitrant pityriasis rubra pilaris. *Case Rep. Dermatol.* 3,85-8.

[151] Strauss, JF, 3rd; Schuler, LA; Rosenblum, MF, Tanaka, T.(1981). Cholesterol metabolism by ovarian tissue. *Adv. Lipid Res.* 18,99-157.

[152] Tavani, DM; Tanaka, T; Strauss, JF, 3rd, Billheimer, JT.(1982). Regulation of acyl coenzyme A: cholesterol acyltransferase in the luteinized rat ovary: observations with an improved enzymatic assay. *Endocrinology* 111,794-800.

[153] Flint, AP, Armstrong, DT.(1971). The compartmentation of non-esterified and esterified cholesterol in the superovulated rat ovary. *Biochem. J.* 123,143-52.

[154] Tuckey, RC, Stevenson, PM.(1980). Cholesteryl esterase and endogenous cholesteryl ester pools in ovaries from maturing and superovulated immature rats. *Biochim. Biophys. Acta.* 618,501-9.

[155] Behrman, HR; Orczyk, GP; Macdonald, GJ, Greep, RO.(1970). Prolactin induction of enzymes controlling luteal cholesterol ester turnover. *Endocrinology* 87,1251-6.

[156] Klemcke, HG, Brinkley, HJ.(1980). Effects of bromocriptine and PRL on luteal and adrenal cholesterol ester hydrolase and serum progesterone concentrations in mature pseudopregnant rats. *Biol. Reprod.* 22,1029-39.

[157] Azhar, S; Khan, I, Gibori, G.(1989). The influence of estradiol on cholesterol processing by the corpus luteum. *Biol. Reprod.* 40,961-71.

[158] Behrman, HR; Moudgal, NR, Greep, RO.(1972). Studies with antisera to luteinizing hormone in vivo and in vitro on luteal steroidogenesis and enzyme regulation of cholesteryl ester turnover in rats. *J. Endocrinol.* 52,419-26.

[159] Boyd, GSa, Oliver, MF.The physiology of the circulating cholesterol and lipoproteins.In: Cook RP, editor.Cholesterol. New York:Academic Press;1958. p.182.

[160] Dyer, AR; Stamler, J; Paul, O; Shekelle, RB; Schoenberger, JA; Berkson, DM; Lepper, M; Collette, P; Shekelle, S, Lindberg, HA.(1981). Serum cholesterol and risk of death from cancer and other causes in three Chicago epidemiological studies. *J. Chronic Dis.* 34, 249-60.

[161] Howson, CP; Kinne, D, Wynder, EL.(1986). Body weight, serum cholesterol, and stage of primary breast cancer. *Cancer* 58,2372-81.

[162] White, A; Handler, Pa, Smith, EL. Princliples of biochemsitry. New York: McGraw-Hil; 1973.

[163] Allegra, CJ.Antifolates.In: Chabner BA, Collins JM, editors.Cancer Chemotherapy: Principles and Practice.Philadelphia:Lippincott Williams and Wilkins;1990. p.109.

[164] Mineeva, EN.(1988). Effect of estrogens on the lipid composition of the plasma membranes of the uterine cells in ovariectomized rats. *Farmakol. Toksikol.* 51,51-2.

[165] Ignar-Trowbridge, DM; Hughes, AR; Putney, JW, Jr.; McLachlan, JA, Korach, KS.(1991). Diethylstilbestrol stimulates persistent phosphatidylinositol lipid turnover by an estrogen receptor-mediated mechanism in immature mouse uterus. *Endocrinology* 129,2423-30.

[166] Tanaka, T, Strauss, JF, 3rd.(1982). Stimulation of luteal mitochondrial cholesterol side-chain cleavage by cardiolipin. *Endocrinology* 110,1592-8.

In: Methotrexate
Editors: V. S. Castillo and L. A. Moyano

ISBN: 978-1-62100-596-4
© 2012 Nova Science Publishers, Inc.

Chapter II

Acute Toxicity of High Doses of Methotrexate in the Treatment of Linfoblastic Leukemia in Children: A Case Report

L. Periáñez Párraga[1,], O. Pérez-Rodríguez[1], F. do Pazo-Oubiña[2], M. Crespí Monjo[1] and F. Comas Gallardo[1]*

[1]Hospital Universitari Son Espases. Palma de Mallorca, Illes Balears, Spain
[2]Hospital Clínic. Barcelona, Spain

Abstract

Background and objective. High-dose methotrexate (HD-MTX) is frequently used in various malignancies. With leucovorin rescue and standard supportive care, HD-MTX carries a low risk for severe treatment-related toxicity. However, some patients experience a delay in methotrexate (MTX) elimination and develop a HD-MTX induced renal failure which may be life threatening.

Glucarpidase cleaves glutamate from MTX resulting in the formation of a non-toxic metabolite and in a rapid reduction in MTX serum concentration.

We describe a case of HD-MTX induced renal failure in a 12 year old boy successfully treated with glucarpidase.

Design. Case report.

Main outcome measures. To evaluate the efficacy of glucarpidase, MTX serum concentration (MTXs) before and after glucarpidase administration were registered. Data related to renal function was also registered.

Results. A 12 year old patient with an acute lymphoblastic leukemia started his first consolidation chemotherapy cycle with HD-MTX ($5g/m2=7.2g$) but during the infusion the patient developed fever and MTX administration was stopped after only 1,1g. Twenty-four hours later, MTXs was 5.50 µM. Leucovorin rescue was started, but MTXs

---

* Contact mail: leonord.perianez@ssib.es.

at 36h was 4.75 µM. Serum creatinine was also increased from initial 53.04 µmol/L to 238.68 µmol/L. The calculated creatinine clearance (18 ml/min/1.73m2) demonstrated a renal failure.

The patient was admitted to the pediatric intensive care unit and treated with rasburicase, hyperhidratation and furosemide, but MTXs and serum creatinine were still high: 38 h post-infusion concentration was 3.91 µM and creatinine was 256.36 µmol/L. Glucarpidase was then administered at a dose of 2000UI (50 UI/kg). A pronounced and rapid reduction in circulating MTX was observed: 0.53 µM (56h), 0.26 µM (68h), 0.13 µM (80h), 0.09 µM (92h) and renal function was normalised.

Conclusions. In this case, glucarpidase was effective in reducing serum MTX levels and in normalizing renal function after intoxication with HD-MTX.

1. Introduction

Methotrexate (MTX), a classical antifolate, is one of the most extensively used and studied anticancer agents [1–4]. Unlike other anticancer agents, MTX can be safely administered over a wide dose range, ranging from 20 mg/m2 per week in maintenance chemotherapy for acute lymphoblastic leukemia (ALL) and treatment of non-oncologic diseases including rheumatoid arthritis (RA) or psoriasis [4–6], and when combined with leucovorin (LV) rescue, to doses of 1,000–33,000 mg/m2 [7]. The termed high-dose methotrexate (HDMTX) is usually administered as a prolonged i.v. infusion and is an important component in the treatment regimens for a variety of cancers, including acute lymphoblastic leukemia, lymphoma, osteosarcoma, breast cancer, and head and neck cancer [3, 8– 11]. HDMTX can be safely administered to patients with normal renal function by vigorously hydrating and alkalinizing the patient to enhance the solubility of MTX in urine and through the use of pharmacokinetically guided LV rescue to prevent potentially lethal MTX toxicity [2, 12].

Despite these preventive measures, MTX-induced nephrotoxicity continues to occur, although infrequently. As MTX is primarily cleared by renal excretion, MTX induced renal dysfunction leads to delayed elimination of MTX, and the resulting sustained, elevated plasma MTX concentration may lead to ineffective rescue by LV and a marked enhancement of MTX's other toxicities [3, 9, 13–15]. Since the introduction of HDMTX with LV rescue more than 25 years ago by Djerassi et al. [16], our ability to safely administer this regimen to patients has improved, and there have been a number of advances in the treatment of HDMTX-induced renal dysfunction over the past 20 years.

2. Pharmacology

Methotrexate (formerly Amethopterin) is an antimetabolite and chemically methotrexate is N-[4-[[(2,4-diamino-6-pteridinyl)methyl]methylamino]benzoyl]-L-glutamic acid.

The structural formula is:

$$C_{20}H_{22}N_8O_5 \qquad \qquad M.W.: 454.45$$

Knowledge of MTX's mechanism of action and metabolism are important for understanding MTX-associated toxicities and treatment. MTX enters the cell via the reduced folate carrier and undergoes polyglutamation catalysed by folylpolyglutamate synthetase. Once polyglutamated, MTX is retained in cells for prolonged periods of time. Methotrexate and its polyglutamates block de novo nucleotide synthesis primarily by depleting cells of reduced tetrahydrofolate cofactors through inhibition of dihydrofolate reductase (DHFR) [17]. MTX polyglutamates and dihydrofolates that accumulate as a result of DHFR inhibition also inhibit thymidylate synthase and other enzymes involved in the purine biosynthetic pathway (Figure 1) [18, 19].

Similar to other antimetabolites, critical determinants of MTX cytotoxicity are not only drug concentration but also duration of exposure. High concentrations of MTX may be well tolerated for brief periods of time, whereas prolonged exposure to low concentrations can result in life-threatening toxicity. The type of toxicity observed with MTX is also a function of this concentration–time dependence. Exposure to millimolar concentrations of MTX for minutes to hours may lead to acute renal, central nervous system, and liver toxicity; exposure to MTX concentrations as low as 0.01 and 0.005 μM for >24 hours may result in bone marrow and gastrointestinal epithelial toxicity, respectively [20].

Following administration of HDMTX, two metabolites, 7-hydroxy-methotrexate (7-OH-MTX) and 2,4-diamino-N10-methylpteroic acid (DAMPA), are observed in plasma. Within 12-24 hours of the start of a HDMTX infusion, the plasma concentration of 7-OH-MTX, formed by the action of the enzyme aldehyde oxidase, exceeds the concentration of MTX [21, 22]. Intracellular polyglutamation of 7-OHMTX results in prolonged retention and enhanced cytotoxicity [23]. DAMPA, a minor, inactive [24] metabolite of MTX, accounting for <5% of the total dose of drug that is excreted in urine [24], is presumably formed from MTX that is excreted into the intestinal tract, hydrolysed by bacterial carboxypeptidases, and then reabsorbed.

2.1. Pharmacokinetics

Absorption: In adults, oral absorption appears to be dose dependent. Peak serum levels are reached within one to two hours. At doses of 30 mg/m2 or less, MTX is generally well absorbed with a mean bioavailability of about 60%. The absorption of doses greater than 80 mg/m2 is significantly less, possibly due to a saturation effect.

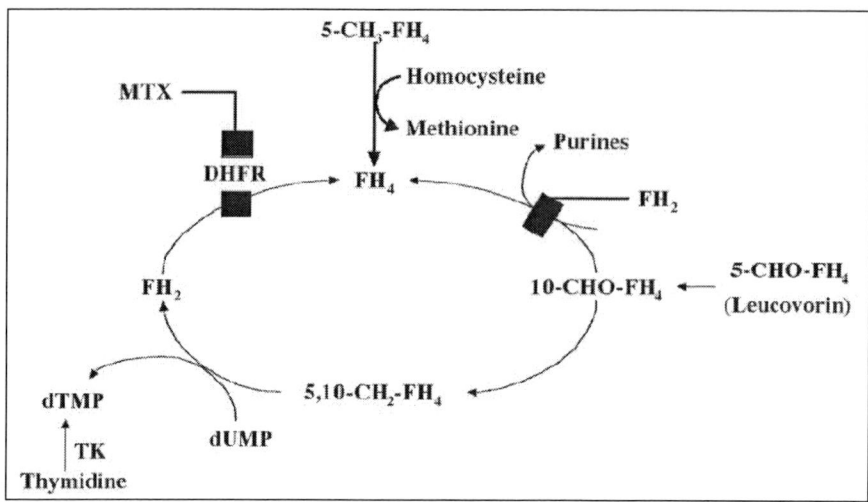

Figure 1. Folate pathway.

In leukemic pediatric patients, oral absorption of MTX also appears to be dose dependent and has been reported to vary widely (23% to 95%). A twenty fold difference between highest and lowest peak levels (Cmax: 0.11 to 2.3 micromolar after a 20 mg/m2 dose) has been reported. Significant interindividual variability has also been noted in time to peak concentration (Tmax: 0.67 to 4 hrs. after a 15 mg/m2 dose) and fraction of dose absorbed. The absorption of doses greater than 40 mg/m2 has been reported to be significantly less than that of lower doses. Food has been shown to delay absorption and reduce peak concentration. Methotrexate is generally completely absorbed from parenteral routes of injection. After intramuscular injection, peak serum concentrations occur in 30 to 60 minutes. As in leukemic pediatric patients, a wide inter-individual variability in the plasma concentrations of MTX has been reported in pediatric patients with JRA. Following oral administration of MTX in doses of 6.4 to 11.2 mg/m2/week in pediatric patients with juvenile rheumatoid arthritis (JRA), mean serum concentrations were 0.59 micromolar (range, 0.03 to 1.40) at 1 hour, 0.44 micromolar (range, 0.01 to 1) at 2 hours, and 0.29 micromolar (range, 0.06 to 0.58) at 3 hours. In pediatric patients receiving MTX for acute lymphocytic leukemia (6.3 to 30 mg/m2), or for JRA (3.75 to 26.2 mg/m2), the terminal half-life has been reported to range from 0.7 to 5.8 hours or 0.9 to 2.3 hours, respectively.

Distribution: After intravenous administration, the initial volume of distribution is approximately 0.18 L/kg (18% of body weight) and steady-state volume of distribution is approximately 0.4 to 0.8 L/kg (40% to 80% of body weight). Methotrexate competes with reduced folates for active transport across cell membranes by means of a single carrier-mediated active transport process. At serum concentrations greater than 100 micromolar, passive diffusion becomes a major pathway by which effective intracellular concentrations can be achieved. Methotrexate in serum is approximately 50% protein bound. Laboratory studies demonstrate that it may be displaced from plasma albumin by various compounds including sulphonamides, salicylates, tetracycline, chloramphenicol, and phenytoin.

Methotrexate does not penetrate the blood-cerebrospinal fluid barrier in therapeutic amounts when given orally or parenterally. High cerebrospinal fluid (CSF) concentrations of the drug may be attained by intrathecal administration.

In dogs, synovial fluid concentrations after oral dosing were higher in inflamed than uninflamed joints. Although salicylates did not interfere with this penetration, prior prednisone treatment reduced penetration into inflamed joints to the level of normal joints.

Metabolism: After absorption, MTX undergoes hepatic and intracellular metabolism to polyglutamated forms which can be converted back to MTX by hydrolase enzymes. These polyglutamates act as inhibitors of dihydrofolate reductase and thymidylate synthetase. Small amounts of MTX polyglutamates may remain in tissues for extended periods. The retention and prolonged drug action of these active metabolites vary among different cells, tissues and tumors. A small amount of metabolism to 7-hydroxyMethotrexate may occur at doses commonly prescribed. Accumulation of this metabolite may become significant at the high doses used in osteogenic sarcoma. The aqueous solubility of 7-hydroxyMethotrexate is 3 to 5 fold lower than the parent compound. Methotrexate is partially metabolized by intestinal flora after oral administration.

Half-Life: The terminal half-life reported for MTX is approximately three to ten hours for patients receiving treatment for psoriasis, or rheumatoid arthritis or low dose antineoplastic therapy (less than 30 mg/m2). For patients receiving high doses of MTX, the terminal half-life is eight to 15 hours.

Excretion: Renal excretion is the primary route of elimination and is dependent upon dosage and route of administration. With IV administration, 80% to 90% of the administered dose is excreted unchanged in the urine within 24 hours. There is limited biliary excretion amounting to 10% or less of the administered dose. Enterohepatic recirculation of MTX has been proposed.

Renal excretion occurs by glomerular filtration and active tubular secretion. Nonlinear elimination due to saturation of renal tubular reabsorption has been observed in psoriatic patients at doses between 7.5 and 30 mg. Impaired renal function, as well as concurrent use of drugs such as weak organic acids that also undergo tubular secretion, can markedly increase MTX serum levels. Excellent correlation has been reported between MTX clearance and endogenous creatinine clearance.

Methotrexate clearance rates vary widely and are generally decreased at higher doses. Delayed drug clearance has been identified as one of the major factors responsible for MTX toxicity. It has been postulated that the toxicity of MTX for normal tissues is more dependent upon the duration of exposure to the drug rather than the peak level achieved. When a patient has delayed drug elimination due to compromised renal function, a third space effusion, or other causes, MTX serum concentrations may remain elevated for prolonged periods.

The potential for toxicity from high dose regimens or delayed excretion is reduced by the administration of leucovorin calcium during the final phase of MTX plasma elimination.

Pharmacokinetic monitoring of MTX serum concentrations may help identify those patients at high risk for MTX toxicity and aid in proper adjustment of leucovorin dosing.

Methotrexate has been detected in human breast milk. The highest breast milk to plasma concentration ratio reached was 0.08:1.

2.2. Use

Actually, the oncology-related uses are: Treatment of trophoblastic neoplasms (gestational choriocarcinoma, chorioadenoma destruens and hydatidiform mole), acute lymphocytic leukemia (ALL), meningeal leukemia, breast cancer, head and neck cancer (epidermoid), cutaneous T-Cell lymphoma (advanced mycosis fungoides), lung cancer (squamous cell and small cell), advanced non-Hodgkin's lymphomas (NHL), osteosarcoma.

Furthermore, the MTX is used in other non-oncology uses like treatment of psoriasis (severe, recalcitrant, disabling) and severe rheumatoid arthritis (RA), including polyarticular-course juvenile rheumatoid arthritis (JRA).

Whereas others think there are anothers unlabeled or investigational uses: Treatment and maintenance of remission in Crohn's disease; ectopic pregnancy; dermatomyositis/polymyositis; bladder cancer, central nervous system tumors (including nonleukemic meningeal cancers), acute promyelocytic leukemia (maintenance treatment), soft tissue sarcoma (desmoid tumors); acute graft-versus-host disease (GVHD) prophylaxis; medical management of abortion; systemic lupus erythematosus; Takayasu arteritis.

2.3. Dosing

Adult

Details concerning dosing in combination regimens should also be consulted.

Note: Doses between 100-500 mg/m2 may require leucovorin calcium rescue. Doses >500 mg/m2 require leucovorin calcium rescue: I.V., I.M., Oral: Leucovorin calcium 10-15 mg/m2 every 6 hours for 8 or 10 doses, starting 24 hours after the start of methotrexate infusion. Continue until the methotrexate level is ≤ 0.1 micromolar (10^{-7}M). Some clinicians continue leucovorin calcium until the methotrexate level is <0.05 micromolar (5×10^{-8}M) or 0.01 micromolar (10^{-8}M).

If the 48-hour methotrexate level is >1 micromolar (10^{-6}M) or the 72-hour methotrexate level is >0.2 micromolar (2×10^{-7}M): I.V., I.M, Oral: Leucovorin calcium 100 mg/m2 every 6 hours until the methotrexate level is ≤ 0.1 micromolar (10^{-7}M). Some clinicians continue leucovorin calcium until the methotrexate level is <0.05 micromolar (5×10^{-8}M) or 0.01 micromolar (10^{-8}M).

Antineoplastic dosage range: I.V.: Range is wide from 30-40 mg/m2/week to 100-12,000 mg/m2 with leucovorin calcium rescue.

Breast cancer: I.V.: 30-60 mg/m2 Day 1 and 8 every 3-4 weeks

Head and neck cancer: Oral, I.M., I.V.: 25-50 mg/m2 once weekly

Lymphoma, non-Hodgkin's: I.V.:

- 30 mg/m2 days 3 and 10 every 3 weeks or
- 120 mg/m2 day 8 and 15 every 3-4 weeks or
- 200 mg/m2 day 8 and 15 every 3 weeks or
- 400 mg/m2 every 4 weeks for 3 cycles or
- 1 g/m2 every 3 weeks or
- 1.5 g/m2 every 4 weeks

Meningeal leukemia: I.T.: Usual dose: 12 mg/dose. Note: Optimal intrathecal chemotherapy dosing should be based on age rather than on body surface area (BSA); CSF volume correlates with age and not to BSA

Mycosis fungoides (cutaneous T-cell lymphoma): Oral, I.M.: Initial (early stages):

- 5-50 mg once weekly or
- 15-37.5 mg twice weekly

Osteosarcoma: I.V.: 8-12 g/m2 weekly for 2-4 weeks

Psoriasis: Some experts recommend concomitant folic acid 1-5 mg/day (except the day of methotrexate) to reduce hematologic, gastrointestinal, and hepatic adverse events related to methotrexate.

Oral: 2.5-5 mg/dose every 12 hours for 3 doses given weekly or

Oral, I.M., SubQ: 10-25 mg/dose given once weekly; titrate to lowest effective dose

Note: An initial test dose of 2.5-5 mg is recommended in patients with risk factors for hematologic toxicity or renal impairment [25].

Rheumatoid arthritis: Some experts recommend concomitant folic acid at a dose of least 5 mg/week (except the day of methotrexate) to reduce hematologic, gastrointestinal, and hepatic adverse events related to methotrexate.

Oral (manufacturer labelling): 7.5 mg once weekly or 2.5 mg every 12 hours for 3 doses/week (dosage exceeding 20 mg/week may cause a higher incidence and severity of adverse events); alternatively, 10-15 mg once weekly, increased by 5 mg every 2-4 weeks to a maximum of 20-30 mg once weekly has been recommended by some experts [26].

I.M., SubQ (unlabeled route): 15 mg once weekly (dosage varies, similar to oral) [27].

Trophoblastic neoplasms:

- Oral, I.M.: 15-30 mg/day for 5 days; repeat in 7 days for 3-5 courses
- I.V.: 11 mg/m2 days 1 through 5 every 3 weeks

Unlabeled Uses

Active Crohn's disease (unlabeled use): Induction of remission: I.M., SubQ: 15-25 mg once weekly; remission maintenance: 15 mg once weekly

Note: Oral dosing has been reported as effective but oral absorption is highly variable. If patient relapses after a switch to oral, may consider returning to injectable.

Bladder cancer (unlabeled use): I.V.:

- 30 mg/m2 day 1 and 8 every 3 weeks or
- 30 mg/m2 day 1, 15, and 22 every 4 weeks

Dermatomyositis/polymyositis (unlabeled uses):

- Oral: Initial: 7.5-15 mg/week, often adjunctively with high-dose corticosteroid therapy; may increase in weekly 2.5 mg increments to target dose of 10-25 mg/week (Note: Administration of folate 5-7 mg/week has been used to reduce side effects).
- I.V., I.M.: Doses of 20-60 mg/week have been employed if failure with oral therapy (doses >50 mg/week may require leucovorin calcium rescue)

Ectopic pregnancy (unlabeled use): I.M.:

- Single-dose regimen: Methotrexate 50 mg/m2 on day 1; Measure serum hCG levels on days 4 and 7; if needed, repeat dose on day 7
- Two-dose regimen: Methotrexate 50 mg/m2 on day 1; Measure serum hCG levels on day 4 and administer a second dose of methotrexate 50 mg/m2; Measure serum hCG levels on day 7 and if needed, administer a third dose of 50 mg/m2
- Multidose regimen: Methotrexate 1 mg/kg on day 1; leucovorin calcium 0.1 mg/kg I.M. on day 2; measure serum hCG on day 2; methotrexate 1 mg/kg on day 3; leucovorin calcium 0.1 mg/kg on day 4; measure serum hCG on day 4; continue up to a total of 4 courses based on hCG concentrations

GVHD (acute) prophylaxis: I.V.: 15 mg/m2/dose on day 1 and 10 mg/m2/dose on days 3 and 6 after allogeneic transplant (in combination with cyclosporine and prednisone) or 15 mg/m2/dose on day 1 and 10 mg/m2/dose on days 3, 6, and 11 after allogeneic transplant (in combination with cyclosporine)

Nonleukemic meningeal cancer (unlabeled uses): I.T.: 10-12 mg/dose twice weekly for 4 weeks, then weekly for 4 weeks, then monthly (NCCN CNS cancer guidelines v.2.2009) or 12 mg/dose twice weekly for 4 weeks, then weekly for 4 doses, then monthly for 4 doses or 10 mg twice weekly for 4 weeks, then weekly for 1 month, then every 2 weeks for 2 months

Takayasu arteritis, refractory or relapsing disease (unlabeled use): Oral: Initial dose: 0.3 mg/kg/week (maximum: 15 mg/week), titrated by 2.5 mg increments every 1-2 weeks until reaching a maximum tolerated weekly dose of 25 mg (use in combination with a corticosteroid)

Pediatric

Details concerning dosing in combination regimens should also be consulted.

Note: Doses between 100-500 mg/m2 may require leucovorin calcium rescue. Doses >500 mg/m2 require leucovorin calcium rescue: I.V., I.M., Oral: Leucovorin calcium 10-15 mg/m2 every 6 hours for 8 or 10 doses, starting 24 hours after the start of methotrexate infusion. Continue until the methotrexate level is ≤0.1 micromolar (10^{-7}M). Some clinicians continue leucovorin calcium until the methotrexate level is <0.05 micromolar (5 x 10^{-8}M) or 0.01 micromolar (10^{-8}M).

If the 48-hour methotrexate level is >1 micromolar (10^{-6}M) or the 72-hour methotrexate level is >0.2 micromolar (2 x 10^{-7}M): I.V., I.M, Oral: Leucovorin calcium 100 mg/m2 every 6 hours until the methotrexate level is ≤0.1 micromolar (10^{-7}M). Some clinicians continue leucovorin calcium until the methotrexate level is <0.05 micromolar (5 x 10^{-8}M) or 0.01 micromolar (10^{-8}M).

Dermatomyositis (unlabeled use): Oral: 15-20 mg/m2/week as a single dose once weekly or 0.3-1 mg/kg/dose once weekly

GVHD (acute) prophylaxis (unlabeled use): I.V.: Refer to adult dosing.

Juvenile rheumatoid arthritis: Oral, I.M.:10 mg/m2 once weekly, then 5-15 mg/m2/week as a single dose or as 3 divided doses given 12 hours apart

Antineoplastic dosage range:

- Oral, I.M.: 7.5-30 mg/m2/week or every 2 weeks
- I.V.: 10-18,000 mg/m2 bolus dosing or continuous infusion over 6-42 hours

Pediatric solid tumors (high-dose): I.V.:

- <12 years: 12-25 g/m2
- ≥12 years: 8 g/m2

Acute lymphocytic leukemia (intermediate-dose): I.V.: Loading: 100 mg/m2 bolus dose, followed by 900 mg/m2/day infusion over 23-41 hours.

Meningeal leukemia: I.T.: 6-12 mg/dose based on age. Note: Optimal intrathecal chemotherapy dosing should be based on age rather than on body surface area (BSA); CSF volume correlates with age and not to BSA

- <1 year: 6 mg/dose
- 1 year: 8 mg/dose
- 2 years: 10 mg/dose
- ≥3 years: 12 mg/dose

Geriatric

Meningeal leukemia: I.T.: Consider a dose reduction (CSF volume and turnover may decrease with age)

Rheumatoid arthritis/psoriasis: Oral: Initial: 5-7.5 mg/week, not to exceed 20 mg/week

Renal Impairment

The FDA-approved labelling does not contain dosage adjustment guidelines.
The following guidelines have been used by some clinicians:

- Clcr 61-80 mL/minute: Administer 75% of dose
- Clcr 51-60 mL/minute: Administer 70% of dose
- Clcr 10-50 mL/minute: Administer 30% to 50% of dose
- Clcr <10 mL/minute: Avoid use
- Hemodialysis: Not dialyzable (0% to 5%); supplemental dose is not necessary
- Peritoneal dialysis effects: Supplemental dose is not necessary
- CAVH effects: Unknown

Hepatic Impairment

The FDA-approved labelling does not contain dosage adjustment guidelines. The following guidelines have been used by some clinicians (Floyd, 2006):

- Bilirubin 3.1-5 mg/dL or transaminases >3 times ULN: Administer 75% of dose
- Bilirubin >5 mg/dL: Avoid use

2.4. Adverse Reactions

An adverse reaction to a drug has been defined as any noxious or unintended reaction to a drug that is administered in standard doses by the proper route for the purpose of prophylaxis, diagnosis, or treatment. Some drug reactions may occur in everyone, whereas others occur only in susceptible patients. A drug allergy is an immunologically mediated reaction that exhibits specificity and recurrence on re-exposure to the offending drug.

Adverse reactions vary by route and dosage. The hematologic and/or gastrointestinal toxicities may be common at dosages used in chemotherapy. These reactions are much less frequent when used at typical dosages for rheumatic diseases.

The adverse reactions related MTX are:

Frequency	System	Toxicity	Comments
Frequency >10%	Central nervous system (with I.T. administration or very high-dose therapy)	Arachnoiditis	Acute reaction manifested as severe headache, nuchal rigidity, vomiting, and fever; may be alleviated by reducing the dose
		Subacute toxicity	10% of patients treated with 12-15 mg/m2 of I.T. methotrexate may develop this in the second or third week of therapy; consists of motor paralysis of extremities, cranial nerve palsy, seizure, or coma. This has also been seen in pediatric cases receiving very high-dose I.V. methotrexate.
		Demyelinating encephalopathy	Seen months or years after receiving methotrexate; usually in association with cranial irradiation or other systemic chemotherapy
	Dermatologic	Reddening of skin	
	Endocrine and metabolic	Hyperuricemia, defective oogenesis or spermatogenesis	
	Gastrointestinal	Ulcerative stomatitis, glossitis, gingivitis, nausea, vomiting, diarrhea, anorexia, intestinal perforation, mucositis	(dose dependent; appears in 3-7 days after therapy, resolving within 2 weeks)
	Hematologic	Leukopenia, myelosuppression (nadir: 7-10 days), thrombocytopenia	
	Renal	Renal failure, azotaemia, nephropathy	
	Respiratory	Pharyngitis	
Frequency 1% to 10%	Cardiovascular	Vasculitis	
	Central nervous system	Dizziness, malaise, encephalopathy, seizure, fever, chills	
	Dermatologic	Alopecia, rash, photosensitivity, depigmentation or hyperpigmentation of skin	
	Endocrine and metabolic	Diabetes	
	Genitourinary	Cystitis	
	Hematologic	Haemorrhage	

Frequency	System	Toxicity	Comments
	Hepatic	Cirrhosis and portal fibrosis have been associated with chronic methotrexate therapy; acute elevation of liver enzymes are common after high-dose methotrexate, and usually resolve within 10 days.	
	Neuromuscular and skeletal	Arthralgia	
	Ocular	Blurred vision	
	Renal	Renal dysfunction	Manifested by an abrupt rise in serum creatinine and BUN and a fall in urine output; more common with high-dose methotrexate, and may be due to precipitation of the drug.
	Respiratory	Pneumonitis	Associated with fever, cough, and interstitial pulmonary infiltrates; treatment is to withhold methotrexate during the acute reaction; interstitial pneumonitis has been reported to occur with an incidence of 1% in patients with RA (dose 7.5-15 mg/week)
Frequency <1%		Acute neurologic syndrome (at high dosages - symptoms include confusion, hemiparesis, transient blindness, and coma); anaphylaxis, alveolitis, cognitive dysfunction (has been reported at low dosage), decreased resistance to infection, erythema multiforme, hepatic failure, leukoencephalopathy (especially following craniospinal irradiation or repeated high-dose therapy), lymphoproliferative disorders, osteonecrosis and soft tissue necrosis (with radiotherapy), pericarditis, plaque erosions (psoriasis), seizure (more frequent in pediatric patients with ALL), Stevens-Johnson syndrome, thromboembolism	

2.5. Contraindications

- Pregnant women with psoriasis or rheumatoid arthritis; use in treatment of neoplastic diseases only when potential benefit outweighs risk to fetus.
- Nursing women
- Excessive alcohol consumption, alcoholic liver disease, or other chronic liver disease in patients with psoriasis or rheumatoid arthritis.
- Overt or laboratory evidence of immunodeficiency syndromes in patients with psoriasis or rheumatoid arthritis.

- Preexisting blood dyscrasias (e.g., bone marrow hypoplasia, leukopenia, thrombocytopenia, clinically important anemia) in patients with psoriasis or rheumatoid arthritis.
- Known hypersensitivity to methotrexate.

2.6. Drug Interactions

Preventing a reduction in renal elimination of methotrexate is the key to minimizing consequences from drug interactions.

The most frequently interactions are:

- Acitretin: May enhance the hepatotoxic effect of Methotrexate. Risk X: Avoid combination
- BCG: Immunosuppressant may diminish the therapeutic effect of BCG. Risk X: Avoid combination
- Bile Acid Sequestrants: May decrease the absorption of Methotrexate. Risk C: Monitor therapy
- Cardiac Glycosides: Antineoplastic Agents may decrease the absorption of Cardiac Glycosides. This may only affect digoxin tablets. Exceptions: Digitoxin. Risk C: Monitor therapy
- Ciprofloxacin: May increase the serum concentration of Methotrexate. Risk C: Monitor therapy
- Ciprofloxacin (Systemic): May increase the serum concentration of Methotrexate. Risk C: Monitor therapy
- Cyclosporine: Methotrexate may increase the serum concentration of Cyclosporine. This may result in nephrotoxicity. Cyclosporine may increase the serum concentration of Methotrexate. This may result in nausea, vomiting, oral ulcers, hepatotoxicity and/or nephrotoxicity. Risk D: Consider therapy modification
- Cyclosporine (Systemic): May increase the serum concentration of Methotrexate. This may result in nausea, vomiting, oral ulcers, hepatotoxicity and/or nephrotoxicity. Methotrexate may increase the serum concentration of Cyclosporine (Systemic). This may result in nephrotoxicity. Risk D: Consider therapy modification
- Denosumab: May enhance the adverse/toxic effect of Immunosuppressant. Specifically, the risk for serious infections may be increased. Risk C: Monitor therapy
- Echinacea: May diminish the therapeutic effect of Immunosuppressant. Risk D: Consider therapy modification
- Eltrombopag: May increase the serum concentration of OATP1B1/SLCO1B1 Substrates. Management: According to eltrombopag prescribing information, consideration of a preventative dose reduction may be warranted. Risk D: Consider therapy modification
- Leflunomide: Immunosuppressant may enhance the adverse/toxic effect of Leflunomide. Specifically, the risk for hematologic toxicity such as pancytopenia, agranulocytosis, and/or thrombocytopenia may be increased. Management: Consider

not using a leflunomide loading dose in patients receiving other immunosuppressant. Patients receiving both leflunomide and another immunosuppressant should be monitored for bone marrow suppression at least monthly. Risk D: Consider therapy modification

- Leflunomide: Methotrexate may enhance the adverse/toxic effect of Leflunomide. Particular concerns are an increased risk of pancytopenia and/or hepatotoxicity. Risk C: Monitor therapy
- Natalizumab: Immunosuppressant may enhance the adverse/toxic effect of Natalizumab. Specifically, the risk of concurrent infection may be increased. Risk X: Avoid combination
- Nonsteroidal Anti-Inflammatory Agents: May decrease the excretion of Methotrexate. Risk D: Consider therapy modification
- Penicillins: May decrease the excretion of Methotrexate. Risk C: Monitor therapy
- P-Glycoprotein Inducers: May decrease the serum concentration of P-Glycoprotein Substrates. P-glycoprotein inducers may also further limit the distribution of p-glycoprotein substrates to specific cells/tissues/organs where p-glycoprotein is present in large amounts (e.g., brain, T-lymphocytes, testes, etc.). Risk C: Monitor therapy
- P-Glycoprotein Inhibitors: May increase the serum concentration of P-Glycoprotein Substrates. P-glycoprotein inhibitors may also enhance the distribution of p-glycoprotein substrates to specific cells/tissues/organs where p-glycoprotein is present in large amounts (e.g., brain, T-lymphocytes, testes, etc.). Risk C: Monitor therapy
- Pimecrolimus: May enhance the adverse/toxic effect of Immunosuppressant. Risk X: Avoid combination
- Probenecid: May increase the serum concentration of Methotrexate. Management: Avoid concomitant use of probenecid and methotrexate if possible. If used together, consider lower methotrexate doses and monitor for evidence of methotrexate toxicity. Risk D: Consider therapy modification
- Proton Pump Inhibitors: May decrease the excretion of Methotrexate. Antirheumatic doses of methotrexate probably hold minimal risk. Risk C: Monitor therapy
- Salicylates: May increase the serum concentration of Methotrexate. Salicylate doses used for prophylaxis of cardiovascular events are not likely to be of concern. Risk D: Consider therapy modification
- Sapropterin: Methotrexate may decrease the serum concentration of Sapropterin. Specifically, methotrexate may decrease tissue concentrations of tetrahydrobiopterin. Risk C: Monitor therapy
- Sipuleucel-T: Immunosuppressant may diminish the therapeutic effect of Sipuleucel-T. Risk C: Monitor therapy
- Sulfonamide Derivatives: May enhance the adverse/toxic effect of Methotrexate. Management: Consider avoiding concomitant use of methotrexate and either sulfamethoxazole or trimethoprim. If used concomitantly, monitor for the development of signs and symptoms of methotrexate toxicity (eg, bone marrow suppression). Risk D: Consider therapy modification

- Tacrolimus (Topical): May enhance the adverse/toxic effect of Immunosuppressant. Risk X: Avoid combination
- Theophylline Derivatives: Methotrexate may increase the serum concentration of Theophylline Derivatives. Risk C: Monitor therapy
- Trastuzumab: May enhance the neutropenic effect of Immunosuppressant. Risk C: Monitor therapy
- Trimethoprim: May enhance the adverse/toxic effect of Methotrexate. Management: Consider avoiding concomitant use of methotrexate and either sulfamethoxazole or trimethoprim. If used concomitantly, monitor for the development of signs and symptoms of methotrexate toxicity (e.g., bone marrow suppression). Risk D: Consider therapy modification
- Vaccines (Inactivated): Immunosuppressant may diminish the therapeutic effect of Vaccines (Inactivated). Risk C: Monitor therapy
- Vaccines (Live): Methotrexate may enhance the adverse/toxic effect of Vaccines (Live). Risk D: Consider therapy modification
- Vitamin K Antagonists (eg, warfarin): Antineoplastic Agents may enhance the anticoagulant effect of Vitamin K Antagonists. Antineoplastic Agents may diminish the anticoagulant effect of Vitamin K Antagonists. Risk C: Monitor therapy

Ethanol/Nutrition/Herb Interactions
- Ethanol: Avoid ethanol (may be associated with increased liver injury).
- Food: Methotrexate peak serum levels may be decreased if taken with food. Milk-rich foods may decrease methotrexate absorption. Folate may decrease drug response.
- Herb/Nutraceutical: Avoid echinacea (have immunostimulant properties).

2.7. Pregnancy Risk Factor: X

Overdosage
Leucovorin is indicated to decrease the toxicity and counteract the effect of inadvertently administered overdosages of MTX. Leucovorin administration should begin as promptly as possible. As the time interval between MTX administration and leucovorin initiation increases, the effectiveness of leucovorin in counteracting toxicity decreases. Monitoring of the serum MTX concentration is essential in determining the optimal dose and duration of treatment with leucovorin.

In cases of massive overdosage, hydration and urinary alkalinization may be necessary to prevent the precipitation of MTX and/or its metabolites in the renal tubules. Generally speaking, neither hemodialysis nor peritoneal dialysis have been shown to improve MTX elimination. However, effective clearance of MTX has been reported with acute, intermittent hemodialysis using a high-flux dialyzer [28].

In postmarketing experience, overdose with MTX has generally occurred with oral and intrathecal administration, although intravenous and intramuscular overdose have also been reported.

Reports of oral overdose often indicate accidental daily administration instead of weekly (single or divided doses). Symptoms commonly reported following oral overdose include those symptoms and signs reported at pharmacologic doses, particularly hematologic and gastrointestinal reaction. For example, leukopenia, thrombocytopenia, anaemia, pancytopenia, bone marrow suppression, mucositis, stomatitis, oral ulceration, nausea, vomiting, gastrointestinal ulceration, gastrointestinal bleeding. In some cases, no symptoms were reported. There have been reports of death following overdose. In these cases, events such as sepsis or septic shock, renal failure, and aplastic anaemia were also reported.

3. Pharmacogenetic Origin

Methylenetetrahydrofolate reductase (MTHFR) has a pivotal role in the metabolism of folate and methionine, both important factors in DNA methylation and synthesis in humans. C677T is a common polymorphism; the incidence of this mutation in homozygous or heterozygous state is 18–20% and 40% in the Italian population, respectively, which is higher compared with other Northern European Caucasian ethnicity.

In fact in the Northern European Caucasian population, the incidence of this polymorphism in the homozygous state is 10% [29, 30]. As a result of this mutation, homozygotes have 30% of the normal MTHFR enzyme activity, while heterozygotes have 60% of normal MTHFR activity, causing impaired remethylation of homocysteine to methionine and subsequent hyperomocysteinemia. This polymorphism has been associated in the last few years with cancerogenesis, neural tube defect or cardiovascular disease secondary to mild hyperhomocysteinemia in combination with low folate status [31, 32]. Treatment with antimetabolites such as methotrexate (MTX) can increase homocysteinemia, causing additional toxicity. In fact, more recently this polymorphism has been associated with MTX toxicity in transplanted patients receiving a short course of MTX as graft-versus-host disease (GvHD) prophylaxis [33].

When MTHFR C677T was considered, further evidence of correlation between MTHFR genotype and MTX intolerance were demonstrated. Patients reported were submitted to prolonged administration of MTX as part of their therapeutic program for at least 2 years. The vast majority of homozygous patients experienced MTX intolerance more frequently, requiring dose modification and temporary MTX withdrawal leading to overall poor compliance with maintenance. Time to completion of maintenance chemotherapy was also prolonged, although it was not significant (28.5 versus 26.5 months) in homozygous patients. Heterozygous did not show any difference in terms of toxicity compared with wild-type patients. Combined toxicity on liver and bone marrow function was encountered more frequently in patients with the homozygous genotype.

After MTX dosage adjustments, patients who developed toxicity were subsequently treated with full doses of other chemotherapy.

Currently, an empirical treatment approach is taken in most diseases, although at least nine enzymes metabolizing anticancer agents exhibit genetic polymorphisms [34]. It is probable that in the near future a panel of disease-specific genotypes will be utilized to identify subsets of patients who are genetically predisposed to develop toxicity from specific drugs.

Recently, MTHFR polymorphism has been associated with higher risk of toxicity after very low doses of MTX given for GvHD prevention in patients submitted to allogeneic stemcell transplantation [33]. The attribution of MTX toxicity to MTHFR genotype could be difficult in this setting [35], where toxicity is the result of conditioning regimen, GvHD occurrence and infections. In our study, maintenance chemotherapy that includes administration of small and continuous doses of chemotherapy allowed us to ascertain the role of MTHFR genotype in the development of toxicity during MTX administration.

4. Pathogenesis of MTX-Induced Renal Dysfunction

Acute renal insufficiency following HDMTX is an uncommon complication in the era of hydration therapy and urinary alkalinization [36].

The aetiology of MTX-induced renal dysfunction is believed to be mediated by the precipitation of MTX and its metabolites in the renal tubules [21, 22, 37] or a direct toxic effect of MTX on the renal tubules [17]. More than 90% of MTX is cleared by the kidneys [13]. MTX is poorly soluble at acidic pH, and its metabolites, 7-OH-MTX and DAMPA, are six- to tenfold less soluble than MTX, respectively [21, 24]. An increase in the urine pH from 6.0 to 7.0 results in a five- to eightfold greater solubility of MTX and its metabolites, a finding that underlies the recommendation of i.v. hydration (2.5–3.5 litters of fluid per m2 per 24 h, beginning 12 hours before MTX infusion and continuing for 24–48 hours) and urine alkalinization (40–50 mEq sodium bicarbonate per litter of i.v. fluid) during, and after the administration of HDMTX.

Shorter durations of HDMTX infusions with resultant higher plasma and urinary MTX concentrations may carry an increased risk for renal dysfunction. Several drugs have been associated with increased toxicity when coadministered with MTX. The most significant interactions involve agents that interfere with MTX excretion, primarily by competing for renal tubular secretion, such as probenecid, salicylates, sulfisoxazole, penicillin, and nonsteroidal anti-inflammatory agents [38–41].

Widemann et al. reviewed 3887 patients with osteosarcoma treated with HDMTX and found 68 (1.8%) patients affected with grade 2 or worse nephrotoxicities [42]. The number dropped to 23 (0.6%) if only grade 3 and 4 toxicities were counted, and 3 patients died from the complication. The incidence of HDMTX-associated nephropathy is unknown in other cancer patients. The reason why an individual patient comes down with acute renal insufficiency after HDMTX therapy was not a focus in the Widemann et al. report [42]. A review of the 15 patients described in 11 case reports [43-45] reveals a variety of primary malignancies, different ages of presentation (from 2 to 79 years), and different doses of methotrexate used (1.5–12 g/m2) (Table 1). Most of the patients were suffering from either osteosarcoma or non-Hodgkin lymphoma. Only 6 of the 15 patients were aged less than 18 years [44, 45]. A closer look at the 9 cases in which clinical details were available suggests that compromised renal function may be an important predisposing factor to HDMTX-associated nephropathy. The presence of pre-existing renal impairment [46], inadequate urinary alkalinization [47], and concomitant exposure to nephrotoxic agents, including indomethacin [48] and ifosfamide.

Maiche et al. [49] also noted an adverse association of concomitant drugs used close to the time of HDMTX infusion. Of 60 patients with osteosarcoma and non-Hodgkin lymphoma treated with HDMTX, 12 (20%) developed renal insufficiency of grade 2 severity or worse. Renal insufficiency affected only those patients (12 out of 30) who had concomitant drug treatments. The drugs of exposure included nonsteroidal anti-inflammatory agents (n=6), sulphonamide (n=1), iopamidol (n=1), cefotaxime (n=2), pindalol (n=1), and carbamazepine (n=1). However, such an adverse association may not be apparent in other cases. In the most recent report [45], in which a 14-year-old boy was receiving HDMTX infusions alternating with courses of ifosfamide and etoposide, the methotrexate clearance had been observed to be deteriorating following the fourth and fifth infusions—a likely consequence of prior exposure to ifosfamide [50]. The patient developed acute renal failure following the sixth HDMTX infusion, but the authors considered that the aetiology of delayed methotrexate elimination remains unknown because he did not receive medication known to be nephrotoxic or to alter the clearance of methotrexate.

MTX induced renal dysfunction results in sustained, elevated plasma MTX concentrations, which in turn may lead to ineffective rescue by LV and a marked enhancement of MTX's other toxicities, especially myelosuppression, mucositis, hepatitis, and dermatitis [43]. Vomiting and diarrhea during or shortly after the administration of MTX have been observed in patients who developed MTX toxicity [51], but the majority of patients with renal dysfunction are initially asymptomatic, and most present with nonoliguric renal dysfunction [46,51]. An abrupt rise in serum creatinine during or shortly after MTX infusion indicates the development of renal dysfunction and can result in significantly elevated plasma MTX concentrations. Although the risk for MTX toxicity is dependent upon the dose and schedule of administration, plasma MTX concentrations should be ≤ 1.0 µM at 42 h after the start of the HDMTX infusion, and plasma MTX concentrations ≥ 10 µM at this time point are associated with a high risk for the development of toxicities [43,51]. In the absence of early diagnosis based on urine output, serum creatinine, and plasma MTX determination, coupled with intervention that includes pharmacokinetically guided increase in leucovorin rescue, patients present following a delay of several days with severe mucositis, profound bone marrow suppression, and less commonly, dermatitis.

4.1. Conventional Treatment Approaches

The objective of preventing HDMTX toxicity (alkalinization, maintaining urine output, monitoring serum creatinine and plasma MTX concentrations, and pharmacokinetically guided leucovorin rescue) are also the cornerstones of management of the patient who develops early signs of renal dysfunction.

Renal dysfunction recognized by a rise in serum creatinine and elevated plasma MTX concentrations should be initially addressed by promptly increasing the leucovorin dose or schedule based on the time-dependent concentration of MTX based on Bleyer's normogram (Figure 2) [2]. Similar to MTX, leucovorin (5-formyltetrahydrofolate) enters the cell via the reduced folate carrier and is converted to its active metabolite 5-methyltetrahydrofolate (5-mTHF). The reversal of MTX by leucovorin is competitive, with relatively higher concentrations of leucovorin required as the MTX concentration increases [2, 4]. Hydration and alkalinization should be continued or increased, provided that adequate urine output can be maintained. Other supportive care measures include administering antibiotics, management of fluid and electrolytes, and transfusion of blood products as necessary. The concern that patients remain at risk for severe MTX toxicity as long as elevated concentrations of MTX persist in the circulation is reflected in the scientific literature, in which methods that attempt to address the underlying problem of impaired MTX elimination have been reported.

Other supportive care to decrease the MTX level is the dialysis methods. However, a major limitation on the use of dialysis-based methods is the marked rebound in plasma MTX concentrations that can occur when the dialysis is stopped. Rebound increases in the post dialysis plasma MTX concentration were in the range of 10%–221% of the postprocedure MTX level [52] and 90%–100% of the preprocedure MTX level [53]. Further limitations of these methods are the accompanying risks for complications from these invasive procedures. Reported complications include cardiac arrest in one patient after plasma exchange [54], bleeding from the catheter exit site [55], anaemia [55], thrombocytopenia [55], and hypokalaemia and severe hypophosphatemia [56].

4.2. Investigational Treatment Approaches

Thymidine (Thd) is an endogenous nucleoside that can effectively circumvent MTX toxicity in patients with normal renal function [57]. Unlike leucovorin, Thd does not compete with MTX for transport into the cell but is directly converted to thymidine monophosphate by the salvage enzyme thymidine kinase, thereby circumventing blockade of the de novo pathway by MTX (Figure 3) [58]. Repletion of deoxythymidine monophosphate (dTMP) and consequently of thymidine triphosphate pools allows restoration of DNA synthesis.

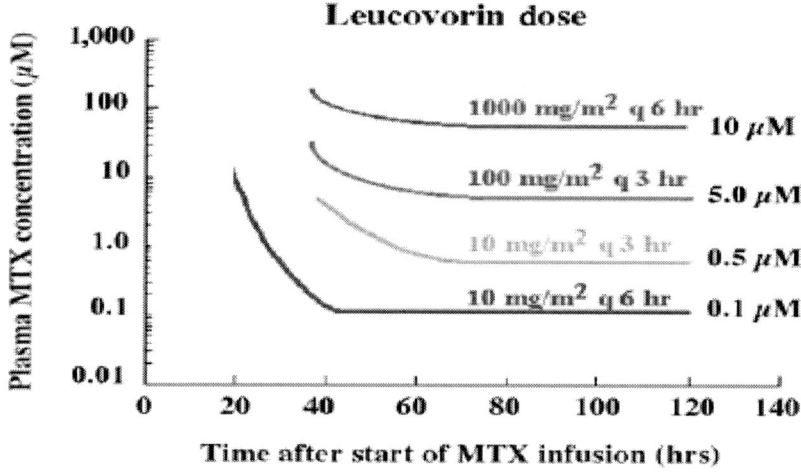

Figure 2. Normogram adapted from Bleyer WA.

In humans, the half-life of Thd is approximately 10 minutes, and thus this investigational drug needs to be administered as a continuous i.v. infusion in order to maintain effective plasma concentrations [59]. Thd has been used in 16 patients with MTX-induced renal dysfunction as a rescue agent in combination with leucovorin [14, 58]. Severe toxicity was observed in only three patients, in whom Thd was initiated 5, 12, and 13 days after the start of MTX infusion. The development of Thd as an investigational agent by the National Cancer Institute (NCI) Cancer Therapy Evaluation Program (CTEP) was discontinued, and thus Thd is currently not available for investigational use.

Other molecule which is in investigation is the carboxypeptidase-G class of enzymes hydrolyze the terminal glutamate from naturally occurring folates and folate analogs, such as MTX [60]. Carboxypeptidase-G rapidly converts MTX to the inactive metabolites DAMPA and glutamic acid, thus providing an alternate route of elimination to renal excretion. In the 1970s carboxypeptidase-G1, extracted from *Pseudomonas stutzeri* [61, 62], effectively lowered plasma MTX concentrations in a small number of patients with brain tumors who had been treated with HDMTX [63]. The bacterial source of CPDG1, however, was lost, and no additional patients were treated [64]. Subsequently, carboxypeptidase-G2 (CPDG2, glucarpidase), a recombinant form of the bacterial enzyme CPDG2, cloned from *Pseudomonas* strain RS-16, has become available and is being developed by CTEP and by Protherics Inc. (Brentwood, TN). It hydrolyzes the glutamate residue from naturally occurring and synthetic folate analogues [65]. When administered to patients with HDMTX-induced renal dysfunction, CPDG2 metabolizes circulating MTX to the inactive metabolite DAMPA (Figure 3), thus providing an alternative route of elimination to renal excretion. In 21 patients with MTX-induced renal dysfunction treated on a "compassionate-use" protocol of the NCI, CPDG2 lowered plasma MTX concentrations within 15 minutes of administration by >98% [66]. This group of patients received Thd in addition to CPDG2, because of the concern that CPDG2 could hydrolyze both LV and its active metabolite, 5-mTHF.

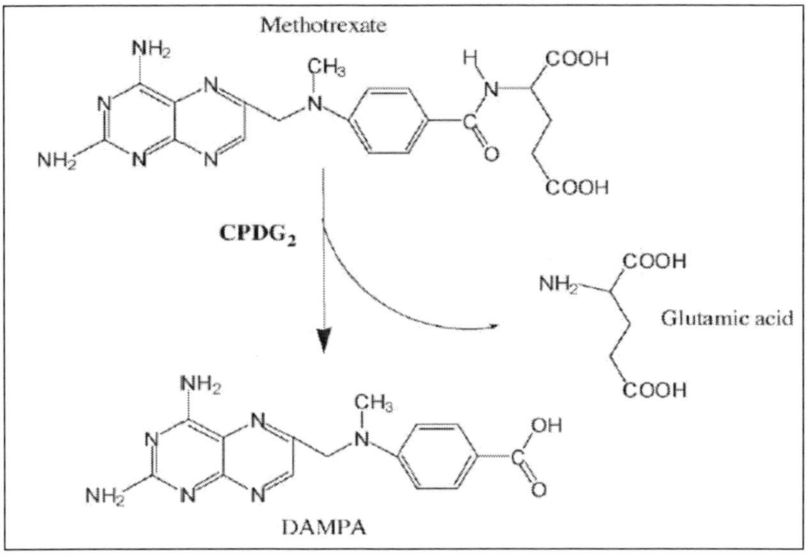

Figure 3. CPDG2 hydrolyses MTX.

CPDG2 and Thd rescue were well tolerated in these patients, and MTX-related toxicities were mild to moderate. To assess the role of Thd in these patients, this study was subsequently amended to restrict Thd administration to patients with prolonged (>96 hours) exposure to MTX or with severe toxicity at study entry. MTX-associated toxicities and outcome were compared in 44 patients who did and 56 patients who did not receive Thd. That study demonstrated that CPDG2 and LV rescue without Thd effectively rescued patients with HDMTX-induced renal dysfunction, provided CPDG2 was administered within 96 hours of the start of the MTX infusion [67].

The efficacy in rapidly lowering plasma MTX concentrations was confirmed in a European study [68], in which LV and CPDG2 were administered to 82 patients with HDMTX-induced renal dysfunction. CPDG2 was administered at a median of 52 hours (range:25–178h) following the start of the MTX infusion and resulted in a 97% (range:73–99%) reduction in plasma MTX concentrations. While CPDG2 preferentially hydrolyzes MTX (Km of 8 μ M), it can also hydrolyze LV (Km of 120 μ M) and its active metabolite 5-mTHF (Km of 35 μ M). The effect of CPDG2 on MTX, LV, and 5-mTHF plasma concentrations was assessed in 11 patients using reverse-phase high-performance liquid chromatography. Although LV concentrations were maintained following CPDG2 administration, LV was likely in the form of the inactive d-isomer. The active metabolite of LV, 5-mTHF, was indeed a substrate for CPDG2 and was effectively hydrolyzed. These findings formed the basis for the recommendation to continue with the administration of high doses of LV (250 mg/m2 every 6 hours) for 48 hours after CPDG2 to allow for restoration of the intracellular reduced folate pool. Hempel et al. [69] recently evaluated the effect of CPDG2 on the inactive disomer and the active l-isomer of LV in vitro, and demonstrated that the active l-isomer was degraded much faster than the d-isomer.

After systemic CPDG2 administration, DAMPA plasma concentrations are similar to pre-CPDG2 MTX concentrations. Persistently high concentrations of the poorly water soluble DAMPA could theoretically lead to further renal toxicity by precipitation in the renal tubules. Interestingly, following administration of CPDG2 for MTX-induced renal dysfunction, plasma DAMPA concentrations decline more rapidly than MTX concentrations, suggesting a nonrenal elimination of DAMPA [70].

The most commonly reported adverse reaction considered to be related to treatment with CPDG2 was paraesthesia which occurred in 2.1 % patients. The next most common adverse reactions were flushing, burning sensation, feeling hot, headache, tremor, hypotension, and nausea which were all reported in more than one patient. None of these reactions were classed as serious [71].

In a nonhuman primate study of DAMPA metabolism, DAMPA was found to be metabolized to hydroxy-DAMPA, DAMPA-glucuronide, and hydroxy-DAMPA-glucuronide [72]. These metabolites were also identified in patients who received CPDG2 for MTX-induced renal toxicity.

4.3. Risk Versus Benefits of Glucarpidase

Usual treatment for patients who develop HDMTX induced renal dysfunction relies on high doses of leucovorin to reduce the risk for toxicity, and with markedly elevated plasma MTX concentrations, the use of a dialysis-based methods of drug removal is often attempted. These hemodialysis/filtration-based methods must be continuously applied, or repeated on a daily basis in order to reduce plasma MTX concentrations to a range in which standard doses of oral LV can be administered. The risks associated with hemodialysis/filtration-based methods include the risks associated with the insertion of vascular access devices, the risk for bleeding secondary to heparinization and thrombocytopenia, and the risks associated with multiple transfusions of blood products.

The benefits of CPDG2 administration include a >98% decrease in plasma MTX concentration within minutes of enzyme administration. Patients can then be safely managed with LV rescue alone. Early administration of CPDG2 may diminish the risk for serious to life-threatening MTX toxicity. Furthermore, patients avoid the risks associated with hemodialysis/filtration-based methods of MTX removal, which may not be readily available outside of major medical centers.

The risks of CPDG2 administration appear to be infrequent and minor in nature. Four of 21 patients treated with CPDG2 described readily reversible side effects consisting of a feeling of warmth (n=2), tingling in the fingers (n=1), flushing (n=2), shaking (n=1), and head pressure (n=1) [70], and only 2 of 82 patients in a European study of CPDG2 for HDMTX-induced renal dysfunction described mild and completely reversible symptoms of flushing (n=2) and shaking (n=1) [68]. The theoretical risk for a worsening of renal function secondary to accumulation of the poorly water soluble MTX metabolite DAMPA has not been borne out, as the time to renal recovery is no different than that of historical controls treated with hemodialysis/filtration-based methods [73]. Even though CPDG2 hydrolyses MTX preferentially, 5-mTHF, the active metabolite of leucovorin, is also hydrolysed. Continuing to administer higher doses of leucovorin for 48 hours after administration of CPDG2 is therefore currently recommended and appears effective.

5. Case Report

Acute lymphocytic leukemia (ALL) is a heterogeneous disease, both in terms of its pathology and the populations that it affects.

Disease pathogenesis involves a number of deregulated pathways controlling cell proliferation, differentiation, and survival that are important determinants of treatment response [74]. Recent data extracted from the Surveillance, Epidemiology and End Results (SEER) registry have demonstrated a statistically significant improvement in survival for older adolescent and adults with ALL (ages 15–59 years) during the past two decades from 1980 to 2004 [75]. The greatest survival improvements occurred in the 15- to 19-year-old age bracket, for whom 5-year relative survival improved from 41.0% to 62.1%, with lower rates of improvement achieved for patients 20 to 59 years of age [75]. Nevertheless, survival for even the most favorable "young adult" group (the older adolescents) falls short of the outstanding results now achieved in children between the ages of 2 and 10 years, in which nearly 90% are long-term survivors [76].

Case Report

A 12-year-old boy (53 kg, 1.6 m2) was admitted to the Department of Pediatric Oncology for exploration of high risk ALL-B (Cytogenetic translocation t(9;22) and more than 5 % blast cells on day +14/+21). He was treated according to "Sociedad Española de Oncología

Pediátrica" (SEOP) 2005 [77] induction recommendations without incidence. He had no other relevant history or receive concomitant mediation interact with MTX.

The day +36, as haematological criteria, began the first consolidation from ALL-SEOP 2005, consisting of MTXHD 5g/m2 infusion over 24 h, treated oral adjuvant (50 mg/24 mercaptopurine and imatinib 400 mg/24 h) and intrathecal (MTX-AraC-hydrocortisone).

Routine HD-MTX drug monitoring consists in determining serum MTX level by FPIA every 24 h after the HD-MTX infusion, until 0.2 µmol/l is reached. During HDMTX courses and elimination, patients receive intensive hydration, urine alkalization and leucovorin rescue.

During the first administration of the consolidation phase the patient had a maximum febrile (39.1 ° C), so that infusion stopped after 3 h of the start and having given 1.1 g of 7.2 g MTX scheduled. After establishment of empirical antibiotic with teicoplanin and ceftazidime, MTX concentration (MTXs) at 24 h after the infusion was 5.5 µmol/l. Folinic rescue was started (30 mg/m2/6 h) as Bleyer normogram, and hyperhydration of 3 l/m2/day with urinary alkalinization to facilitate the removal of drug.

The patient developed deterioration of his general status. Twenty-four hours after the end of infusion serum creatinine level was 2.24 mg/dL and developed hyperuricemia (5.3 mg/dl) and hyperphosphatemia (8.5 mg/dl). After 36h the creatinine level was 2.7 mg/dl (4.5 times the basal value) with renal function impaired to 18 ml/min/1,73 m2, determined by urine 24 h. The patient presented a renal toxicity grade II and liver grade IV from WHO classification. The value obtained for MTXs was of 4.75 µmol.

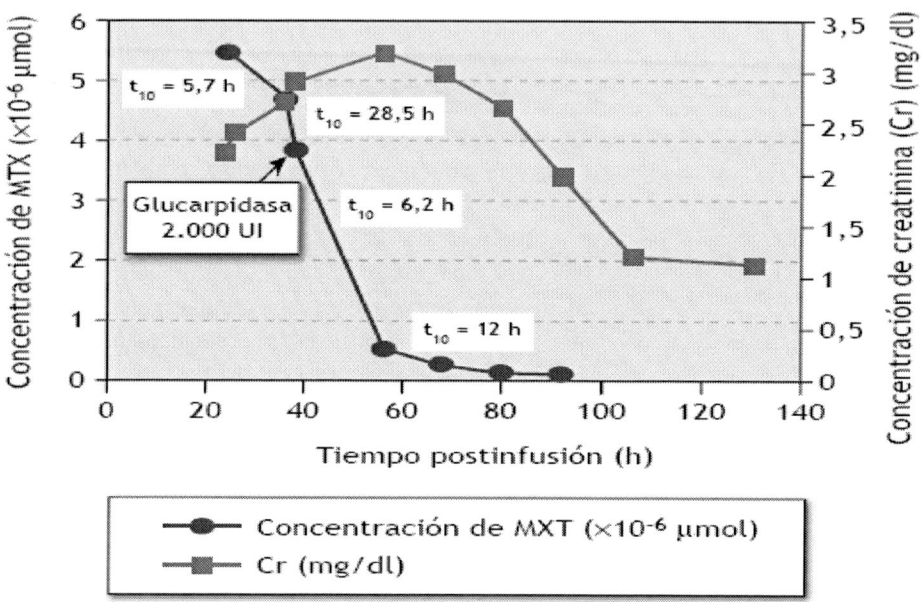

Figure 4. Analytics parameters evolution.

Due to worsening kidney function, decided enter the patient in the intensive pediatric care unit. During the physical examination, the patient referred paresthesias in his hands. In the intensive care unit the patient started rasburicase treatment (12 mg/24 h), aluminium hydroxide, perfusion without potassium and calcium folinic (100 mg/m2/6 h), hyperhydration

5 l/m2/day, maintenance of urinary alkalinization (bicarbonate 6 ml/100 ml), furosemide infusion (0.2 mg/kg/h) and prior antibiotic therapy, adjusted to kidney failure.

The MTX level determined at 38h after stopping infusion was 3.91 µmol, biochemically expressed by creatinine level 2.9 mg/dl and ALT of 66 UI/l. Forty hours post-infusion and lack of effectiveness of corrective measures, according to the overdose scheme to MTXHD from ALL-SEOP 2005, we decided to administer carboxypeptidase G2 (CPDG2), 50 U/kg/day, the pharmacy department handles the drug acquisition under the heading "off label use". CPDG2 (50 U/kg) was administered to the patient at 40 h, according to ALL-SEOP 2005 recommendations. Given the lack of availability of CPDG2 in our country, 2000 IU/24 h was given in 5 min at 40 h. Leucovorin was discontinued 2 h before and 2 h later of the CPDG2 administration.

FPIA-determined dosages indicated a decrease in MTX level: 0.53 µmol (56 h), 0.26 µmol (68 h), 0.13 µmol (80 h), 0.09 µmol (92 h); a decrease of 84% compared to previous values. DAMPA is known to cross-react with MTX when quantified by FPIA [78, 79], which becomes an unreliable method after CPDG2 administration. Thus, MTX levels following CPDG2 administration had to be assessed by an HPLC method. For technical reasons, determination of serum MTX concentrations by the HPLC method had to be delayed. After CPDG2 administration, an aliquot of the serum of each blood sample was frozen after CPDG2 inactivation.

After recovery of kidney function (45 ml/min/1,73m2) and MTX level, the patient was discharged to intensive care unit to general pediatric service. The kidney and liver function gradually returned to normal, with uraemia of 2.1 mg/dl, creatinine value 0.83 mg/dl and bilirubin 0.3 mg/dl at day 6 post-infusion (Figure 4).

One week after the patient was discharged without incidence.

Discussion

We report here the case of a patient affected by ALL, who developed MTX intoxication after administration of the first consolidation of HD-MTX. The patient was administered one dose of CPDG2, an enzyme that hydrolyzes MTX and its main toxic metabolite to inactive metabolites [80]. DAMPA is eliminated faster than MTX by an extra renal route [72]. Administration of CPDG2 has become an essential part of the rescue of patients with MTX intoxication [80].

The toxicity reduction depends on adequate leucovorin rescue and a quickly elimination of cytostatic.

Delaying this action can trigger an acute renal failure resulting from the precipitation of MTX or its metabolites in the renal tubules [80]. The FPIA-determined MTX dosage, which is unreliable after CPDG2 administration owing to a cross-reaction between MTX and DAMPA [81, 82], was the only available data concerning MTX levels at the time of intoxication. Given the rarity of the situation and the severity of the intoxication, it was difficult for clinicians to know if the remaining side effects should have been attributed to high serum MTX levels or to the accumulation of metabolites. Furthermore, although DAMPA is non-toxic, it is less soluble and a large amount of DAMPA could lead to additional toxicity [80].

Thus, determination of MTX concentration by an HPLC method after administration of the enzyme is essential for patient monitoring. A real-time determination will provide a better evaluation of MTX elimination and of the necessity of a second administration of the enzyme (due to the high cost of the drug) as compared with dialysis, in order to eliminate the remaining non-toxic metabolites, and to reduce hyperhydration-induced hypervolemia.

Possible causes of delay in the MTX elimination referred: a deteriorated renal dysfunction, the presence of mutated genotypes, in which there is greater tendency toxicity [83], and inadequate hydration and alkalinization [84].

Subsequently, the patient has made a genetic polymorphism study of TPMT and MTHFR genes, both involved in the metabolism of MTX, and found to be heterozygous to C677T in the MTHFR gene. This genetic alteration is a trend to increased toxicity, so advised for next treatments a reduction in dose and including its suspension [83].

Single nucleotide polymorphisms are commonly occurring single variations in the order of the nucleotides that constitute DNA [85]. Such variations can dramatically alter the synthesis of proteins important to the metabolism of or response to many pharmacologic agents [86]. Thus, the emerging field of pharmacogenetics, which explores the contribution of genetic differences to drug response, has provided insight into the origin of many adverse drug reactions [87]. These considerations are particularly important when drugs with narrow therapeutic indexes or those typically administered at or near their maximum tolerated doses are prescribed.

The second consolidation treatment was performed at MTX 3g/m2 and was well tolerated. Subsequent administrations doses were full and uneventful. Once the scheduled was finished the patient was programmed for haematological transplant.

In the present case, we have confirmed that CPDG2 is essential for rescue after severe acute intoxication by HDMTX. However, FPIA for MTX level determination is unreliable after administration of CPDG2. HPLC appears to be an effective method to determine the true remaining serum MTX level, and to assess the necessity for a second administration of CPDG2. In spite of its toxic potential, HD-MTX remains a very efficient drug for the treatment of ALL. The use of an MTX test-dose would appear to be a valuable tool to help clinicians to decide whether further HD-MTX should be administered. Prospective evaluation of an MTX test-dose in this context in more patients will be required to confirm our initial finding.

References

[1]   Allegra CJ. Antifolates. In: Chabner BA, Collins JM, eds. Cancer Chemotherapy. Philadelphia: Lippincott Company, 1990:110–153.

[2]   Bleyer WA. Methotrexate: clinical pharmacology, current status and therapeutic guidelines. *Cancer Treat. Rev.* 1977;4:87–101.

[3]   Djerassi I. High-dose methotrexate (NSC-740) and citrovorum factor (NSC-3590) rescue: background and rationale. *Cancer Chemother. Rep.* 1975;6:3–6.

[4]   Jolivet J, Cowan KH, Curt GA et al. The pharmacology and clinical use of methotrexate. *N. Engl. J. Med.* 1983;309:1094–1104.

[5]   Albertioni F, Flato B, Seideman P et al. Methotrexate in juvenile rheumatoid arthritis. Evidence of age dependent pharmacokinetics. *Eur. J. Clin. Pharmacol.* 1995;47:507–511.

[6]   Bright RD. Methotrexate in the treatment of psoriasis. *Cutis* 1999;64: 332–334.

[7]   Balis FM, Savitch JL, Bleyer WA et al. Remission induction of meningeal leukemia with high-dose intravenous methotrexate. *J. Clin. Oncol.* 1985;3:485–489.

[8]   Ackland SP, Schilsky RL. High-dose methotrexate: a critical reappraisal. *J. Clin. Oncol.* 1987;5:2017–2031.

[9]   Frei E 3rd, Blum RH, Pitman SW et al. High dose methotrexate with leucovorin rescue. Rationale and spectrum of antitumor activity. *Am. J. Med.* 1980;68:370–376.

[10]   Djerassi I. Methotrexate infusions and intensive supportive care in the management of children with acute lymphocytic leukemia: follow-up report. *Cancer Res.* 1967;27: 2561–2564.

[11]   Yap HY, Blumenschein GR, Yap BS et al. High-dose methotrexate for advanced breast cancer. *Cancer Treat. Rep.* 1979;63:757–761.

[12]   Stoller RG, Hande KR, Jacobs SA et al. Use of plasma pharmacokinetics to predict and prevent methotrexate toxicity. *N. Engl. J. Med.* 1977;297: 630–634.

[13]   Bleyer WA. The clinical pharmacology of methotrexate: new applications of an old drug. *Cancer* 1978;41:36–51.

[14]   Abelson HT, Fosburg MT, Beardsley GP et al. Methotrexate-induced renal impairment: clinical studies and rescue from systemic toxicity with high-dose leucovorin and thymidine. *J. Clin. Oncol.* 1983;1:208–216.

[15]   Stark AN, Jackson G, Carey PJ et al. Severe renal toxicity due to intermediate-dose methotrexate. *Cancer Chemother. Pharmacol.* 1989;24:243–245.

[16]   Djerassi I, Kim JS, Nayak NP et al. High-dose methotrexate with citrovorum factor rescue: a new approach to cancer chemotherapy. Recent advances in cancer treatment. Tagnon HJ, Staquet MJ, ed. New York: Raven Press, Monograph Series of the European Organization for Research on Treatment of Cancer 1977;3:3–6.

[17]   Messmann R, Allegra C. Antifolates. In Chabner B, Longo D, eds. Cancer Chemotherapy and Biotherapy. Philadelphia: Lippincott Williams and Wilkins, 2001:139–184.

[18]   Chabner BA, Allegra CJ, Curt GA et al. Polyglutamation of methotrexate: Is methotrexate a prodrug? *J. Clin. Invest.* 1985;76:907–912.

[19]   Allegra CJ, Chabner BA, Drake JC et al. Enhanced inhibition of thymidylate synthase by methotrexate polyglutamates. *J. Biol. Chem.* 1985;260:9720–9726.

[20]   Chabner BA, Young RC. Threshold methotrexate concentration for in vivo inhibition of DNA synthesis in normal and tumorous target tissues. *J. Clin. Invest.* 1973;52:1804–1811.

[21]   Jacobs SA, Stoller RG, Chabner BA et al. 7-Hydroxymethotrexate as a urinary metabolite in human subjects and rhesus monkeys receiving high dose methotrexate. *J. Clin. Invest.* 1976;57:534–538.

[22]   Lankelma J, van der Klein E, Ramaekers F. The role of 7-hydroxymethotrexate during methotrexate anti-cancer therapy. *Cancer Lett.* 1980;9: 133–142.

[23]   Sholar PW, Baram J, Seither R et al. Inhibition of folate-dependent enzymes by 7-OH-methotrexate. *Biochem. Pharmacol.* 1988;37:3531–3534.

[24] Donehower RC, Hande KR, Drake JC et al. Presence of 2,4-diamino-N10-methylpteroic acid after high-dose methotrexate. *Clin. Pharmacol. Ther.* 1979;26:63–72.

[25] Kalb RE, Strober B, Weinstein G, et al, "Methotrexate and Psoriasis: 2009 National Psoriasis Foundation Consensus Conference," *J. Am. Acad. Dermatol*, 2009, 60(5):824-7.

[26] Visser K, Katchamart W, Loza A, et al, "Multinational Evidence-Based Recommendations for the Use of Methotrexate in Rheumatic Disorders With a Focus on Rheumatoid Arthritis: Integrating Systematic Literature Research and Expert Opinion of a Broad International Panel of Rheumatologists in the 3E Initiative," *Ann. Rheum. Dis,* 2009, 68(7):1086–93.

[27] Braun J, Kästner P, Flaxenberg P, et al, "Comparison of the Clinical Efficacy and Safety of Subcutaneous Versus Oral Administration of Methotrexate in Patients With Active Rheumatoid Arthritis: Results of a Six-Month, Multicenter, Randomized, Double-Blind, Controlled, Phase IV Trial," *Arthritis Rheum*, 2008, 58(1):73-81.

[28] Wall SM, Johansen MJ, Molony DA et al. Effective clearance of methotrexate using high-flux hemodialysis membranes. *Am. J. Kidney Dis.* 1996; 28:846-54.

[29] De Stefano V, Chiusolo P, Paciaroni K et al. Prevalence of the 677C to T mutation in the methylenetetrahydrofolate reductase gene in Italian patients with venous thrombotic disease. *Thromb. Haemost.* 1998; 79: 686–687.

[30] Ueland PM, Hustad S, Schneede J et al. Biological and clinical implications of the MTHFR C677T polymorphism. *Trends Pharmacol. Sci.* 2001; 22: 195–201.

[31] Payne DA, Chamoun AJ, Seifert SL, Stouffer GA. MTHFR C677T mutation. A predictor of early-onset coronary artery disease risk. *Thromb. Res.* 2001; 103: 275–279.

[32] Shields DC, Kirke PN, Mills JL et al. The 'thermolabile' variant of methylenetetrahydrofolate reductase and neural tube defects: an evaluation of genetic risk and the relative importance of the genotypes of the embryo and the mother. *Am. J. Hum. Genet.* 1999; 64: 1045–1055.

[33] Ulrich CM, Yasui Y, Storb R et al. Pharmacogenomics of methotrexate: toxicity among marrow transplantation patients varies with the methylenetetrahydrofolate reductase C677T polymorphism. *Blood* 2001; 98: 231–234.

[34] Sekine I, Saijo N. Polymorphism of metabolizing enzymes and transport proteins involved in the clearance of anticancer agents. *Ann. Oncol.* 2001; 12: 1515–1525.

[35] Matsuo K, Suzuki R, Morishima Y, Hamajima N. Attribution of posttransplantation toxicity to methotrexate regarding genotype of methylenetetrahydrofolate reductase gene (MTHFR) polymorphism needs further clarification (letter). *Blood* 2001; 98: 2283.

[36] Pitman SW, Frei E III. Weekly methotrexate-calcium leucovorin rescue: effect of alkalinization on nephrotoxicity; pharmacokinetics in the CNS; and use in CNS non-Hodgkin's lymphoma. *Cancer Treat. Rep.* 1977;61:695–701.

[37] Smeland E, Fuskevag OM, Nymann K et al. High-dose 7-hydroxymethotrexate: acute toxicity and lethality in a rat model. *Cancer Chemother. Pharmacol.* 1996;37:415–422.

[38] Balis FM. Pharmacokinetic drug interactions of commonly used anticancer drugs. *Clin. Pharmacokinet.* 1986;11:223–235.

[39] Basin KS, Escalante A, Beardmore TD. Severe pancytopenia in a patient taking low dose methotrexate and probenecid. *J. Rheumatol.* 1991;18: 609–610.

[40] Cassano WF. Serious methotrexate toxicity caused by interaction with ibuprofen. *Am. J. Pediatr. Hematol. Oncol.* 1989;11:481–482.

[41] Furst DE, Herman RA, Koehnke R et al. Effect of aspirin and sulindac on methotrexate clearance. *J. Pharm. Sci.* 1990;79:782–786.

[42] Widemann BC, Balis FM, Kempf-Bielack B, et al. High-dose methotrexate-induced nephrotoxicity in patients with osteosarcoma: incidence, treatment, and outcome. *Cancer* 2004;100:2222–2232.

[43] Ahmad S, Shen FH, BleyerWA. Methotrexate-induced renal failure and ineffectiveness of peritoneal dialysis. *Arch. Intern. Med.* 1978;138:1146–1147.

[44] Widemann BC, Hetherington ML, Murphy RF, Balis FM, Adamson PC. Carboxypeptidase-G2 rescue in a patient with high dose methotrexate-induced nephrotoxicity. *Cancer* 1995;76:521–526.

[45] Peyriere H, Cociglio M, Margueritte G, Vallat C, Blayac JP, Hillaire-Buys D. Optimal management of methotrexate intoxication in a child with osteosarcoma. *Ann. Pharmacother.* 2004;36:422–427.

[46] Krackhardt A, Schwartz S, Korfel A, Thiel E. Carboxypeptidase G2 resuce in a 79-year-old patient with cranial lymphoma after high-dose methotrexate induced acute renal failure. *Leukemia Lymph.* 1999;35:631–635.

[47] van den Bongard HJ, Mathot RA, BoogerdW, et al. Successful rescue with leucovorin and thymidine in a patient with high-dose methotrexate induced acute renal failure. *Cancer Chemother. Pharmacol.* 2001;47:237–240.

[48] Maiche AG. Acute renal failure due to concomitant action of methotrexate and indomethacin. *Lancet* 1986;1:1390.

[49] Maiche AG, Lappalainen K, Teerenhovi L. Renal insufficiency in patients treated with high dose methotrexate. *Acta Oncol.* 1988;27:73–74.

[50] Crews KR, Liu T, Rodriguez-Galindo C, et al. High-dose methotrexate pharmacokinetics and outcome of children and young adults with osteosarcoma. *Cancer* 2004; 100:1724–1733.

[51] Lawrenz-Wolf B, Wolfrom C, Frickel C et al. [Severe renal impairment of methotrexate elimination after high dose therapy]. *Klin. Padiatr.* 1994;206:319–326. German.

[52] Greil J, Wyss PA, Ludwig K et al. Continuous plasma resin perfusion for detoxification of methotrexate. *Eur. J. Pediatr.* 1997;156:533–536.

[53] Jambou P, Levraut J, Favier C et al. Removal of methotrexate by continuous venovenous hemodiafiltration. *Contrib. Nephrol.* 1995;116:48–52.

[54] Bouffet E, Frappaz D, Laville M et al. Charcoal haemoperfusion and methotrexate toxicity. *Lancet* 1986;1:1497.

[55] Relling MV, Stapleton FB, Ochs J et al. Removal of methotrexate, leucovorin, and their metabolites by combined hemodialysis and hemoperfusion. *Cancer* 1988;62:884–888.

[56] Saland JM, Leavey PJ, Bash RO et al. Effective removal of methotrexate by high-flux hemodialysis. *Pediatr. Nephrol.* 2002;17:825–829.

[57] Howell SB, Herbst K, Boss GR et al. Thymidine requirements for the rescue of patients treated with high-dose methotrexate. *Cancer Res.* 1980;40:1824–1829.

[58] Grem JL, King SA, Sorensen JM et al. Clinical use of thymidine as a rescue agent from methotrexate toxicity. *Invest. New Drugs* 1991;9:281–290.

[59] Ensminger WD, Frei E 3rd. The prevention of methotrexate toxicity by thymidine infusions in humans. *Cancer Res.* 1977;37:1857–1863

[60] Albrecht AM, Boldizsar E, Hutchison DJ. Carboxypeptidase displaying differential velocity in hydrolysis of methotrexate, 5-methyltetrahydrofolic acid, and leucovorin. *J. Bacteriol.* 1978;134:506–513.

[61] McCullough JL, Chabner BA, Bertino JR. Purification and properties of carboxypeptidase G 1. *J. Biol. Chem.* 1974;246:7207–7213.

[62] Chabner BA, Johns DG, Bertino JR. Enzymatic cleavage of methotrexate provides a method for prevention of drug toxicity. *Nature* 1972;239: 395–397.

[63] Abelson HT, Ensminger W, Kufe D et al. High-dose methotrexate-carboxypeptidase G1 - a selective approach to the therapy of central nervous system tumors. In: Kisliuk RL, Brown GM, eds. Chemistry and Biology of Pteridines. New York: Elsevier North Holland, Inc., 1979:629–633.

[64] Adamson PC, Balis FM, McCully CL et al. Methotrexate pharmacokinetics following administration of recombinant carboxypeptidase-G2 in rhesus monkeys. *J. Clin. Oncol.* 1992;10:1359–1364.

[65] Sherwood RF, Melton RG, Alwan SM et al. Purification and properties of carboxypeptidase G2 from Pseudomonas sp. strain RS-16. Use of a novel triazine dye affinity method. *Eur. J. Biochem.* 1985;148:447–453.

[66] Widemann BC, Hetherington ML, Murphy RF et al. Carboxypeptidase-G2 rescue in a patient with high dose methotrexate-induced nephrotoxicity. *Cancer* 1995;76:521–526.

[67] Adamson P, Balis F, Boron M, et al. Carboxypeptidase-G2 (CPDG2) and leucovorin (LV) rescue with and without addition of thymidine (Thd) for high-dose methotrexate (HDMTX) induced renal dysfunction *Proc. Am. Soc. Clin. Oncol.* 2005;23:153s.

[68] Buchen S, Ngampolo D, Melton RG et al. Carboxypeptidase G2 rescue in patients with methotrexate intoxication and renal failure. *Br. J. Cancer* 2005;92:480–487.

[69] Hempel G, Lingg R, Boos J. Interactions of carboxypeptidase G2 with 6S-leucovorin and 6R-leucovorin in vitro: implications for the application in case of methotrexate intoxications. *Cancer Chemother. Pharmacol.* 2005;55:347–353.

[70] Widemann BC, Balis FM, Murphy RF et al. Carboxypeptidase-G2, thymidine, and leucovorin rescue in cancer patients with methotrexate-induced renal dysfunction. *J. Clin. Oncol.* 1997;15:2125–2134.

[71] Prod Info VoraxazeTM. Protherics Laboratory. UK Limited. June, 2007.

[72] Widemann BC, Sung E, Anderson L et al. Pharmacokinetics and metabolism of the methotrexate metabolite, 2,4-diamino-N10-methylpteroic acid. *J. Pharmacol. Exp. Ther.* 2000;294:894–901.

[73] Widemann BC, Balis FM, Kempf-Bielack B et al. High-dose methotrexate- induced nephrotoxicity in patients with osteosarcoma. *Cancer* 2004;100:2222–2232.

[74] Pui CH, Robison LL, Look AT. Acute lymphoblastic leukaemia. *Lancet* 2008;371:1030 –1043.

[75] Pulte D, Gondos A, Brenner H. Trends in survival after diagnosis with hematologic malignancy in adolescence or young adulthood in the United States, 1981–2005. *Cancer* 2009;115:4973– 4979.

[76] Smith MA, Seibel NL, Altekruse SF, et al. Outcomes for children and adolescents with cancer: challenges for the twenty first century. *J. Clin. Oncol.* 2010;28:2625–2634.

[77] Sociedades Españolas de Hematología y Oncología Pediátricas. Protocolo de estudio y tratamiento de la leucemia aguda linfoblástica en pediatría (niños mayores de 1 año) (LAL/SHOP- 2005). Versión final: enero, 2006.

[78] Donehower RC, Hande KR, Drake JC, Chabner BA (1979) Presence of 2,4-diamino-N10-methylpteroic acid after high-dose methotrexate. *Clin. Pharmacol. Ther.* 26:63–72.

[79] Donehower RC (1980) Metabolic conversion of methotrexate in man. *Recent Results Cancer Res.* 74:37–41.

[80] Buchen S, Ngampolo D, Melton RG, Hasan C, Zoubek A, Henze G et al (2005) Carboxypeptidase G2 rescue in patients with methotrexate intoxication and renal failure. *Br. J. Cancer* 92:480–487.

[81] Donehower RC, Hande KR, Drake JC, Chabner BA (1979) Presence of 2,4-diamino-N10-methylpteroic acid after high-dose methotrexate. *Clin. Pharmacol Ther.* 26:63–72.

[82] Donehower RC (1980) Metabolic conversion of methotrexate in man. *Recent Results Cancer Res.* 74:37–41.

[83] Przekop PR, TulganH, Przekop AA, Glantz M. Adverse drug reaction to methotrexate: pharmacogenetic origin. *JAOA* 2006;106: 706-7.

[84] Flobaum CD, Meyers PA. High-dose leucovorin as sole therapy for methotrexate toxicity. *J. Clin. Oncol.* 1999;17:1589-94.

[85] Evans WE, Relling MV. Pharmacogenomics: translating functional genomics into rational therapeutics [review]. *Science* 1999;286:487–491.

[86] Weinshilboum R. Inheritance and drug response [review]. *N. Engl. J. Med.* 2003;348: 529–537.

[87] Ingelman-Sundberg M, Rodriguez-Antona C. Pharmacogenetics of drug metabolizing enzymes: implications for a safer and more effective drug therapy [review]. *Philos. Trans. R. Soc. Lond B. Biol. Sci.* 2005;360:1563–1570.

In: Methotrexate
Editors: V. S. Castillo and L. A. Moyano

ISBN: 978-1-62100-596-4
© 2012 Nova Science Publishers, Inc.

Chapter III

Pharmacogenetics Update on MTHFR and Methotrexate Toxicity

Elixabet Lopez-Lopez, Nerea Bilbao and Africa Garcia-Orad
Department of Genetics, Physic Anthropology and Animal Physiology,
University of the Basque Country, Leioa, Spain

Abstract

Methotrexate (MTX) is an important component of therapy in several immune diseases (rheumatoid arthritis, psoriasis…) and cancers (acute lymphoblastic leukaemia, osteosarcoma, ovarian cancer…). Despite its clinical success, treatment with MTX often causes toxicity, dose reduction or treatment cessation being necessary. Several toxicities have been reported, including nodulosis, hypersensitive pneumonitis, central nervous system toxicity, postdosing reactions, gastrointestinal symptoms such as nausea, vomiting, abdominal pain, and diarrhoea, hepatitis with elevated transaminase levels, hematologic abnormalities, rash, alopecia and osteopathy.

For drugs such as MTX, with a very narrow therapeutic index, every effort should be made to minimize interpatient variability in drug exposure in order to maximize the benefit while keeping the risk of serious adverse effects at an acceptable level. Therefore, for appropriate use of MTX, it would be useful to identify predictors of the MTX adverse effects.

In this context, pharmacogenetics is gaining relevance. Pharmacogenetics studies the inherited genetic variations involved in drug response, with the aim to prospectively individualize the selection of medications and their doses to enhance efficacy and safety.

MTHFR is a key enzyme for intracellular folate homeostasis and metabolism. The non-synonymous C677T and A1298C variants in the 5,10-methylenetetrahydrofolate reductase (MTHFR) gene are among the most studied genetic polymorphisms for identifying predictors of response to methotrexate. An alteration in reduced folate pools, derived from inherited changes in MTHFR activity, may have a significant effect on the response to methotrexate, whose activity depends on cellular composition of folate.

The MTHFR 677T allele encodes proteins with decreased enzymatic activity, so people with the CT genotype exhibit only 60% of the MTHFR activity and those with the

TT genotype demonstrate 30% bioactivity. MTHFR 1298C allele is responsible for a milder decrease in MTHFR activity, CC individuals having 60% of the normal activity.

In this chapter, we perform an extensive review of the studies that analyze the association of these two MTHFR polymorphisms with MTX toxicity in different diseases. We find that there is a great heterogeneity among studies but, after a deep analysis of the literature data, we conclude that MTHFR C677T and A1298C polymorphisms do not appear to be good MTX toxicity markers in most of the cases.

Introduction

Methotrexate (MTX) is an important component of the therapy in several immune diseases (rheumatoid arthritis, psoriasis...) and malignant diseases (acute lymphoblastic leukemia, osteosarcoma, ovarian cancer...). Despite its clinical success, treatment with high-dose MTX often causes toxicity, requiring a dose reduction or cessation of treatment. Several toxicities have been reported, including nodulosis, hypersensitive pneumonitis, central nervous system toxicity, postdosing reactions, gastrointestinal symptoms such as nausea, vomiting, abdominal pain and diarrhoea, hepatitis with elevated transaminase levels, hematologic abnormalities, rash, alopecia and osteopathy. Therefore, for appropriate use of MTX, it would be useful to find a predictor of the adverse effects of MTX that identified which patients are going to suffer from these adverse effects. (Imanishi et al, 2007).

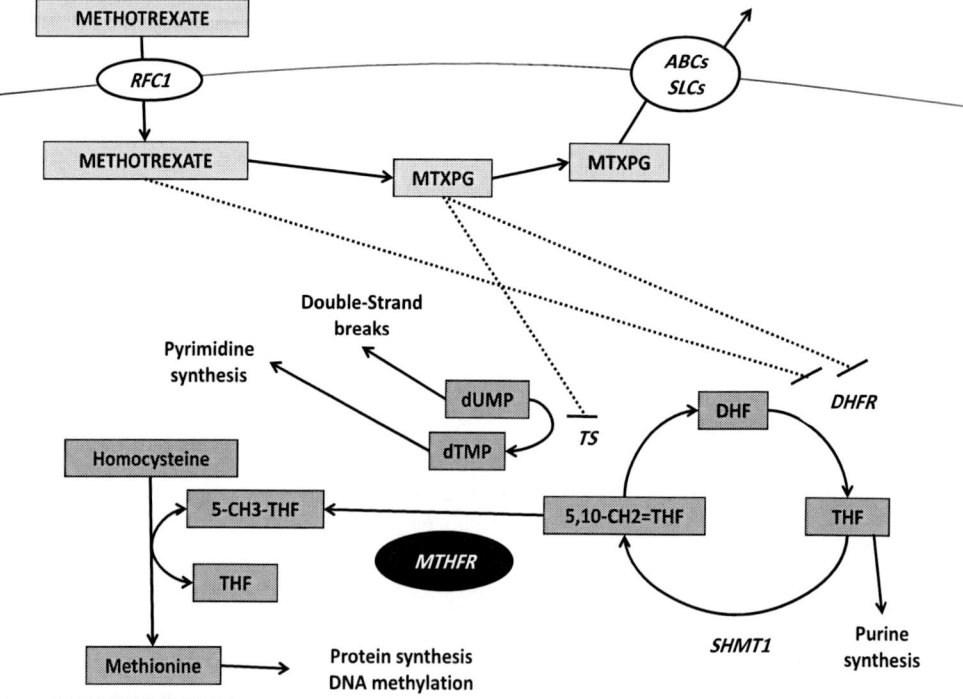

Figure 1. Methotrexate pathway. Methotrexate and its metabolites are indicated. Enzymes and transporters are in italics. MTHFR is in black.

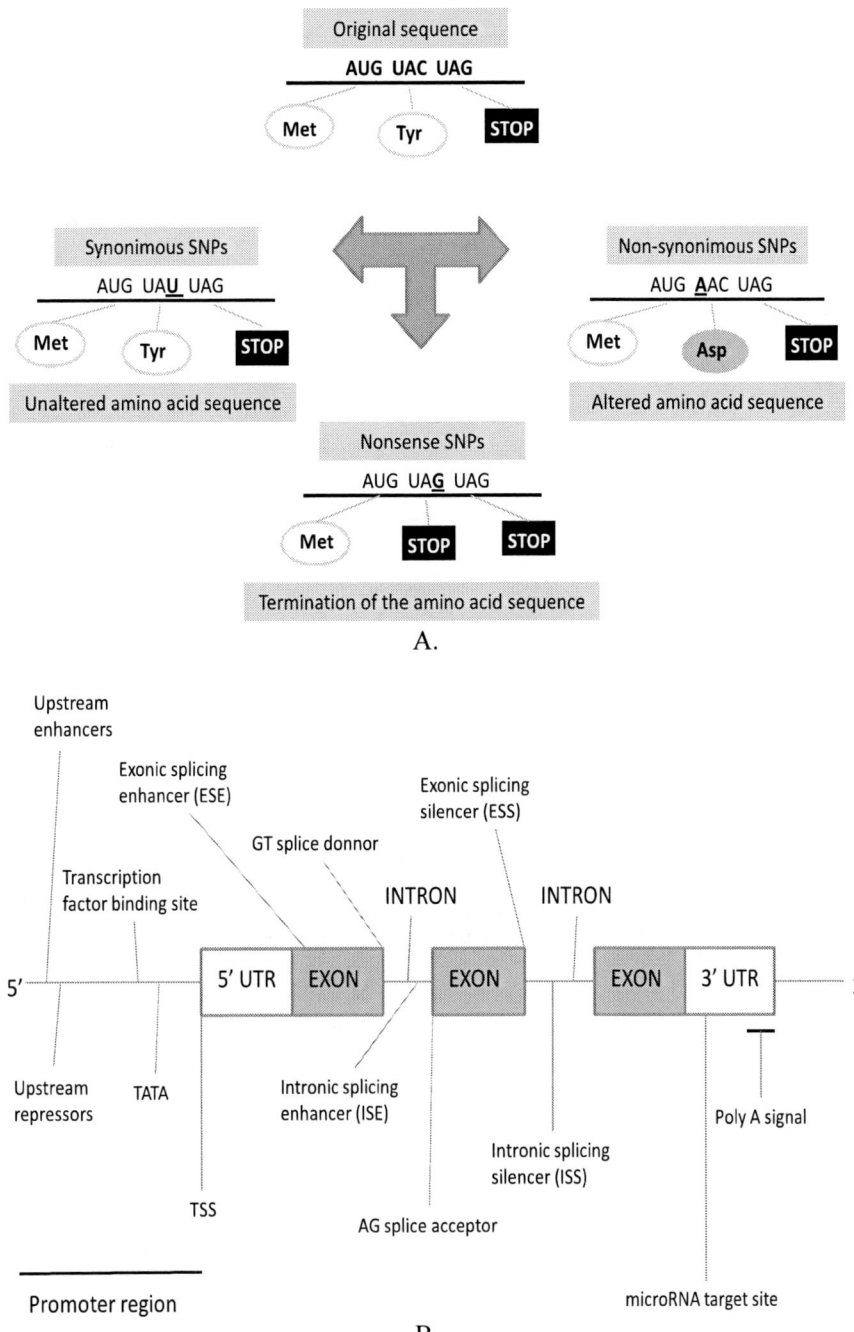

Figure 2. A) Exonic SNPs with possible functional effect on the amino acid sequence. B) SNPs with other possible functional effect on the gene.

MTX enters the cell via active transport mediated by the reduced folate carrier (RFC1) (Goldman et al, 1985; Gorlick et al). MTX acts by inhibiting two enzymes. MTX directly inhibits dihydrofolate reductase (DHFR), which converts folates (DHF) to their active form tetrahydrofolate (THF), affecting other important enzymes, such as methylenetetrahydrofolate reductase (MTHFR) and serine hydromethyl transferase (SHMT1). On the other hand, the conversion of MTX to its polyglutamated forms (MTXPG) results in the inhibition of thymidylate synthase (TS).These combined mechanisms interfere with nucleic acid synthesis, favouring cell death (Krajinovic et al, 2004a). Effective cellular levels of MTX are reduced by different transporters that pump MTX out of the organism. These transporters include ABC transporters, such as the multidrug resistance protein (ABCB1) and the breast cancer resistance protein (ABCG2) (Swerts et al, 2006), and organic anion transporters, such as SLCO1B1 (Treviño et al, 2009; Abe et al, 2001) (Figure 1).

MTHFR is a key enzyme for intracellular folate homeostasis and metabolism. MTHFR catalyses the irreversible conversion of 5,10-methylentetrahydrofolate (5,10-CH2-THF), required for purine and thymidine synthesis, to 5-methyltetrahydrofolate (5-CH-THF), the primary methyl donor for the remethylation of homocysteine to methionine which is required for protein synthesis and the synthesis of S-Adenosyl-methionine, the methyl group donor for nucleic acid methylation. Alterations in reduced folate pools, as a consequence of inherited changes in MTHFR activity, may have a significant effect on the responsiveness of malignant and non-malignant cells to antifolates, whose activity depends on the composition of cellular folate pools (Figure 1). Therefore, modifications in the intracellular folates pool could increase the toxic effect of MTX (De Mattia and Toffoli, 2009). In this context, pharmacogenetic studies could be very useful.

Pharmacogenetics studies the inherited genetic polymorphisms involved in drug response, with the aim to prospectively individualize the selection of medications and their doses to enhance efficacy and safety.

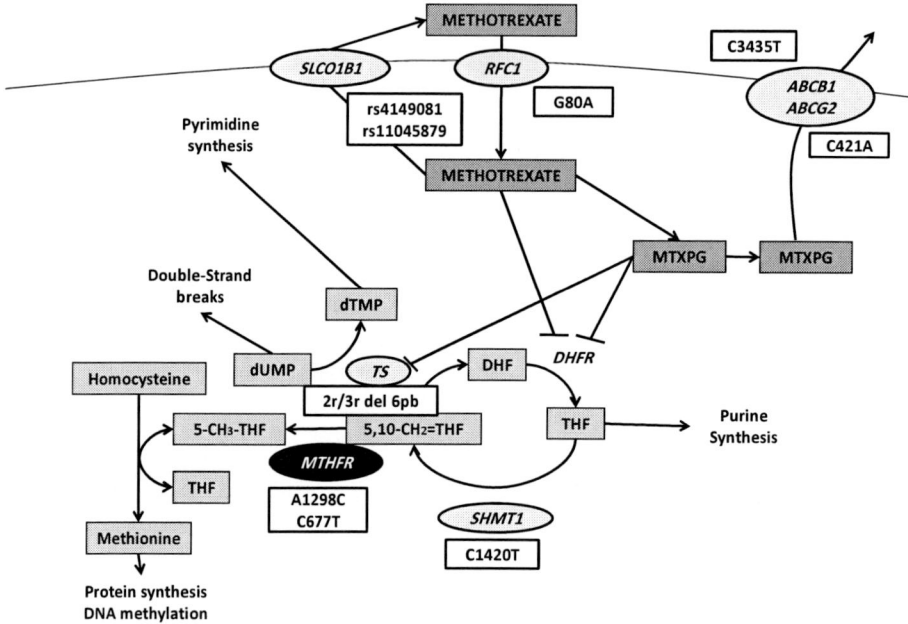

Figure 3. Polymorphisms analyzed in association with MTX toxicity. Genes are encircled and polymorphisms are framed in white. MTHFR is in black.

The most common genetic polymorphisms are SNPs. SNPs or single nucleotide polymorphisms are single base substitutions of a single nucleotide with another, observed in the general population at a frequency greater than 1%. SNPs can be found throughout the human genome in non-genic regions, as well as in genes. Within a gene, SNPs located in coding regions are called coding SNPs (cSNPs). Among cSNPs, those that give place to a change in the coded amino acid are referred to as non-synonymous SNPs. Even though cSNPs have been the most studied polymorphisms in the past years, SNPs in regulatory regions, including splicing regions microRNAs target sequences, CpG sites and other non-genic regions have also gained importance, due to their potential functional effects. The different types of SNPs with possible functional effect are illustrated in the figure below (Figure 2).

Polymorphisms of the methotrexate transporters, methotrexate targets and folate-metabolizing enzymes that could influence the toxic effects of methotrexate have been studied (Figure 3).

Among the most studied genetic polymorphisms for identifying predictors of response to methotrexate are the non-synonymous C677T (Ala222Val) and A1298C (Glu429Ala) SNPs in the 5,10-methylenetetrahydrofolate reductase (MTHFR) gene.

The MTHFR 677T allele encodes proteins with decreased enzymatic activity, so people with the CT genotype exhibit only 60% of the normal MTHFR activity and those with the TT genotype demonstrate 30% bioactivity (Cheok et al, 2006; Frosst et al, 1995). MTHFR 1298C allele is responsible for a milder decrease in MTHFR activity, CC individuals having 60% of the normal activity (Weisberg et al, 2001).

Due to the functional effect of these two polymorphisms, a large body of published studies has investigated the potential role of MTHFR polymorphisms on toxicity to MTX in several diseases, specially in paediatric acute lymphoblastic leukaemia and rheumatoid arthritis. However, the results are controversial.

In this review, we critically evaluated the relationship of genetic variants of MTHFR with the cytotoxic effect of treatment with MTX in different diseases.

MTHFR C677T and A1298C Polymorphism and Toxicity in Paediatric Acute Lymphoblastic Leukaemia

Acute lymphoblastic leukaemia (ALL) is the most common childhood cancer, accounting for 30% of all paediatric malignancies. During the last 20 years, survival rates for ALL have improved dramatically due to advances in specific chemotherapy for childhood ALL, with expected cure rates higher than 80%. Methotrexate (MTX) is an important component of this therapy.

When we performed a thorough review of the literature (Table 1), in spite of what is expected for the functional effect of the MTHFR polymorphisms, in paediatric acute lymphoblastic leukaemia, most of the published studies do not find significant association between the MTHFR 677T low functional variant and higher MTX toxicity (Shimasaki et al, 2006; Karathanasis et al, 2011; Chatzidakis et al, 2006; Kishi et al, 2003; Pakakasama et al,

2007; Huang et al, 2008; Lopez-Lopez et al, 2011; Kishi et al, 2007; Horinouchi et al, 2010; Krajinovic et al, 2004b; Aplenc et al, 2005). Three studies even showed a protective effect of the 677T variant. Van Kooten Niekerk et al (2008) found an association between the TT genotype and less neutropenia after high-dose MTX. Costea et al (2006) also found a correlation between CT/TT genotype and less leucopoenia and fewer weeks with toxicity during low dose maintenance therapy. Finally, Kantar et al find that individuals with CT/TT genotypes had less thrombocytopenia and hyperbilirubinemia (Kantar et al, 2009).

Table 1. Association of MTHFR C677T polymorphism and toxicity in cancer

Paediatric ALL					
Patients (n)	MTX dose	Ethnicity	Toxicity	Main results	References
ALL/LBL (15)	high	Japanese	NA	No association with MTX levels at 48h, hematologic and hepatic toxicity, mucositis or vomits	Shimasaki et al, 2006
ALL/LBL (24)	low	Japanese	NA	No association with hepatic toxicity	Horinouchi et al, 2010
ALL (35)	high	Cretan	NA	No association with anaemia, thrombocytopenia, leucopoenia, hepatic toxicity or mucositis	Karathanasis et al, 2011
ALL (46)	high	Greek	NA	No association with anaemia, leucopoenia or hepatic toxicity	Chatzidakis et al, 2006
ALL (53)	high	White (38) and non-white (15)	NA	No association with homocysteine levels, fever or thrombosis	Kishi et al, 2003
ALL (76)	high	Thai	NA	No association with myelosupression, mucositis or febrile neutropenia	Pakakasama et al, 2007
ALL (81)	high	European	NA	No association with MTX levels at 48h and 72h, treatment delay, mucositis, hospital admissions, transfusions, hepatic toxicity, skin toxicity or hematologic toxicity	Huang et al, 2008
ALL (115)	high	Spanish	NA	No association with MTX levels at 72h	Lopez-Lopez et al, 2011
ALL (240)	high	North American	NA	No association with MTX clearance, gastrointestinal toxicity, infection, hyperbilirubinemia or neurotoxicity	Kishi et al, 2007
ALL (201)	low	French-Canadian	NA	No association with weeks without MTX due to toxicity and average MTX dose	Krajinovic et al, 2004b
ALL (520)	low	African-American (28), Asian (13), Caucasian (396), Hispanic (58), other (25)	NA	No association with CNS toxicity, diarrhoea, hiperbilirubinemia, neuropathy, mucositis, hepatic toxicity or infections	Aplenc et al, 2005
ALL/NHL (37)	high	Turkish	-T	CT+TT associated with less thrombocytopenia and hyperbilirubinemia but not with anaemia, leucopoenia, febrile neutropenia, hepatic and renal toxicity.	Kantar et al, 2009

Paediatric ALL					
Patients (n)	MTX dose	Ethnicity	Toxicity	Main results	References
				MTX levels are increased at 24h but are significantly decreased at 36h and there is no significant association at 42, 48, 72h	
ALL (88)	high	European	-T	Association with less neutropenia. No association with leucopoenia, thrombocytopenia, hepatic toxicity, fever or treatment interruption	van Kooten et al, 2008
ALL (186)	low	European descent	-T	CT+TT are associated with less leucopoenia and less weeks with toxicity. No association with thrombocytopenia, neutropenia or hepatic toxicity	Costea et al, 2006
ALL/LBL (20)	low	Japanese	+T	Association with MTX interruption	Shimasaki et al, 2008
ALL/ML (26)	high	Japanese	+T	Higher MTX levels at 48h but no association with hepatotoxicity	Imanishi et al, 2007
ALL (40)	high	Egyptian	+T	Association with diarrhoea, mucositis, hepatic toxicity and neutropenia but not with infections	Tantawy et al, 2010
ALL/ML (64)	high	Central European	+T	Association with mucositis and MTX clearance but no association with leucopoenia, thrombocytopenia, neurotoxicity	Faganel Kotnik et al, 2011
ALL (151)	high	Caucasian	+T	Association with higher toxicity	D'Angelo et al, 2011
ALL (181)	high	Chinese	+T	Association with thrombocytopenia but no association with anaemia, neutropenia, hepatic toxicity, mucositis, skin toxicity, hematologic toxicity, non-hematologic toxicity or MTX plasma levels at 48h	Liu et al, 2011
Adult ALL					
ALL (55)	Low	Italian	+T	Association with increased toxicity	Chiusolo et al, 2002
ALL/APL (61)	Low	Italian	+T	Association with increased toxicity	Chiusolo et al, 2007
ALL (122)	Low	Italian	+T	Association with increased leucopoenia, gastrointestinal and hepatic toxicity	Ongaro et al, 2009
Other					
CNS-L (68)	High	Caucasian	+T	TT genotype associated with CNS toxicity	Linnebank et al, 2009
Adult NHL (68)	Low	Italian	+T	TT genotype associated with increased risk of mucositis and hepatic toxicity and not with haematologic toxicity	Gemmati et al, 2007
Paediatric NHL (484)	High	Caucasian	NA	No association with toxicity	Seidemann et al, 2006
Ovarian (43)	Low	Italian	+T	TT associated with increased G3/G4 toxicity	Toffoli et al, 2003

Table 1. (Continued)

Paediatric ALL					
Patients (n)	MTX dose	Ethnicity	Toxicity	Main results	References
Urothelial (40)	High	Japanese	NA	No association with toxicity.	Tsuchiya et al, 2008
OS (96)	high	Spanish	+T	TT associated with haematological toxicity but not with gastrointestinal toxicity.	Patiño et al, 2009
Transplant receivers (89)	Low	German	NA	No association with mucositis and aplasia	Pihusch et al, 2004
Transplant receivers (82)	Low	Turkish	NA	No association with extramedullary toxicity.	Soydan et al, 2008
Transplant receivers (159)	Low	Japanese	NA	No association with toxicity.	Sugimoto et al, 2008
Other					
Transplant receivers (84)	Low	Caucasian	NA	No association with hepatic toxicity.	Goekkurt et al 2007
Transplant receivers (72)	Low	Korean	+T	Association of TT genotype with hepatic toxicity.	Kim et al, 2007
Transplant receivers (220)	Low	White (196) non-white (24)	+T	TT associated with toxicity	Ulrich et al, 2001
Transplant receivers (172)	Low	Caucasian	+T	T allele associated with mucositis	Robien et al, 2006
Transplant receivers (133)	Low	White (120) non-white (13)	+T	TT genotype associated with mucositis.	Robien et al, 2004

High MTX dose: 1.5-8g/m2; Low dose: 15-300mg/m2.

When we further analyzed the six studies where a positive association was found, we observed several problems such as differences in treatment protocols among studies, small or non-homogeneous populations, the use of different toxicity criteria and even errors in the conclusions of one of such studies.

The first study (Shimasaki et al, 2008) reports an association between the T allele and an increase in MTX treatment interruption during maintenance therapy. But this study was carried out with a small and heterogeneous population (20 ALL or LBL) and only one patient with the TT genotype was reported. As a consequence, consistent conclusions cannot be reached, due to the low statistical power of the study. In addition, the only work that analyzed a similar toxicity criterion, carried out in a larger population of 201 ALL patients, does not find any association with MTX treatment interruption (Krajinovic et al, 2004b) (Table 1).

Imanishi and collaborators studied 26 children with ALL or ML (Imanishi et al, 2007) and concluded that patients with the TT genotype had higher MTX plasma levels 48h after infusion. No one else has reported this association, as far as we know. We consider that the statistical power of the study is low, due to the low number of patients included. In addition, supporting the lack of association, several studies did not find association with MTX plasma levels 48h after infusion (Shimasaki et al, 2006; Huang et al, 2008; Kantar et al, 2009; Liu et al, 2011). Two other studies that analyze a parameter related to MTX plasma levels, MTX clearance, again show conflicting results. While one of them, carried out with 64 children with LLA or ML (Faganel Kotnik et al, 2011), describes an association between the TT genotype and a decrease in MTX clearance, the larger study of Kishi et al with 240 paediatric ALL patients do not find any association with MTX clearance (Kishi et al, 2007).

Association between the TT genotype and higher risk of diarrhoea was described in an only study with 40 paediatric ALL patients (Tantawy et al, 2010). Two studies carried out with 240 and 520 paediatric ALL patients, respectively, did not find this correlation (Kishi et al, 2007; Aplenc et al, 2005). Accordingly, 677TT genotype cannot be considered a good predictor of severe diarrhoea.

Two different studies have found an association with higher risk of mucositis when they analyzed, respectively, 40 and 64 children with ALL (Tantawy et al, 2010; Faganel Kotnik et al, 2011). Other six studies have not found this association (Shimasaki et al, 2006; Karathanasis et al, 2011; Pakakasama et al, 2007; Huang et al, 2008; Aplenc et al, 2005; Liu et al, 2011). Most of these studies included larger samples and different populations. This lack of replication in most of the studies does not support a effect of the 677TT polymorphism in the risk of mucositis.

Tantawy and collaborators also found an association with hepatic toxicity (Tantawy et al, 2011). Given that, as mentioned above, this study has not a very high statistical power and that the other 10 studies that analyzed this parameter did not find association with hepatic toxicity (Shimasaki et al, 2006; Karathanasis et al, 2011; Chatzidakis et al, 2006; Huang et al, 2008; Horinouchi et al, 2010; Aplenc et al, 2005; van Kooten et al, 2008; Costea et al, 2006; Imanishi et al, 2007; Liu et al, 2011), we can conclude that 677TT genotype does not appear to be either a good predictor of hepatic toxicity.

The same conclusion applies to the reported association of the TT genotype with higher risk of neutropenia (Tantawy et al, 2011). Studies with larger samples do not find this association with neutropenia (Costea et al, 2006; Liu et al, 2011). Furthermore, another study even found the opposite effect, association with a lower risk of neutropenia (Van Kooten et al, 2008) (Table 1).

The association of the CT and TT genotypes with an increased risk in thrombocytopenia has also been reported (Liu et al, 2011), but it is only statistically significant for the CT genotype, which makes difficult to explain the effect from a functional point of view. Other studies do not find any association with this parameter (Karathanasis et al, 2011; van Kooten et al, 2008; Costea et al, 2006; Faganel Kotnik et al, 2011; Liu et al, 2011). Again another study reports a correlation of the CT and TT genotypes with less thrombocytopenia (Kantar et al, 2009). In conclusion, the available data do not support a clear association of the 677T variant with a higher risk of thrombocytopenia.

Finally, the work by D'Angelo and collaborators, reports an association between the TT genotype and an increase in toxicity (D'Angelo et al, 2011). However, when the data provided are reanalysed, we could not see the association. From the re-analysis, we drew the opposite conclusion to what the authors conclude, in the group treated with 5 g of MTX, the TT genotype seems to be protective against toxicity and not a risk factor.

In summary, despite the great heterogeneity among studies, including the size of their samples and the toxicity criteria selected, when we analyzed in depth the different studies published, most of them did not find association of MTHFR C677T polymorphism and toxicity. When association is reported, it is not replicated by other studies. As a consequence we can reach the conclusion that the MTHFR C677T polymorphism is not a good marker of MTX-related toxicity in paediatric ALL.

Regarding the role of MTHFR A1298C polymorphism in MTX-induced adverse events, less controversial results are available until now for paediatric ALL (Table 2). No association between the polymorphism and toxicity has been found in six studies (Tantawy et al, 2010; Lopez-Lopez et al, 2011; D'Angelo et al, 2011; Krajinovic et al, 2004b; Kishi et al, 2007; Aplenc et al, 2005). In other 5 studies, the authors report a protective effect for the 1298C variant against different kinds of toxicity: leucopoenia (Faganel Kotnik et al, 2011), myelosupression (Pakakasama et al, 2007), transfusions (Huang et al, 2008), thrombocytopenia (van Kooten et al, 2008) and skin toxicity (Liu et al, 2011).

We only found 2 studies in which the AC/CC genotypes were associated with higher toxicity (Kantar et al, 2009; Karathanasis et al, 2011). Both studies show an association with hepatic toxicity in 37 children with LLA or NHL and 35 paediatric LLAs, respectively.

Table 2. Association of MTHFR A1298C polymorphism and toxicity in cancer

Paediatric ALL					
Patients (n)	MTX dose	Ethnicity	Toxicity	Main results	References
ALL (40)	high	Egyptian	NA	No association with diarrhoea, mucositis, hepatic toxicity, neutropenia or infections	Tantawy et al, 2010
ALL (115)	high	Spanish	NA	No association with MTX levels at 72h	Lopez-Lopez et al, 2011
ALL (151)	high	Caucasian European	NA	No association with global toxicity, haematological and non-haematological toxicity	D'Angelo et al, 2011
ALL (201)	low	French-Canadian	NA	No association with weeks without MTX due to toxicity and average MTX dose	Krajinovic et al, 2004b
ALL (240)	high	North American	NA	No association with MTX clearance, gastrointestinal toxicity, infection, hyperbilirubinemia or neurotoxicity	Kishi et al, 2007
ALL (520)	low	African-American (28), Asian (13), Caucasian (396), Hispanic (58), other (25)	NA	No association with CNS toxicity, diarrhoea, hiperbilirubinemia, neuropathy, mucositis, hepatic toxicity or infections	Aplenc et al, 2005
ALL/ML (64)	high	Central European	-T	Association with less leucopoenia. No association with thrombocytopenia, neurotoxicity, mucositis or MTX clearance.	Faganel Kotnik et al, 2011
ALL (76)	high	Thai	-T	CC is associated with less myelosupression. No association with mucositis or febrile neutropenia.	Pakakasama et al, 2007
ALL (81)	high	European	-T	AC+CC associated with less transfusions but not with MTX levels at 48h and 72h, treatment delay, mucositis, hospital admissions, hepatic toxicity, skin toxicity or hematologic toxicity	Huang et al, 2008
ALL (88)	high	European	-T	Association with less thrombocytopenia but not with neutropenia, leucopoenia, fever or MTX interruption	van Kooten et al, 2008
ALL (181)	high	Chinese	-T	AC+CC showed less skin toxicity but were not associated with thrombocytopenia, anaemia, neutropenia, hepatic toxicity, mucositis, hematologic or non-hematologic toxicity or MTX levels at 48h	Liu et al, 2011

Paediatric ALL					
Patients (n)	MTX dose	Ethnicity	Toxicity	Main results	References
ALL (35)	high	Cretan	+T	Association with hepatic toxicity but not with hematologic toxicity or mucositis	Karathanasis et al, 2011
ALL/NHL (37)	high	Turkish	+T	AC+CC were associated with higher MTX plasma levels at 48h, anaemia, thrombocytopenia, leucopoenia, hepatic toxicity and febrile neutropenia but not with renal toxicity or hyperbilirubinemia	Kantar et al, 2009
Adult ALL					
ALL/APL (61)	Low	Italian	NA	No association with toxicity (haematological or hepatic)	Chiusolo et al, 2007
ALL (122)	Low	Italian	-T	AC+CC genotypes were associated with decreased leucopoenia and hepatic toxicity but not with gastrointestinal toxicity-	Ongaro et al, 2009
Other					
CNS-L (68)	High	Caucasian	-T	AC/CC genotypes had a protective effect against CNS white matter changes.	Linnebank et al, 2009
Other					
Adult NHL (68)	Low	Italian	+T	CC genotype was associated with increased risk of mucositis but not with hepatic or hematologic toxicity.	Gemmati et al, 2007
Urothelial (40)	High	Japanese	NA	No association with toxicity	Tsuchiya et al, 2008
OS (96)	High	Spanish	NA	No association with haematological or gastrointestinal toxicity.	Patiño et al, 2009
Transplant receivers (72)	Low	Korean	NA	No association of the A1298C polymorphism	Kim et al, 2007
Transplant receivers (84)	Low	Caucasian	+T	1298C increases hepatic toxicity	Goekkurt et al 2007
Transplant receivers (172)	Low	Caucasian	-T	1298C associated with less mucositis.	Robien et al, 2006

High MTX dose: 1.5-8g/m2; Low dose: 15-300mg/m2.

This association was not replicated by other four studies that analyzed the same parameter in larger populations with higher statistical power (Tantawy et al, 2010; Aplenc et al, 2005; Huang et al, 2008; Liu et al, 2011). Consequently, MTHFR A1298C does not seem to be a good marker of hepatic toxicity.

In the report by Kantar and collaborators, an association is found with higher MTX plasma levels at 48h, anaemia, thrombocytopenia, leucopoenia and febrile neutropenia. Other studies that analyse these parameters do not find association with toxicity (Huang et al, 2008; Liu et al, 2011; Faganel Kotnik et al, 2011; van Kooten et al, 2008; Pakakasama et al, 2007). Given the limited statistical power of the positive study, carried out with 37 children with ALL or NHL, we can safely conclude that MTHFR A1298C does not appear to be a good predictor of all those types of toxicity.

According to the published data analyzed above and our previous results (Lopez-Lopez et al, 2011), MTHFR 1298C variant does not seem either to be a good MTX toxicity marker in paediatric ALL patients. In fact, we can consider that it seems to be more likely a protective factor rather than a toxicity marker.

Finally, according to what we propose, two works have analysed the summation effect of the haplotype of these polymorphisms on toxicity. Krajinovic et al did not find differences between individuals with or without the T677A1298 haplotype with regard to missed weeks of MTX due to toxicity or average drug dose received weekly in 201 children with ALL (Krajinovic et al, 2004b). Liu et al found a protective effect of the C677C1298 haplotype against anaemia in 181 paediatric ALL patients (Liu et al, 2011).). This haplotype includes the 1298C allele, that had been proposed as a toxicity risk factor because of its functional effect. These results agree with what we have already discussed, although the 1298C allele encodes a protein with less enzyme activity, different studies repeatedly report a small protective effect against toxicity for this allele.

We also want to point that it has been argued that associations of the MTHFR C677T and A1298C polymorphisms with toxicity may be different in different population groups (De Matia and Toffoli, 2009). When the different populations studied are taken into account, we could not observe that the differences in results could be attributable to differences in the ethnic origin of the patients under study (Table 1-2).

After a thorough review of the literature, taking into account the heterogeneity among studies, including patient sample size and the toxicity criteria selected, we can draw the conclusion that most of the studies reported until now do not find associations between MTHFR polymorphisms and toxicity in paediatric ALL. Additionally, none of the associations reported has been replicated by other, usually larger, studies. In conclusion, the MTHFR C677T and A1298C polymorphisms are not good markers of MTX-related toxicity in paediatric ALL, and could have a protective effect that should be analyzed.

MTHFR Polymorphisms and Toxicity in Adult Acute Lymphoblastic Leukaemia

Adults with ALL are also treated with MTX, but unlike paediatric ALL, there are few reports that study the involvement of MTHFR C677T and A1298C polymorphisms in toxicity.

To our knowledge, only two groups have analyzed the implication of MTHFR C677T polymorphism in toxicity in three studies with 55 ALL, 61 ALL or acute promyelocytic leukaemia (APL) and 122 ALL patients respectively (Chiusolo et al, 2002; Chiusolo et al, 2007; Ongaro et al, 2009) (Table 1). Surprisingly, in this case, it has been observed a correlation between the MTHFR 677T allele and increased toxicity during low-dose MTX therapy in all the studies. This could be attributable to the difference in treatment, as proposed by Ongaro and collaborators (Ongaro et al, 2009).

The effect of MTHFR A1298C polymorphism on toxicity after MTX treatment has been analyzed in only two of the above mentioned studies with adult ALL patients. Chiusolo et al (2007) did not find association with the presence of any toxicity, hematologic or hepatic, in 61 ALL or APL patients. Ongaro et al, in a larger sample of 122 ALL patients, found an association between AC/CC genotypes and decreased leucopoenia and hepatic toxicity (Ongaro et al, 2009) (Table 2). These results are more similar to those found in paediatric ALL, where, in some cases, the C allele is also associated with decreased toxicity against what was expected for its functional effect.

In conclusion, MTHFR C677T could have a predictive role for MTX toxicity in adult ALL with low dose treatment but more studies with larger samples and in different populations should be carried out in order to draw consistent conclusions. However, MTHFR A1298C polymorphism does not seem to be a good toxicity marker, similar to what was observed in paediatric ALL.

MTHFR Polymorphisms in other Malignant Diseases

Methotrexate is also used in the therapy of other malignancies, both lymphomas (Central Nervous System [CNS] lymphoma, Non Hodgkin Lymphoma [NHL]) and solid tumours (ovarian cancer, urothelial cancer and osteosarcoma).

In lymphomas, we can observe the same tendency as in ALL when MTHFR C677T and A1298C polymorphisms are analyzed in association with MTX toxicity. In a study with 484 paediatric NHL patients, the authors could not find any association between MTHFR C677T polymorphism and toxicity (Seidemann et al, 2006). While in adults, in two works with 68 primary CNS lymphoma patients and 68 adult NHLs respectively MTHFR 677TT genotypes were associated with toxicity (Linnebank et al, 2009; Gemmati et al, 2007) (Table 1). MTHFR 1298C was only studied in adults and variant showed contradictory results. It was associated with less toxicity in one of the studies (Linnebank et al, 2009) and with increased toxicity in the other study (Gemmati et al, 2007) (Table 2).

In solid tumours, in adults, Toffoli et al found a significant association between toxicity and MTHFR 677TT genotype in 43 ovarian cancer patients treated with low doses of MTX (Toffoli et al, 2003). On the other hand, in 40 urothelial cancer patients, MTHFR C677T and A1298C polymorphisms were not associated with toxicity (Tsuchiya et al, 2008). In this case, the results are contradictory and the number of patients analyzed is limited. In 96 children with osteosarcoma (OS), MTHFR 677TT genotype was associated with increased hematologic toxicity but A1298C polymorphism showed no association (Patiño et al, 2009), which opposes to that observed in paediatric ALL (Table 1-2).

It must be remarked that, in these pathologies, the number of studies reported is reduced and that, as most studies have been carried out with small samples, their statistical power is reduced. In addition, there is a great heterogeneity among therapeutic approaches for each disease, so it is not accurate to draw a general conclusion. Further studies with larger samples would be necessary.

MTHFR Polymorphisms in Transplants Receivers

Patients undergoing bone marrow transplants also receive methotrexate as graft-versus-host disease prophylaxis (GVHD).

Regarding the role of the MTHFR C677T polymorphism, eight studies have been published. Four studies performed with 82, 89, 159 and 84 patients, treated with low doses of MTX, have not found any association with toxicity (Soydan et al, 2008; Pihusch et al, 2004;

Sugimoto et al, 2008; Goekkurt et al, 2007). The other four studies, carried out with 72, 220, 172 and 133 patients, with similar treatment, find an association between the 677TT genotype and an increased risk of toxicity (Kim et al, 2007; Ulrich et al, 2001; Robien et al, 2006; Robien et al, 2004) (Table 1). Consequently, the role of MTHFR C677T polymorphism is still controversial but it does not seem to be a good toxicity marker.

The MTHFR A1298C polymorphism has been analyzed in three studies. One study carried out with 72 patients does not find association with MTX related toxicity (Kim et al, 2007). Another study finds an association of the 1298C allele with increased toxicity in a group of 84 patients (Goekkurt et al, 2007). And the last one, by contrast, finds an association between the 1298C allele and less toxicity in 172 patients (Robien et al, 2006) (Table 2). With these clearly contradictory results, MTHFR A1298C polymorphism does not seem to be either a good marker.

We can conclude that, according to the reported data, in GVHD treatment, MTHFR polymorphisms do not appear to be good MTX toxicity predictors.

Table 3. Association of MTHFR C677T polymorphism and toxicity in immune diseases

Rheumatoid arthritis					
Patients (n)	MTX dose	Ethnicity	Toxicity	Main results	References
RA (218)	Low	Caucasian and African American	+T	T allele associated with alopecia in African American.	Ranganathan et al, 2008
RA (106)	Low	Japanese	+T	T allele associated with a higher rate of overall MTX toxicity.	Urano et al, 2002
RA (110)	Low	Chinese	+T	The patients with CT or TT genotype had higher risks of adverse events than those with CC genotype.	Xiao et al, 2010
RA (113)	Low	European	+T	T allele associated with adverse events.	Van Ede et al, 2002
RA (159)	Low+ folic acid	Japanese	+T	T allele associated with overall adverse events.	Taniguchi et al, 2007
RA (214)	Low+ folic acid	North American	+T	TT associated with CNS toxicity. No association with GI, alopecia or overall toxicity.	Weisman et al, 2006
RA (385)	Low	Korean	+T	T allele associated with the risk of toxicity.	Kim et al, 2006
200 RA	Low+ folic acid	New Zealander	NA	No association with adverse effects.	Stamp et al, 2010
RA (100)	Low	Japanese	NA	No association with MTX serum levels	Fukino et al, 2007
RA (150)	Low+ folic acid	Indian	NA	No association with toxicity.	Aggarwal et al, 2006
RA (150)	Low	Central European	NA	No association with overall MTX toxicity	Bohanec et al, 2008
RA (167)	Low	Japanese	NA	No association with toxicity.	Kumagai et al, 2003
RA (205)	Low+ folic acid	White (n=191), Asian (n=5), Black (n=2), others (n=7)	NA	No association with adverse events.	Wessels et al, 2006
RA (223)	Low+ folic acid	Caucasian (n=193) and African-American (n=30)	NA	No association with toxicity.	Hughes et al, 2006

Rheumatoid arthritis					
Patients (n)	MTX dose	Ethnicity	Toxicity	Main results	References
RA (34)	Low	Indian	NA	No association with adverse events	Ghodke et al, 2008
RA (45)	Low	North American	NA	No association with toxicity	Dervieux et al, 2006
RA (612)	Low+ folic acid	Spanish	NA	No association with cardiovascular events	Palomino-Morales et al, 2010
RA (70)	Low	Mexican	NA	No association with elevation of transaminases.	Mena et al, 2010
RA (731)	Low	Japanese	NA	No association with fracture risk.	Urano et al, 2009
RA (93)	Low+ folic acid	Israeli	NA	No association with toxicity.	Berkun et al, 2004
RA (79), PsA (4), AS (1)	Low+ folic acid	Italian	NA	No association with toxicity.	Taraborelli et al, 2009
Other					
JIA (92)	Low	Japanese	NA	No association with toxicity.	Yanagimachi et al, 2011
JIA (58)	Low	Caucasian	+T	CT patients had more adverse events than CC patients.	Schmeling et al, 2005
JIA (69)	Low	European	+T	TT associated with adverse effects.	Tukova et al, 2010
PsA (203)	Low+ folic acid	Caucasian	NA	No association with toxicity	Campalani et al, 2007
PsA (119)	Low	North American	+T	TT associated with more liver toxicity.	Chandran et al, 2010
IBD (102)	Low	Caucasian	NA	No association with toxicity.	Herrlinger et al, 2005
Psoriasis (374)	Low+ folic acid	Various	NA	No association with toxicity	Warren et al, 2009

High MTX dose: 1.5-8g/m2; Low dose: 15-300mg/m2.

MTHFR Polymorphisms and Immune Diseases

Several immune diseases are also treated with methotrexate, including rheumatoid arthritis (RA), juvenile idiopathic arthritis (JIA), psoriatic arthritis (PsA), psoriasis and inflammatory bowel disease (IBD). MTHFR polymorphisms have also been analyzed (table 3 and 4).

In RA, when we analyzed in depth the results published in the bibliography, we could observe that, from the 21 reported studies, seven find an association with an increase in adverse events in RA patients (Ranganathan et al, 2008; Urano et al, 2002; Xiao et al, 2010; van Ede et al, 2002; Taniguchi et al, 2007; Weisman et al, 2006; Kim et al, 2006), while fourteen studies do not find associations between MTHFR C677T polymorphisms and toxicity (Stamp et al, 2010; Fukino et al, 2007; Aggarwal et al, 2006; Bohanec et al, 2008; Kumagai et al, 2003; Wessels et al, 2006; Hughes et al, 2006; Ghodke et al, 2008; Dervieux et al, 2006; Palomino-Morales et al, 2010; Mena et al, 2010; Urano et al, 2009; Berkun et al, 2004; Taraborelli et al, 2009) (Table 3). We could not find any characteristic that defined the group of studies that show an association with toxicity, including ethnicity, treatment or toxicity criteria. These resultsdo not make clear, once again, the usefulness of MTHFR C677T polymorphism in MTX toxicity.

Regarding the efficacy of MTHFR A1298C polymorphism, the results in RA are similar to that observed in paediatric acute lymphoblastic leukemia. Most studies do not find an association with toxicity (Fukino et al, 2007; Urano et al, 2002; Xiao et al, 2010; Taniguchi et al, 2007; Kumagai et al, 2003; Wessels et al, 2006; Ghodke et al, 2008; Urano et al, 2009; Taraborelli et al, 2009).

Table 4. Association of MTHFR A1298C polymorphism and toxicity in immune diseases

Rheumatoid arthritis					
Patients (n)	MTX dose	Ethnicity	Toxicity	Main results	References
IBD (102)	Low	Caucasian	+T	C allele associated with toxicity.	Herrlinger et al, 2005
RA (45)	low	North American	+T	AC+CC genotypes associated with toxicity	Dervieux et al, 2006
RA (612)	Low+folic acid	Spanish	+T	Association with cardiovascular events	Palomino-Morales et al, 2010
RA (70)	Low	Mexican	+T	Association with elevation of transaminases.	Mena et al, 2010
RA (100)	low	Japanese	NA	No association with MTX serum levels	Fukino et al, 2007
RA (106)	Low	Japanese	NA	No association with toxicity	Urano et al, 2002
RA (110)	Low	Chinese	NA	No association with adverse events.	Xiao et al, 2010
RA (159)	Low+folic acid	Japanese	NA	No association with adverse events.	Taniguchi et al, 2007
RA (167)	115 low +52 without MTX	Japanese	NA	No association with toxicity.	Kumagai et al, 2003
RA (205)	White (n=191), Asian (n=5), Black (n=2), others (n=7)	European	NA	AC+CC genotypes associated with adverse events.	Wessels et al, 2006
RA (34)	low	Indian	NA	No association with adverse events	Ghodke et al, 2008
RA (731)	Low/ corticosteroids	Japanese	NA	No association with fracture risk.	Urano et al, 2009
RA (79), PA (4), AS (1)	Low+folic acid	Italian	NA	No association with toxicity.	Taraborelli et al, 2009
RA (150)	Low	Central European	-T	C allele protective effect on overall MTX toxicity	Bohanec et al, 2008
RA (223)	Low +folic acid	Caucasian (n=193) and African-American (n=30)	-T	A allele associated with an increase in MTX-related adverse effects in caucasian.	Hughes et al, 2006
RA (93)	Low+folic acid	Israeli	-T	CC genotype associated with less MTX-related adverse effects.	Berkun et al, 2004
PsA (203)	Low+folic acid	Caucasian	-T	C allele is protective towards hepatic toxicity.	Campalani et al, 2007
Other					
PsA (119)	Low	North American	NA	No association with toxicity.	Chandran et al, 2010

Rheumatoid arthritis					
Patients (n)	MTX dose	Ethnicity	Toxicity	Main results	References
Psoriasis (374)	Low+folic acid	Various	NA	No association with toxicity	Warren et al, 2009
JIA (58)	Low	Caucasian	NA	No association with adverse events.	Schmeling et al, 2005
JIA (69)	Low	European	NA	No association with adverse events.	Tukova et al, 2010
JIA (92)	Low	Japanese	NA	No association with toxicity.	Yanagimachi et al, 2011

High MTX dose: 1.5-8g/m2; Low dose: 15-300mg/m2.

Four studies report an association with higher toxicity (Herrlinger et al, 2005; Dervieux et al, 2006; Palomino-Morales et al, 2010; Mena et al, 2010) and other three studies even find the opposite, a protective effect against toxicity (Bohanec et al, 2008; Hughes et al, 2006; Berkun et al, 2004) (Table 4).

Two meta-analyses have been published to analyze the role of MTHFR polymorphisms on MTX toxicity in RA. According, to what we can observe from the above mentioned studies, none of them shows association between MTHFR A1298C polymorphism and toxicity. However, the results for MTHFR C677T polymorphism are opposed: while one of them reports an increased risk of toxicity for the 677T allele (Fisher et al, 2009), the other one does not find any association (Lee et al, 2010). As a result, the function of MTHFR C677T in MTX toxicity remains controversial.

In other immune diseases, there are few published reports and are in line with this because when, in the same pathology, two or more jobs are recorded, results are inconclusive.

In JIA, a work carried out with 92 patients did not show association of the C677T polymorphism with toxicity (Yanagimachi et al, 2011). Another study carried out with 58 patients reported an increase of adverse events in the patients with the CT genotype, which is difficult to explain from a functional point of view (Schmeling et al, 2005). And a third work, found association between the TT genotype and toxicity (Tukova et al, 2010) (Table 3). Once again, all these contradictory results, do not allow considering MTHFR C677T a good toxicity marker. In addition, none of these studies found an association between the A1298C polymorphism and toxicity (Table 4).

In PsA, a study performed with 203 patients reported no association between C677T polymorphism and toxicity and a protective effect for the MTHFR 1298CC genotype against toxicity (Campalani et al, 2007). By contrast, another study with 119 patients found an association between the 677TT genotype and liver toxicity and did not find any association between the A1298C polymorphism and toxicity (Chandran et al, 2010) (Table 3-4).

In IBD, the only study reported to date, with 102 patients, did not show an association between MTHFR C677T polymorphism and toxicity (Herrlinger et al, 2005). And, in psoriasis, no association was found between any of the two polymorphisms and toxicity in a study carried out with 374 patients (Warren et al, 2009) (Table 3-4).

In short, in rheumatoid arthritis, the role of MTHFR C677T polymorphism is still controversial and A1298C polymorphism does not appear to be a good MTX toxicity predictor. In other immune disease, there is a shortage of pharmacogenetic data, in those diseases in which two or more studies have been published, the results observed are also controversial, and in pathologies in which an only study has been carried out, no association has been found. We can conclude that, according to the above mentioned data, MTHFR polymorphisms do not seem good MTX toxicity predictors.

Conclusion

On the basis of the clinical data obtained so far, the MTHFR C677T and A1298C polymorphisms cannot be considered good markers of MTX-related toxicity in paediatric ALL, in spite of their functional effect on MTHFR protein function. In rheumatoid arthritis and transplant receivers on GVHD prophylaxis treatment with MTX, these polymorphisms do not seem to be either good toxicity. In other pathologies, there are not conclusive results: or the number of studies is scarce or results are controversial, but we can observe the same tendency towards no association. The only disease in which the association between MTHFR 677T allele and toxicity seems to have some consistence is adult acute lymphoblastic leukaemia, as it is replicated in the three reported studies. But these studies were carried out with quite small samples and the results should be replicated.

References

Abe T, Unno M, Onogawa T, et al. LST-2, a human liver-specific organic anion transporter, determines methotrexate sensitivity in gastrointestinal cancers. *Gastroenterology* 2001; 120:1689–1699.

Aggarwal P, Naik S, Mishra KP, et al. Correlation between methotrexate efficacy and toxicity with C677T polymorphism of the methylenetetrahydrofolate gene in rheumatoid arthritis patients on folate supplementation. *Indian J. Med. Res*. 2006;124:521-526.

Aplenc R, Thompson J, Han P, et al. Methylenetetrahydrofolate reductase polymorphisms and therapy response in pediatric acute lymphoblastic leukemia. *Cancer Res*. 2005;65: 2482-2487.

Berkun Y, Levartovsky D, Rubinow A, Methotrexate related adverse effects in patients with rheumatoid arthritis are associated with the A1298C polymorphism of the MTHFR gene. *Ann. Rheum. Dis*. 2004;63:1227-1231.

Bohanec Grabar P, Logar D, Lestan B, et al. Genetic determinants of methotrexate toxicity in rheumatoid arthritis patients: a study of polymorphisms affecting methotrexate transport and folate metabolism. *Eur. J. Clin. Pharmacol*. 2008;64:1057-1068.

Bone Marrow Transplant. 2008 Sep;42(6):429-30. Epub 2008 Jun 30. No abstract available.

Campalani E, Arenas M, Marinaki AM, et al. Polymorphisms in folate, pyrimidine, and purine metabolism are associated with efficacy and toxicity of methotrexate in psoriasis. *J. Invest. Dermatol*. 2007;127:1860-1867.

Chandran V, Siannis F, Rahman P, et al. Folate pathway enzyme gene polymorphisms and the efficacy and toxicity of methotrexate in psoriatic arthritis. *J. Rheumatol*. 2010;37: 1508-1512.

Chatzidakis K, Goulas A, Athanassiadou-Piperopoulou F, Fidani L et al. Methylenetetrahydrofolate reductase C677T polymorphism: association with risk for childhood acute lymphoblastic leukemia and response during the initial phase of chemotherapy in greek patients. *Pediatr. Blood Cancer* 2006;47:147-151.

Cheok MH, Lugthart S, Evans WE. Pharmacogenomics of acute leukemia. *Annu. Rev. Pharmacol. Toxicol.* 2006;46:317–353.

Chiusolo P, Reddiconto G, Casorelli I, et al. Preponderance of methylenetetrahydrofolate reductase C677T homozygosity among leukemia patients intolerant to methotrexate. *Ann. Oncol.* 2002;13:1915-1918.

Chiusolo P, Reddiconto G, Farina G et al. MTHFR polymorphisms' influence on outcome and toxicity in acute lymphoblastic leukemia patients. *Leuk. Res.* 2007;31: 1669-1774.

Costea I, Moghrabi A, Laverdiere C, et al. Folate cycle gene variants and chemotherapy toxicity in pediatric patients with acute lymphoblastic leukemia. *Haematologica* 2006;91: 1113-1116.

D'Angelo V, Ramaglia M, Ianotta A, et al. Methotrexate toxicity and efficacy during the consolidation phase in paediatric acute lymphoblastic leukaemia and MTHFR polymorphisms as pharmacogenetic determinants. *Cancer Chemother. Pharmacol.* 2011 doi:10.1007/s00280-011-1665-1 [Epub ahead of print].

De Mattia E, Toffoli G. C677T and A1298C MTHFR polymorphisms, a challenge for antifolate and fluoropyrimidine-based therapy personalisation. *Eur. J. Cancer* 2009;45: 1333-1351.

Decreased risk of acute graft-versus-host disease following allogeneic hematopoietic stem cell transplantation in patients with the 5,10-methylenetetrahydrofolate reductase 677TT genotype.

Dervieux T, Greenstein N, Kremer J. Pharmacogenomic and metabolic biomarkers in the folate pathway and their association with methotrexate effects during dosage escalation in rheumatoid arthritis. *Arthritis Rheum.* 2006;54:3095-3103.

Faganel Kotnik B, Grabnar I, Bohanec Grabar P, et al. Association of genetic polymorphism in the folate metabolic pathway with methotrexate pharmacokinetics and toxicity in childhood acute lymphoblastic leukaemia and malignant lymphoma. *Eur. J. Clin. Pharmacol.* 2011. doi: 10.1007/s00228-011-1046-z [Epub ahead of print]

Frosst P, Blom HJ, Milos R, et al. A candidate genetic risk factor for vascular disease: A common mutation in methylenetetrahydrofolate reductase. *Nat. Genet.* 1995;10:111–113.

Fukino K, Kawashima T, Suzuki M, et al. Methylenetetrahydrofolate reductase and reduced folate carrier-1 genotypes and methotrexate serum concentrations in patients with rheumatoid arthritis. *J. Toxicol. Sci.* 2007;32:449-452.

Gemmati D, Ongaro A, Tognazzo S, et al. Methylenetetrahydrofolate reductase C677T and A1298C gene variants in adult non-Hodgkin's lymphoma patients: association with toxicity and survival. *Haematologica* 2007;92:478-485.

Ghodke Y, Chopra A, Joshi K, et al. Are Thymidylate synthase and Methylene tetrahydrofolate reductase genes linked with methotrexate response (efficacy, toxicity) in Indian (Asian) rheumatoid arthritis patients? *Clin. Rheumatol.* 2008;27:787-789.

Goekkurt E, Stoehlmacher J, Stueber C, et al. Pharmacogenetic analysis of liver toxicity after busulfan/cyclophosphamide-based allogeneic hematopoietic stem cell transplantation. *Anticancer Res.* 2007;27:4377-4380.

Goldman ID, Matherly LH. The cellular pharmacology of methotrexate. *Pharmacol. Ther.* 1985;28:77–102.

Gorlick R, Goker E, Trippett T, et al. Intrinsic and acquired resistance to methotrexate in acute leukemia. *N. Engl. J. Med.* 1996;335:1041–1048.

Herrlinger KR, Cummings JR, Barnardo MC, et al. The pharmacogenetics of methotrexate in inflammatory bowel disease. *Pharmacogenet Genomics* 2005;15:705-711.

Horinouchi M, Yagi M, Imanishi H, et al. Association of genetic polymorphisms with hepatotoxicity in patients with childhood acute lymphoblastic leukemia or lymphoma. *Pediatr. Hematol. Oncol.* 2010;27:344-354.

Huang L, Tissing WJ, de Jonge R, et al. Polymorphisms in folate-related genes: association with side effects of high-dose methotrexate in childhood acute lymphoblastic leukemia. *Leukemia* 2008;22:1798-1800.

Hughes LB, Beasley TM, Patel H, et al. Racial or ethnic differences in allele frequencies of single-nucleotide polymorphisms in the methylenetetrahydrofolate reductase gene and their influence on response to methotrexate in rheumatoid arthritis. *Ann. Rheum. Dis.* 2006;65:1213-1218.

Imanishi H, Okamura N, Yagi M, et al. Genetic polymorphisms associated with adverse events and elimination of methotrexate in childhood acute lymphoblastic leukemia and malignant lymphoma. *J. Hum. Genet.* 2007;52: 166–171.

Int. J. Hematol. 2008 Jun;87(5):451-8. Epub 2008 Mar 26.

Johnston WT, Lightfoot TJ, Simpson J, et al. Childhood cancer survival: A report from the United Kingdom Childhood Cancer Study. *Cancer Epidemiol.* 2010;34:659–666.

Kantar M, Kosova B, Cetingul N, et al. Methylenetetrahydrofolate reductase C677T and A1298C gene polymorphisms and therapy-related toxicity in children treated for acute lymphoblastic leukemia and non-Hodgkin lymphoma. *Leuk. Lymphoma* 2009;50:912-917.

Karathanasis NV, Stiakaki E, Goulielmos GN, et al. The role of the methylene tetrahydrofolate reductase 677 and 1298 polymorphisms in Cretan children with acute lymphoblastic leukemia. *Genet. Test Mol. Biomarkers* 2011;15:5-10.

Kim I, Lee KH, Kim JH, et al. Polymorphisms of the methylenetetrahydrofolate reductase gene and clinical outcomes in HLA-matched sibling allogeneic hematopoietic stem cell transplantation. *Ann. Hematol.* 2007;86:41-48.

Kim SK, Jun JB, El-Sohemy A, et al. Cost-effectiveness analysis of MTHFR polymorphism screening by polymerase chain reaction in Korean patients with rheumatoid arthritis receiving methotrexate. *J. Rheumatol.* 2006;33:1266-1274.

Kishi S, Cheng C, French D, et al. Ancestry and pharmacogenetics of antileukemic drug toxicity. *Blood* 2007;109:4151-4157.

Kishi S, Griener J, Cheng C, et al. Homocysteine, pharmacogenetics, and neurotoxicity in children with leukemia. *J. Clin. Oncol.* 2003;21:3084-3091.

Koppen IJ, Hermans FJ, Kaspers GJ. Folate related gene polymorphisms and susceptibility to develop childhood acute lymphoblastic leukaemia. *Br. J. Haematol.* 2010;148:3–14.

Krajinovic M, Lemieux-Blanchard E, Chiasson S, et al. Role of polymorphisms in MTHFR and MTHFD1 genes in the outcome of childhood acute lymphoblastic leukemia. *Pharmacogenomics J.* 2004b;4:66-72.

Krajinovic M, Moghrabi A. Pharmacogenetics of methotrexate. *Pharmacogenomics* 2004a; 5:819–834.

Kumagai K, Hiyama K, Oyama T, et al. Polymorphisms in the thymidylate synthase and methylenetetrahydrofolate reductase genes and sensitivity to the low-dose methotrexate therapy in patients with rheumatoid arthritis. *Int. J. Mol. Med.* 2003;11:593-600.

Linnebank M, Moskau S, Jürgens A, et al. Association of genetic variants of methionine metabolism with methotrexate-induced CNS white matter changes in patients with primary CNS lymphoma. *Neuro Oncol.* 2009;11:2-8.

Liu SG, Li ZG, Cui L, et al. Effects of methylenetetrahydrofolate reductase gene polymorphisms on toxicities during consolidation therapy in pediatric acute lymphoblastic leukemia in a Chinese population. *Leuk. Lymphoma* 2011;52:1030-1040.

Lopez-Lopez E, Martin-Guerrero I, Ballesteros J, et al. Polymorphisms of the SLCO1B1 gene predict methotrexate-related toxicity in childhood acute lymphoblastic leukemia. *Pediatr. Blood Cancer* 2011. doi: 10.1002/pbc.23074. [Epub ahead of print]

Mena JP, Salazar-Páramo M, González-López L, et al. Polymorphisms C677T and A1298C in the MTHFR gene in Mexican patients with rheumatoid arthritis treated with methotrexate: implication with elevation of transaminases. *Pharmacogenomics J.* 2010. doi:10.1038/tpj.2010.32. [Epub ahead of print]

Ongaro A, De Mattei M, Della Porta MG, et al. Gene polymorphisms in folate metabolizing enzymes in adult acute lymphoblastic leukemia: effects on methotrexate-related toxicity and survival. *Haematologica* 2009;94:1391-1398.

Pakakasama S, Kanchanakamhaeng K, Kajanachumpol S, et al. Genetic polymorphisms of folate metabolic enzymes and toxicities of high dose methotrexate in children with acute lymphoblastic leukemia. *Ann. Hematol.* 2007;86:609-611.

Palomino-Morales R, Gonzalez-Juanatey C, Vazquez-Rodriguez TR, et al. A1298C polymorphism in the MTHFR gene predisposes to cardiovascular risk in rheumatoid arthritis. *Arthritis Res. Ther.* 2010;12:R71.

Patiño-García A, Zalacaín M, Marrodán L, et al. Methotrexate in pediatric osteosarcoma: response and toxicity in relation to genetic polymorphisms and dihydrofolate reductase and reduced folate carrier 1 expression. *J. Pediatr.* 2009;154:688-693.

Pihusch M, Lohse P, Reitberger J, et al. Impact of thrombophilic gene mutations and graft-versus-host disease on thromboembolic complications after allogeneic hematopoietic stem-cell transplantation. *Transplantation* 2004;78:911-918.

Pui CH, Robinson LL, Look AT. Acute lymphoblastic leukemia. *Lancet* 2008; 371:1030–1043.

Ranganathan P, Culverhouse R, Marsh S, et al. Methotrexate (MTX) pathway gene polymorphisms and their effects on MTX toxicity in Caucasian and African American patients with rheumatoid arthritis. *J. Rheumatol.* 2008;35:572-579.

Robien K, Bigler J, Yasui Y, et al. Methylenetetrahydrofolate reductase and thymidylate synthase genotypes and risk of acute graft-versus-host disease following hematopoietic cell transplantation for chronic myelogenous leukemia. *Biol. Blood Marrow Transplant* 2006;12:973-980.

Robien K, Schubert MM, Bruemmer B, et al. Predictors of oral mucositis in patients receiving hematopoietic cell transplants for chronic myelogenous leukemia. *J. Clin. Oncol.* 2004;22:1268-1675.

Schmeling H, Biber D, Heins S, et al. Influence of methylenetetrahydrofolate reductase polymorphisms on efficacy and toxicity of methotrexate in patients with juvenile idiopathic arthritis. *J. Rheumatol.* 2005;32:1832-1836.

Seidemann K, Book M, Zimmermann M, et al. MTHFR 677 (C-->T) polymorphism is not relevant for prognosis or therapy-associated toxicity in pediatric NHL: results from 484 patients of multicenter trial NHL-BFM 95. *Ann. Hematol.* 2006;85:291-300.

Shimasaki N, Mori T, Samejima H, et al. Effects of methylenetetrahydrofolate reductase and reduced folate carrier 1 polymorphisms on high-dose methotrexate-induced toxicities in children with acute lymphoblastic leukemia or lymphoma. *J. Pediatr. Hematol. Oncol.* 2006; 28:64-68.

Shimasaki N, Mori T, Torii C, et al. Influence of MTHFR and RFC1 polymorphisms on toxicities during maintenance chemotherapy for childhood acute lymphoblastic leukemia or lymphoma. *J. Pediatr. Hematol. Oncol.* 2008;30:347-52.

Soydan E, Topcuoglu P, Dalva K, Arat M.

Stamp LK, Chapman PT, O'Donnell JL, et al. Polymorphisms within the folate pathway predict folate concentrations but are not associated with disease activity in rheumatoid arthritis patients on methotrexate. *Pharmacogenet Genomics* 2010;20:367-376.

Sugimoto K, Murata M, Onizuka M, Inamoto Y, Terakura S, Kuwatsuka Y, Oba T, Miyamura K, Kodera Y, Naoe T.

Swerts K, De Moerloose B, Dhooge C, et al. Prognostic significance of multidrug resistance-related proteins in childhood acute lymphoblastic leukaemia. *Eur. J. Cancer* 2006;42: 295–309.

Taniguchi A, Urano W, Tanaka E, et al. Validation of the associations between single nucleotide polymorphisms or haplotypes and responses to disease-modifying antirheumatic drugs in patients with rheumatoid arthritis: a proposal for prospective pharmacogenomic study in clinical practice. *Pharmacogenet Genomics* 200;17:383-390.

Tantawy AA, El-Bostany EA, Adly AA, et al. Methylene tetrahydrofolate reductase gene polymorphism in Egyptian children with acute lymphoblastic leukemia. *Blood Coagul. Fibrinolysis* 2011;21:28-34.

Taraborelli M, Andreoli L, Archetti S, et al. Methylenetetrahydrofolate reductase polymorphisms and methotrexate: no association with response to therapy nor with drug-related adverse events in an Italian population of rheumatic patients. *Clin. Exp. Rheumatol.* 2009;27:499-502.

The impact of methylenetetrahydrofolate reductase (MTHFR) C677T gene polymorphism on transplant-related variables after allogeneic hematopoietic cell transplantation in patients receiving MTX as GVHD prophylaxis.

Toffoli G, Russo A, Innocenti F, et al. Effect of methylenetetrahydrofolate reductase 677C-->T polymorphism on toxicity and homocysteine plasma level after chronic methotrexate treatment of ovarian cancer patients. *Int. J. Cancer* 2003;103:294-299.

Treviño LR, Shimasaki N, Yang W, et al. Germline genetic variation in an organic anion transporter polypeptide associated with methotrexate pharmacokinetics and clinical effects. *J. Clin. Oncol.* 2009;27:5972–5978.

Tsuchiya N, Inoue T, Narita S, et al. Drug related genetic polymorphisms affecting adverse reactions to methotrexate, vinblastine, doxorubicin and cisplatin in patients with urothelial cancer. *J. Urol.* 2008;180:2389-2395.

Tuková J, Chládek J, Hroch M, et al. 677TT genotype is associated with elevated risk of methotrexate (MTX) toxicity in juvenile idiopathic arthritis: treatment outcome, erythrocyte concentrations of MTX and folates, and MTHFR polymorphisms. *J. Rheumatol.* 2010;37:2180-2186.

Ulrich CM, Yasui Y, Storb R, et al. Pharmacogenetics of methotrexate: toxicity among marrow transplantation patients varies with the methylenetetrahydrofolate reductase C677T polymorphism. *Blood* 2001;98:231-234.

Urano W, Furuya T, Inoue E, et al. Associations between methotrexate treatment and methylenetetrahydrofolate reductase gene polymorphisms with incident fractures in Japanese female rheumatoid arthritis patients. *J. Bone Miner. Metab.* 2009;27:574-583.

Urano W, Taniguchi A, Yamanaka H, et al. Polymorphisms in the methylenetetrahydrofolate reductase gene were associated with both the efficacy and the toxicity of methotrexate used for the treatment of rheumatoid arthritis, as evidenced by single locus and haplotype analyses. *Pharmacogenetics* 2002;12:183-190.

van Ede AE, Laan RF, Blom HJ, et al. Homocysteine and folate status in methotrexate-treated patients with rheumatoid arthritis. *Rheumatology* (Oxford) 2002;41:658-665.

van Kooten Niekerk PB, Schmiegelow K, Schroeder H. Influence of methylene tetrahydrofolate reductase polymorphisms and coadministration of antimetabolites on toxicity after high dose methotrexate. *Eur. J. Haematol.* 2008;81:391-398.

Warren RB, Smith RL, Campalani E, et al. Outcomes of methotrexate therapy for psoriasis and relationship to genetic polymorphisms. *Br. J. Dermatol.* 2009;160:438-441.

Weisberg IS, Jacques PF, Selhub J, et al. The 1298A-->C polymorphism in methylenetetrahydrofolate reductase (MTHFR): in vitro expression and association with homocysteine. *Atherosclerosis* 2001; 156:409-415.

Weisman MH, Furst DE, Park GS, et al. Risk genotypes in folate-dependent enzymes and their association with methotrexate-related side effects in rheumatoid arthritis. *Arthritis Rheum.* 2006;54:607-612.

Wessels JA, de Vries-Bouwstra JK, Heijmans BT, et al. Efficacy and toxicity of methotrexate in early rheumatoid arthritis are associated with single-nucleotide polymorphisms in genes coding for folate pathway enzymes. *Arthritis Rheum.* 2006;54:1087-1095.

Xiao H, Xu J, Zhou X, et al. Associations between the genetic polymorphisms of MTHFR and outcomes of methotrexate treatment in rheumatoid arthritis. *Clin. Exp. Rheumatol.* 2010;28:728-733.

Yanagimachi M, Naruto T, Hara T, et al. Influence of polymorphisms within the methotrexate pathway genes on the toxicity and efficacy of methotrexate in patients with juvenile idiopathic arthritis. *Br. J. Clin. Pharmacol.* 2011;71:237-243.

In: Methotrexate   ISBN: 978-1-62100-596-4
Editors: V. S. Castillo and L. A. Moyano   © 2012 Nova Science Publishers, Inc.

Chapter IV

Methotrexate: Pharmacology, Clinical Uses and Adverse Effects

Usha Verma[1] and Nipun Verma[2]

[1]University of Miami Miller School of Medicine, Miami, Florida, US
[2]Weill Cornell Medical College, New York, NY, US

Methotrexate formerly known as amethopterin is an antimetabolite drug. It is a 4-amino substituted folic acid analogue. The mechanism of action of methotrexate is by competitive inhibition of dihydrofolate reductase (DHFR), an enzyme required for the synthesis of tetrahydrofolate. Tetrahydrofolate is essential for the de novo synthesis of DNA and methotrexate inhibits folate-dependent thymidylate production in cells. Thus, methotrexate inhibits DNA synthesis, which is essential for cell replication and repair in cancer and normal cells.

Methotrexate acts specifically during the S phase of the cell cycle when the cell is undergoing synthesis of DNA. Methotrexate is therefore effective in cancers involving rapidly proliferating cells. Although initially used only in cancer, methotrexate is now widely used for several nonmalignant conditions also. The latter has been possible in part with extensive research and understanding of the pharmacotherapeutics of the drug, and effective monitoring of methotrexate therapy in patients. Methotrexate for example is also used as an immunosuppressant and in small doses as an antinflammatory agent in autoimmune and other non-cancerous diseases. Since Methotrexate acts on rapidly dividing cells, the adverse effects of this medication target those tissues, which rapidly replicate with a fast turn over. We review pharmacology, clinical applications and adverse effects of methotrexate in this chapter.

Pharmacology

Folic acid

Methotrexate

Folates (pteroylglutamates) belong to a family of B_9 vitamins that function as essential cofactors within mammalian cells. Naturally occurring folates are composed of three structural components: a pteridine ring system, a p-aminobenzoic acid (PABA) and a glutamate moiety. One form is folic acid, which is used in multivitamin formulations and food fortification. Within most diets, however, the most common form of folates is 5'-methyl-THF (5'-MTHF). Both folic acid and 5'-MTHF are reduced to tetrahydrofolate (THF) within the cell. Folic acid is first intracellularly reduced to dihydrofolate (DHF) and then reduced further into THF; both of these reactions are mediated by dihyrdrofolate reductase (DHFR). 5'-MTHF is converted to THF in a B_{12} dependent reaction that also produces methionine from homocysteine, a reaction catalyzed by methionine synthase. In the cytosol THF and its derivatives function as one-carbon unit donors in a number of metabolic pathways. These reactions are involved in the de novo biosynthesis of purines and thymidylate, synthesis of amino acids (methionine, serine and glycine) as well as the production of S-adenosyl methionine, which promotes methylation of DNA, histones and neurotransmitters. In addition to their multiple roles in the cytosol, folate cofactors are also transported into the mitochondria where they are involved in glycine metabolism and mitochondrial DNA-encoded protein synthesis.

These numerous and essential functions of folates are disrupted by antifolates for beneficial anti-proliferative and anti-metabolic effects in cancer therapy and anti-inflammatory therapy. Once the cell takes them up, antifolates inhibit key enzymes involved in folate metabolism. As a result they disrupt purine and thymidylate biosynthesis, inhibit DNA replication and ultimately lead to cell death. The principle enzymes inhibited are DHFR, β-glycinamide ribonucleotide transformylase (GARFT), 5'-amino-4'-imidazolecarboxamide ribonucleotide transformylase (AICARFT), and thymidylate synthetase (TYMS). DHFR, as described above, is involved in the reduction of DHF to 5', 6', 7', 8'-THF. THF is converted to 5', 10'-methyltertrahydrofolate (5', 10'-MTHF), which is then oxidized to DHF by TYMS during the production of deoxythymidine monophosphate (dTMP), a required precursor for DNA synthesis. Another THF coenzyme, 10'-formyl THF, is the substrate for the formation of the purine imidazole ring catalyzed by GARFT. A subsequent reaction, catalyzed by AICARFT, generates the purine intermediate inosine 5'-monophosphate (IMP), which ultimately is converted to purine nucleotides adenylate (AMP) and guanylate (GMP). These THF coenzyme dependent enzymes are together responsible for the de novo production of purine and thymine nucleotides that are necessary for DNA synthesis. Methotrexate (MTX), one of the first antifolates developed, is a potent cytotoxic drug used extensively in cancer therapy. MTX almost irreversibly inhibits DHFR. It also inhibits, to a lesser extent, GARFT, AICARFT and TYMS [1]. Collectively inhibition of these enzymes leads to purine and thymidylate depletion within the cell. The targeted cells are unable to synthesize DNA and RNA and as a result cannot proliferate and inflict further harm. Furthermore, apoptosis pathways are activated and eventually lead to cell death [2].

MTX and other antifolates use the same transport systems as naturally occurring folates to enter the cells. The principle cell membrane transporters are the reduced folate receptor (RFC), folate receptors (FR-α and FR-β), and the proton coupled folate receptor (PCFT). RFC is the primary pathway for uptake of natural folates as well as antifolates. MTX in particular has a very high affinity for RFC and is transported mainly via this pathway, while FR-α contributes to a lesser extent [3]. RFC is a 85 kDa membrane glycoprotein that is a member of the major facilitator superfamily of transporters (MFS). RFC functions as a facultative carrier, specifically an anion exchanger, which uses the high intracellular gradient of organic phosphates (such as adenine nucleotides) to power the uphill transport of folates and antifolates. FR-α receptor is a glycosylphosphatidylinositol (GPI)-anchored cell surface glycoprotein which transports via a classical mechanism of receptor mediated endocytosis. After transport into the endosome, antifolates enter the intracellular compartment via PCFT, a high-affinity folate-proton symporter [4]. In contrast to RFC, FR-α has much lower affinity for MTX and so transport via FR-α is largely secondary. Another difference is in the expression of RFC compared to FR-α. RFCs are ubiquitously expressed in normal tissue as well as cancer cells, which fundamentally limits the tolerability of antifolates like MTX. FR-α expression is mainly limited to certain epithelial cells and to a number of carcinomas, with the exception of carcinomas of the head and neck; this specificity makes tumors vulnerable to antifolates without harming healthy tissue [5].

Once MTX is taken up by the cell via RFC and FR-α, it undergoes polyglutamation, a reaction that results in the intracellular retention of the MTX as well as increased affinity of MTX to its target enzymes. Polyglutamation is a Mg-ATP dependent sequential addition of glutamic acid, one equivalent at a time, to the gamma-carboxyl group of THF cofactors and polyglutamable antifolates. The resulting MTX polyglutamate has a number of advantages over the parent compound. First it is a polyanion that is impermeable to the lipid bilayer and thus retained within the cell. Secondly polyglutamates of MTX, in addition to inhibiting DHFR, are also potent inhibitors of TS, AICARTF, adenosine deaminase and 5'-adenylate deaminase [6]. Lastly, membrane transport systems that promote efflux of molecules, such as multidrug resistance proteins (MRPs) and breast cancer resistance proteins (BCRPs) are not capable of transporting long chain polyglutamate derivatives of MTX out of the cell [7]. This increased retention and bioavalability allows MTX to be administered to cancer patients with relatively long intervals between the repeated doses. The importance of polyglutamation in increasing the pharmacological activity of MTX, is reflected by the fact that the level and time course of MTX polyglutamate formation, in addition to DHFR levels and MTX transport into cells, is a key determinate of drug efficacy.

Resistance to MTX treatment can arise from a number of cellular changes, including decreased influx of MTX or increased efflux, impaired polyglutamation, increased expression of DHFR or mutations in DHFR that decreases its affinity to MTX, and an increase in the intracellular pool of THF cofactors. MTX- resistance cell lines have shown mutations with in the RFC gene [8]. Osteosarcoma cases have shown mutations at the 4'UTR of RFC as well as increased methylation of the RFC promoter [9]. Mutations within the breast cancer resistant protein (BCRP), which is able to transport polyglutamates out of the cell, have been seen in cells resistant to MTX and other antifolates [10]. Lastly, amplification of the DHFR gene has been found in acute lymphoblastic leukemia (ALL), ovarian cancer, and soft-tissue sarcoma [11].

MTX can be administered orally or via an IV infusion. Absorption of MTX occurs from the gastrointestinal tract by a saturable active transport system. Food does not affect absorption of MTX. Orally administered MTX is absorbed by the GI tract and delivered to the liver via the portal vein. IV administered MTX is delivered to the liver through the hepatic artery. IV administered MTX has been shown to have a lesser frequency of abnormal elevations of transaminase levels than orally administered MTX in the same individuals. Following IV infusion approximately 10% of MTX is hydroxylated to 7-hydroxyMTX (7-OH-MTX) in hepatocytes. MTX distributes throughout the body, with approximately 50% of MTX in serum bound to albumin. MTX is a hydrophillic compound and shows poor ability to cross-intact cellular barriers. Third space fluid collections, such as ascites or pleural effusions, can accumulate high concentrations of MTX. Leakage of MTX into the circulation from these third spaces can lead to prolonged pharmacological action of MTX even after halting administration of the drug, thus leading to delayed toxicity. MTX is capable of crossing the blood brain barrier slowly. The concentration in CSF can range from 3-10% of plasma concentration of MTX. Due to this low efficiency of movement, high doses of MTX are required to achieve therapeutic concentrations in the CSF [12,13].

MTX and 7-OH-MTX both display first order pharmokinetics and both are primarily cleared renally. The half-life of MTX following IV administration is between 8 to 12 hours, 7-OH-MTX is cleared at a slower rate than the parent compound. Because of its longer half-life the serum concentration of 7-OH-MTX can exceed MTX. The majority of MTX is excreted within the first 12 hours of administration, with over 90% excreted into the urine unchanged. The mechanism of MTX clearance in the kidney is not completely known. It is believed that MTX is eliminated by passive glomerular filtration and active secretion in the proximal tubule and subsequent reabsorption in the distal tubule. It is essential to monitor plasma concentrations of MTX after administration to prevent adverse toxicities. Importantly renal clearance of MTX is prolonged in patients with renal impairment or third-space fluid collections. With high dose MTX therapy rapid drug excretion can produce concentrations of MTX in the urine that exceed the drug solubility below pH 7.0, this in turn can lead to the intrarenal precipitation of MTX and 7-OH-MTX and cause acute kidney damage. MTX induced renal toxicity occurs in approximately 2% of patients receiving high dose MTX therapy [14]. Because MTX is renally excreted, renal damage can increase plasma concentration of MTX and enhance cytotoxic effects, leading to severe mucosal toxicity and myelosuppression. The risk of these adverse effects can be minimized by hydration and urinary alkalinization. Possible drug interactions must also be considered as many drugs inhibit renal excretion of MTX and may increase treatment related toxicity. Weak organic acids such as aspirin, nonsteroidal anti-inflammatory drugs (NSAIDs) and piperacillin inhibit the excretion of MTX. Cephalosporins can also inhibit MTX excretion, possibly by competing for tubular secretion. These and other noteworthy drug interactions will be described in more detail below. In addition to renal excretion, a small amount of MTX is excreted unchanged into the bile and undergoes enterohepatic circulation, the clinical relevance of this process is unclear.

Clinical Uses

The dose related properties of Methotrexate defines the clinical use of this medication in certain conditions. Methotrexate has anti-inflammatory and immunosuppressive action in low doses, while in higher doses this medication has anti-proliferative effects on cells. The clinical use of MTX is defined by its dose related properties. The low dose MTX is now widely used in the treatment of some immune related diseases.

Low dose Methotrexate is used in treatment of several diseases, which include rheumatoid arthritis, psoriatic arthritis, inflammatory bowel disease, Wegners granulomatosis, myasthenia gravis, bullous pemphigoid, polymyalgia rhematica, inflammatory muscle disease, and sarcodosis disease. In addition, low dose MTX treatment has been used for the treatment of difficult asthma as a steroid-sparing agent and in the treatment of ectopic pregnancy.

Use of methotrexate as an antinflammatory and immunosuppressive agent:

Rheumatoid Arthritis (RA)

Methotrexate was initially developed in the 1940's to treat leukemia. The first attempt to use methotrexate for the treatment of rheumatoid arthritis occurred in 1951. In the following years, several studies were conducted to determine the effectiveness and safety of MTX for the treatment of rheumatoid arthritis, for which it was considered an experimental drug throughout the 1970's. Finally in 1988 the FDA formally approved MTX for the treatment of rheumatoid arthritis.

MTX is now considered the first-line DMARD (disease modifying antirheumatic drug) agent for most patients with RA. It is the most commonly prescribed DMARD for rheumatoid arthritis and can be considered a gold standard for long term therapy [15]. This treatment is favored because of a relatively rapid onset of action, good efficacy, low toxicity, ease of administration, and relatively low cost. Compared to other DMARDS, the majority of patients continue to take MTX after 5 years, far more than other therapies- reflecting both its efficacy and tolerability. MTX is effective in reducing the signs and symptoms of RA, as well as slowing or stopping further radiographic damage. The anti-inflammatory effects of MTX in rheumatoid arthritis appear to be related at least in part to the interruption of adenosine and possible effects on TNF pro-inflammatory pathways. The immunosuppressive and toxic effects of MTX are due to the inhibition of an enzyme involved in the metabolism of folic acid, dihydrofolate reductase. The onset of action is seen in as early as 4 to 6 weeks. However the dose required to achieve a response is considerably variable in individual patients and thus may require an additional 4-6 weeks after a dose increase to determine if the drug is working. MTX with an aggressive dosing regimen has been reported to be more effective than leflunomide in the treatment of juvenile rheumatoid arthritis [16]. It has also been shown to be an effective and safe treatment for children with resistant juvenile rheumatoid arthritis when given weekly in low doses for a short term [17]. In patients with partial responses to MTX, additional medications are usually a given with MTX.

Psoriatic Arthritis

Psoriasis is an immune mediated chronic inflammatory disease, which results in significant morbidity. Wide ranges of systemic drugs have been developed in recent years for treatment of psoriasis and associated comorbidities. Low-dose MTX is one of the most frequently used systemic treatments for psoriasis. Low-dose MTX is also effective in the treatment of psoriatic arthritis. The mechanism of action is not clear. Methotreaxte appears to act primarily as an anti-inflammatory and immunosuppressant drug. A favorable efficacy and safety profile has been established for MTX in a large number of clinical trials, as well as in clinical practice [18]. It is also a highly cost effective treatment compared to alefacept.

Psoriatic arthritis: Despite a paucity of high quality clinical data, MTX remains one of the most commonly used medications in the treatment of patients with psoriatic arthritis [19]. MTX is of value to most psoriatic polyarthritis patients (60%) and a maximum efficacy is achieved within 6 months of therapy [20].

Crohns Disease

Corticosteroids are often effective for the remission of Crohns disease, but approximately 20% of patients who respond to corticosteroids have a relapse when steroids are withdrawn and ultimately become steroid dependent [21]. Furthermore, corticosteroids exhibit significant adverse effects. The success of MTX as a treatment for rheumatoid arthritis led to its evaluation in patients with refractory Crohns disease and it has become the principal alternative to azathioprine/6-Mercaptopurine therapy.

In patients with refractory Crohns disease, MTX is effective for the induction of remission and allows for the complete withdrawal from steroids [22]. MTX is also beneficial in maintaining remission and steroid-sparing treatment in children with Crohn disease following failure of thiopurine therapy [23].

Wegners Granulomatosis

MTX, given at a dosage of 20–25 mg per week in combination with glucocorticoids, has emerged as the standard remission induction regimen for WG in patients whose disease is classified as "limited," "early systemic," or "non–life or organ threatening. MTX has now even been documented to be comparable to standard cyclophosphamide therapy in that capacity [24].

Myasthenia Gravis

Myasthenia gravis (MG) is a prototypic antibody-mediated neurological autoimmune disorder. Severe cases may benefit from combined immunosuppression with corticosteroids, cyclosporine A, and even with moderate doses of MTX or cyclophosphamide [25]. In chronic autoimmune conditions such as myasthenia gravis (MG), immunosuppression--usually long-term--is often necessary. MTX, mycophenolate mofetil or tacrolimus should be considered in patients who are intolerant of or unresponsive to azathioprine [26]. Corticosteroids and/or immunosuppressive agents are used in severe forms of the disease. The combination of corticosteroids and immunosuppressive agents are recommended early to spare corticosteroids [27].

Bullous Pemphigoid

Bullous pemphigoid (BP) is an autoimmune blistering skin disease. MTX is an effective and safe drug and provides an excellent treatment option in patients with bullous pemphigoid [28]. Eosonophils are abundant in tissue and blood in patients with bullous pemphigoid and they quickly disappear, without signs of necrosis during MTX therapy. This effect is reflected by diminished expression of the adhesion molecules VCAM-1 and E-selectin in skin and serum. Inhibition of apoptosis plays an important role in autoimmune diseases. MTX therapy induces apoptosis of the tissue eosinophils in bullous pemphigoid [29].

Polymyalgia Rheumatica

In polymyalgia rheumatica, glucocorticoid therapy is the treatment of choice. However, additional immunosuppressive treatment is required when there is resistance to glucocorticoid mono-therapy or when there are complications of glucocorticoid therapy. MTX at 10-15 mg/week is effective in reducing relapse rate and lowering the cumulative dose of glucocorticoid therapy in treatment of polymyalgia rheumatica. MTX may thus be considered as adjunctive therapy to glucocorticoid therapy in glucocorticoid-resistance cases or cases with complications [30].

Refractory Polymyositis

MTX combined with cyclosporine A has been shown to be effective in the treatment of refractory polymyositis, an inflammatory muscle disease [31].

Sarcoidosis

Corticosteroids are often used as the first medication for most patients with sarcoidosis. Several steroid-sparing alternatives have been found effective in treating chronic sarcoidosis. MTX is the most commonly used cytotoxic agent for the treatment of chronic disease [32]. Low dose oral MTX treatment has proven to be effective and safe in children with sarcoidosis and allowed tapering of steroid treatment. [33]

Steroid Dependent Asthma

MTX treatment of patients with steroid dependent asthma, allows a modest reduction in the use of oral corticosteroids. The benefit of treatment with MTX is relatively small and its use should be balanced against the potential for side effects associated with the use of MTX [34].

Ectopic Pregnancy

Use of MTX has revolutionized the treatment of unruptured ectopic pregnancy. MTX a folic acid antagonist inhibits DNA synthesis in actively dividing cells, including trophoblasts. In properly selected patients the success rate of MTX in the treatment of ectopic pregnancy is 94% [35]. The success of MTX treatment depends mainly on β-hCG levels, increasing β-hCG levels are associated with high failure rate. Presence of fetal cardiac activity is also associated with failure of MTX treatment [36]. The overall success rate is greater with multiple-dose MTX therapy than with single-dose therapy (93% v. 88%). Single-dose therapy is however effective for most of the women with ectopic pregnancy. With use of single dose MTX the rate of side effects is low (29% v. 48%). It requires less monitoring and does not require folinic acid rescue treatment [36]. Multiple-dose MTX treatment should be preferably given; when serum β-hCG levels is high (≥ 5000 IU/L) and fetal cardiac activity is present.

Other uses of MTX reported in the literature are prevention of graft versus host disease [37, 38] and primary biliary cirrhosis [39]. MTX has also been found to be useful as a steroid-sparing agent in granulomatous conditions such as idiopathic orbital inflammatory syndrome [40] and xanthogranulomas [41].

Methotrexate Use as Chemotherapeutic Agent

MTX was originally developed as chemotherapeutic agent and continues to be used for chemotherapy either alone or in combination with other agents. MTX is one of the most commonly used chemotherapeutic agents. It is an antimetabolite, and acts to inhibit DNA and RNA synthesis. MTX was first introduced for the treatment for leukemia. Soon afterward it was found that MTX is also effective for the treatment of choriocarcinoma a solid tumor. The drug was then investigated further as a treatment for many other cancers, alone or in combination with other drugs. MTX is approved by the FDA for the treatment of gestational trophoblastic diseases. MTX is also approved as a chemotherapeutic agent alone or in combination with other chemotherapeutic agents to treat acute lymphoblastic leukemia, breast cancer, bladder cancer, stomach cancer, head and neck cancer, lung cancer, advanced non Hodgkins lymphoma, and advanced mycosis fungoides (type of cutaneous T-cell lymphoma) and osteosarcoma. In acute lymphocytic leukemia MTX is used as maintenance therapy in the oral form or for CNS prophylaxis as intrathecal chemotherapy.

Gestational Trophoblastic Disease

Single agent chemotherapeutic treatment with MTX is effective in the treatment of non-metastatic and low risk metastatic gestational trophoblastic neoplasia. Patients with nonmetastatic GTN or metastatic low-risk GTN are treated with single-agent chemotherapy [42-44]. Patients with high-risk metastatic GTN are subdivided into 2 groups: those with a WHO score of less than 7 and those with a score of 7 or higher and who are at high risk of therapy failure. In patients with a WHO score of less than 7, treatment with single-agent chemotherapy (MTX or actinomycin) is highly effective [45]. Patients with WHO score more than 7 require a multiple agent combination chemotherapy, a combination of etoposide, MTX, and actinomycin D in the first week and cyclophosphamide and vincristine (Oncovin) in the second week (EMA-CO regimen) [46].

Adverse Effects

MTX regimes are classified as low-dose, intermediate-dose and high dose. The adverse effects of MTX vary greatly depending on the dose administered and route of administration. IV-administered low-dose MTX (<50 mg/m^2) is used for the treatment of bladder and breast cancer, oral administration is given to patients with T-cell large granular lymphocyte (LGL) leukemia, ALL, acute promyelocytic leukemia, mycosis fungoides as well as a variety of nonmalignant immune-mediated illnesses, such as psoriasis and rheumatoid arthritis [47]. In addition to IV and oral administration, low dose MTX is also given intrathecally for treatment of leptomeningeal metastases or CNS prophylaxis in patients with leukemia or lymphoma. In general low dose therapy commonly used for nonmalignant conditions does not produce life threatening adverse reactions [48]. The adverse effects usually become clinically significant when they result in the early termination of MTX, despite its therapeutic advantages for a particular individual. Intermediate doses of MTX are defined generally between 50 and 500 mg/m^2 and are used primarily for malignant gestational trophoblastic disease (GTD) [49]. High dose MTX (HDMTX) is defined as doses that are greater than 500 mg/m^2. High dose regimens are used for a variety of illnesses, including primary CNS lymphoma and the treatment of osteosarcoma.

With the exception of nephrotoxicity and pulmonary toxicity, most explanations for MTX induced toxicity focus on the depletion of folate stores in normal cells. This theory is supported by the findings that many of these adverse reactions can be alleviated or prevented by the addition of supplemental folic acid. Folinic acid, also known as racemic LV (leucovorin), reduces MTX toxicity, although at doses above 7 mg/week it may also diminish the efficacy of MTX. Folinic acid is reduced folate, produced within the body by reduction of folic acid by DHFR. Since MTX targets DHFR, folinic acid is efficient at rescuing the metabolic block in this pathway [50]. The role of MTX induced folate depletion is also supported by evidence that MTX induced toxicities can be predicted by the baseline folate status at the time of initiation of MTX therapy. Furthermore medications that have the potential for depleting folic acid, such as trimethoprim, have been associated with more serious cases of adverse conditions [51]. In the following discussion the most commonly encountered MTX associated toxicities: hepatoxicity, pulmonary toxicity, myelosuppression, nephrotoxicity and gastrointestinal toxicity are presented.

Hepatoxicity

Hepatoxicity is one of the most serious consequences of MTX treatment. MTX has been shown to induce a variety of changes within liver tissue including steatosis, stellate cell hypertrophy, anisonucleosis and fibrosis. In addition use of MTX has been associated with increases in serum alanine aminotransferase and aspartate amino transferase by 14% and 8% respectively [52]. The mechanism of this toxicity is not completely understood, hepatic folate stores are depleted by MTX and it is believed that this could contribute to cellular stress and cytoxicity. However, direct evidence of a relationship between folate depletion and hepatic toxicity has not yet been obtained. Supplementation with either folic acid or folinic acid has been shown to reduce the frequency of abnormal elevation of serum transaminase levels [53]. In addition to direct damage to hepatocytes MTX may enhance viral damage for patients with concomitant viral hepatitis [54].

Current guidelines for monitoring MTX induced hepatoxicity include liver function testing and measurements of serum alanine aminotransferase, in addition liver biopsies are recommended for patients with other risk factors for hepatotoxicity or consistently abnormal laboratory results. Before initiating MTX treatment patients should have a careful history and physical examination. Alcohol intake, potential exposure to viral hepatitis and any family history of liver disease should be noted. Baseline labs should be taken and attention paid to liver enzymes, serum bilirubin, and serum albumin and, for patients at risk for hepatitis, serological testing for hepatitis B and hepatitis C virus. Pretreatment liver biopsy may be advised for patients with chronic alcohol consumption, hepatitis virus infection or consistently abnormal levels of liver enzymes [55].

Pulmonary Toxicity

Pulmonary toxicity occurs with both low dose and high dose MTX treatment. Acute pneumonitis and pulmonary fibrosis are the most common pulmonary toxicities encountered. However MTX-induced pulmonary conditions can also include nonproductive cough, dyspnea, fever, interstitial pneumonitis, asthma, and bronchiolitis obliterans organizing pneumonia [56]. Pneumonitis is an interstitial pulmonary inflammation and usually occurs within 24-32 weeks of MTX treatment. The chief histological features are diffuse alveolar damage and interstitial mononuclear cellular infiltrates. Diagnosis of pneumonitis is based on type II alveolar proliferation and the presence of lymphocyte, macrophages, B cells and T cells pulmonary infiltrate. The presences of fever, eosinophilia and increased CD4+ T cells and other mononuclear cell infiltration support a hypersensitivity reaction to MTX in pneumonitis. Others believe that the immunosuppressive effects of MTX impair the patient's immune system and thus makes the individual susceptible to latent viral infections which in turn produce the pathological pulmonary inflammation [57]. In either case, MTX-induced pneumonitis stimulates the release of IL-8, a major neutrophil chemotactic factor that stimulates neutrophil influx in the lung. In addition chemoattractant and hematopoietic cytokines such as monocyte chemoattractant protein (MCP-1), G-CSF and GMCSF are secreted by airway epithelial cells. This response is amplified by the release of pro-inflammatory cytokines IL-1β and TNF-α, which induce the production of IL-8 via the p38 MAPK kinase signaling cascade [58].

Pulmonary fibrosis is characterized inflammation, fibroblast proliferation and extracellular matrix remodeling. Current theories for the mechanism of MTX-induced pulmonary fibrosis focus on the role of neutrophils. The neutrophil response appears less than 6 months after taking MTX at a cumulative dose of less than 300 mg. Neutrophils release a number of compounds that stimulate the fibrotic process including hepatocyte growth factor which stimulate type 2 alveolar cells and collagenase-2 (MMP-8) and gelatinase B (MMP-9) that are involved in the extracellular remodeling [59]. In addition the release of free oxygen radicals such as NO and various cytokines such as IL-1beta, TNF-alpha, TNF-beta and TGF-beta could stimulate inflammation and subsequent fibrosis [60].

Myelosuppression

Myelosuppression is a major dose limiting side effect of high dose MTX therapy. This occurs because MTX, like most anticancer drugs, has little selectivity for tumor cells. Toxicity to normal tissue, in particular gastrointestinal tissue and bone marrow, limits the efficacy of the drug. The toxic effect of MTX is exacerbated in patients with impaired renal function, as this increases the concentration of serum MTX. Likewise patients with more frequent dosing (daily instead of weekly) are more prone to myelosuppression. Typically with low dose therapy, as in rheumatoid arthirits, hematologic toxicity in association with macrocytic red bloods may be seen. Higher dose MTX treatment is associated with more serious effects. Leukocytopenia and thrombocytopenia are more common than pancytopenia [61] but pancytopenia can be fatal in up to a quarter of those affected [62].

A therapy to rescue normal cells during treatment with MTX was developed by Goldin. Known as leucovorin (LV) rescue, the strategy is to provide reduced folates to normal cells to bypass the metabolic block produced by MTX. It is not completely understood why LV can rescue normal cells but not malignant cells. It is possible that after MTX treatment folate transport in malignant cells may be diminished more than in normal cells. In this case LV will be preferentially transported into normal cells, where it can compete with MTX for binding sites on DHFR and other enzymes involved in folate metabolism. In this case high concentrations of LV can reactivate the inhibited enzyme and resume production of purine and thymidine [63]. A more likely scenario could be due to cellular differences in polyglutamation. Within the cell LV is able to compete with free MTX but not polyglutamated MTX for binding to DHFR. It has been observed that bone marrow precursors and normal gut epithelium display reduced levels of polyglutamated MTX compared to tumor cells in the same conditions [64]. As a result, LV can more effectively compete against MTX in normal cells, and thus reestablish normal metabolism. It is important to note that LV therapy can only rescue cells that have not sustained extensive DNA damage. Thus LV treatment must be initiated within 24 to 36 hours of high dose MTX therapy in order to be effective [65].

Nephrotoxicity

MTX induced nephrotoxicity is a particularly dangerous adverse effect. Methrotrexate for the most part is excreted by the kidneys, thus with renal dysfunction in addition to the acute damage to renal tubules there is also a delayed elimination of MTX. This leads to a marked elevation in plasma levels of MTX and enhancement of MTX's other toxicities, in particular myelosuppression, mucositis, hepatitis and dermatitis. Renal toxicity occurs in approximately 1.8% of patients receiving high dose MTX therapy [66].

The etiology of MTX-induced renal dysfunction is believed to be due to the precipitation of MTX and its metabolites within the renal tubules. The solubility of MTX is dependent on urine pH, with decreased solubility in acidic pH. MTX metabolites, 7-OH-MTX and DAMPA, are six to tenfold less soluble than MTX. And a pH change from 7.0 to 6.0 leads in a five to eightfold less solubility of MTX and its metabolites. MTX increases this risk of precipitation by reducing the urine flow rate, which concentrates MTX and its metabolites [67]. This chemistry underlies the use of hydration therapy and alkalinization of urine in order to increase MTX solubility, prior to, during and after the administration of HDMTX. In addition LV rescue is also used to reestablish folate metabolism in normal cells despite high levels of plasma MTX.

Patients with MTX-induced renal dysfunction are usually asymptomatic initially, although vomiting and diarrhea during or shortly after the administration of MTX has been observed rarely [68]. By observing urine output, serum creatinine and the plasma MTX concentrations one can monitor renal damage. Plasma MTX concentrations should be less than 1.0 µM 42 hours after the start of HDMTX infusion, and plasma concentrations greater than 10 µM are associated with a high risk for development of serious toxicities [69]. In the absence of adequate monitoring and compensatory treatment for nephrotoxicity, patients will usually present with severe mucositis, profound bone marrow suppression and dermatitis after several days of high dose MTX. At this stage, LV rescue is not effective and damage to cells is largely irreversible, thus there is a small likelihood of relieving MTX toxicities.

Gastrointestinal Toxicity

Similar to MTX induced toxicity in bone marrow, gastrointestinal toxicity is thought to primarily result from folate antagonism in normal cells. These toxicities have been shown to be dose dependent effects; they are compounded by the additional antifolate effects of co-trimoxazole or phenytoin and are possibly alleviated by FA or folinic acid [70]. Gastrointestinal effects include nausea, vomiting, abdominal discomfort, anorexia, weight loss and diarrhea and affect 70% of patients receiving low dose MTX [71]. Sore mouth and oral ulceration can also occur. Ulceration typically appears with two weeks of administration but may also develop very late. After their first appearance lesions are exacerbated by further administration of the drug, but can heal within 3 weeks after MTX discontinuation, possibly once there has been complete cellular clearance of MTX polyglutamates. It is believed that stomatitis is related to concentrations of MTX secreted in saliva that has a topical effect. Serum concentrations do not reliably correlate with saliva concentrations, perhaps explaining why the appearance of stomatitis is fairly unpredictable. The severity of stomatis is also very variable; it can be mild, or painful enough to make eating difficult, and it may persist for days or weeks [72].

It is not clear yet whether folic or folinic acid supplements can prevent or decrease the severity of gastrointestal toxicities. A systematic review in 1998 concluded that folic acid or folinic acid reduced the risk of stomatis and other disorders of the gastrointestinal tract [73]. However a randomized study conducted later found no difference in the proportion of patients developing mucositis or diarrhea [74].

Pharmaceutical Interactions

Many of the adverse effects of MTX treatment arise, or are exacerbated by, interactions between MTX and other medications. These drugs can influence the pharmacokinetics of MTX or its mechanism of action. The excretion pathways of MTX, described earlier, will be expanded on here in order to better understand how particular pharmaceuticals can inhibit clearance of MTX and thus produce toxic results. In particular, it is important to note that the clearance of MTX displays significant variation from one patient to another and so it is crucial to consider each patient individually [75]. A principle half-life of approximately 7.1 hours has been observed for the majority of patients on MTX; however, 17% of patients have a more prolonged elimination half-life of about 26 hours [76]. Renal excretion is the most important method of MTX clearance. On average approximately 80% of MTX and its metabolites are recovered in the urine, but this is also significantly variable ranging from 49% to 96% in patients with rheumatoid arthiritis treated with MTX [77]. The significance of renal excretion for MTX advises against MTX treatment in patients with impaired renal function. In addition because polyglutamation of MTX leads to high tissue distribution, hemodialysis and peritoneal dialysis are not effective methods for removing MTX.

Biliary excretion is responsible for a small but possibly significant portion of MTX excretion. MTX exretion through the bile in a patient with normal renal function could account for 10-30% of total clearance, as measured in several patients. This biliary excretion could provide an alternate and significant mechanism of MTX excretion in patients with severely impaired renal function. In addition it suggests that an interruption of the enterohepatic recirculation may increase MTX elimination [78]. This was verified to an extent by the observation that administration of cholestyramine, a drug that binds bile acids in the gastrointestinal tract and prevents their reabsorption, produced a steep drop in serum MTX levels [79]. Probeneicid, in contrast inhibits both biliary excretion and tubular renal secretion of organic acids, including MTX. After administration of porbenecid and MTX (50-200 mg/m2 intravenously), the serum concentrations of MTX increased by 200-300% at selected time points [80]. Although both cholestyramine and probenecid display significant effects on MTX clearance, further test are needed before the results can be applied clinically.

In addition to probenecid and cholestyramine, penicillin and nonsteriodal anti-inflammatory drugs (NSAIDs) also affect the pharmacokinetic parameters of MTX. The potential sites for NSAIDs and MTX interactions have been proposed to be: a decrease in glomerular filtration of MTX due to a reduction in renal blood flow with inhibition of prostaglandin synthesis, inhibition of MTX tubular secretion and an increase in the unbound fraction of MTX as a result of competition for protein binding sites [81]. MTX and NSAIDs are both organic anions and so it is believed that there could be competition between these two drugs for renal uptake transporters, specifically organic anion transporters OAT1, OAT3, OAT3, and OAT-K1, and reduced folate carrier 1 (RFC-1) [82]. Human organic anion transporter 3 (hOAT3) is expressed in the basolateral membrane of proximal tubule epithelial cells. These cells uptake MTX from the vascular supply via hOAT3, MTX is then secreted by the cells into the proximal tubule lumen. hOAT3 has the highest expression level of the organic anion transporters and it has been shown to be significantly inhibited by NSAIDs such as salicylate and loxoprofen [83].

An important complication is that different NSAIDs produce varying severity of MTX-induced toxicities. Indomethacin and tolmetin have been reported to increase the AUC (area under plasma concentration time curve) of MTX [84]. Etodolac is reported to increase MTX half-life by 38%, although it doesn't produce a change in AUC [85], and ibuprofen may decrease MTX clearance by up to 50% [86]. Overall the appearance of severe adverse effects as a result of NSAID-MTX interactions is rare. But severe complications such as myelosuppression, mucositis, renal dysfunction and CNS toxicity have been reported.

In addition to affecting the pharmacokinetic parameters of MTX, other drugs can also affect the mechanism of MTX either increasing or decreasing MTX activity. Trimethoprim-sulphamethoxazole (TS), trimethoprim and sulphasalazine (SASP) may act as anti-folates and thus when they are administered together with MTX can lead to severe depletion of folate stores in cells [87]. Methotrexate and sulfasalazine have the potential for synergistic toxic effects. Bone marrow suppression, folate depletion and gastrointestinal side effects have been reported with the concomitant use of methotrexate and sulfasalazine [88]. Lastly there has been a well-established interaction between folic acid and MTX. This was described earlier when discussing the cause of many MTX adverse effects and the strategy of LV rescue. Folate supplementation may reduce some of the adverse effects and allow a longer treatment with MTX.

In conclusion, MTX is an antimetabolite and antifolate drug with wide spectrum of clinical usage. In low doses this medication has immunosuppressant and anti-inflammatory effect. In higher doses it is a chemotherapeutic agent for use in certain cancers. The majority of the side effects of this medication are due to folate antagonism. Certain medications have an effect on the pharmacokinetics of MTX and concurrent use of some of these drugs may potentiate the adverse effects of MTX.

References

[1]   Hagner N, Joerger M. Cancer chemotherapy: targeting folic acid synthesis. *Cancer Mang. Res.* 2010; 2:293-301.

[2]   Longley DB, Allen WL, McDermott U, Wilson TR, Latif T, Boyer J, Lynch M, Johnston PG.The roles of thymidylate synthase and p53 in regulating Fas-mediated apoptosis in response to antimetabolites. *Clin. Cancer Res.* 2004; 10:3562-71.

[3]   Wang X, Shen F, Freisheim JH, Gentry LE, Ratnam M. Differential stereospecificities and affinities of folate receptor isoforms for folate compounds and antifolates. *Biochem. Pharmacol.* 1992; 44:1898-1901.

[4]   Qiu A, Jansen M, Sakaris A, Min SH, Chattopadhyay S, Tsai E, Sandoval C, Zhao R, Akabas MH, Goldman ID. Identification of an intestinal folate transporter and the molecular basis for hereditary folate malabsorption. *Cell* 2006; 127:917–28.

[5]   Ross JF, Chaudhuri PK, Ratnam M. Differential regulation of folate receptor isoforms in normal and malignant tissues in vivo and in established cell lines: Physiologic and clinical implications. *Cancer* 1994; 73:2432–43.

[6]   Baggott JE, Vaughn WH, and Hudsonet BB. Inhibition of 5-aminoimidazole-4-carboxamide-ribotide transformylase, adenosine deaminase and 5-adenylate deaminase by polyglutamates of methotrexate and oxidized folates and by 5-aminoimidazole-4-carboxamide-riboside and ribotide. *Biochemical Journal* 1986; 236:193–200.

[7]   Zeng H, Chen ZS, Belinsky MG, Rea PA, Kruh GD. Transport of methotrexate and folates by multidrug resistance protein (MRP) 3 and MRP1: Effect of polyglutamylation on methotrexate transport. *Cancer Research* 2001; 61:7225–32.

[8]   Drori S, Jansen G, Mauritz R, Peters GJ, Assaraf YG. Clustering of mutations in the first transmembrane domain of the human reduced folate carrier in GW1843U89-resistant leukemia cells with impaired antifolate transport and augmented folate uptake. *J. Biol. Chem.* 2000; 275:30855–63.

[9]   Yang R, Qin J, Hoang BH, Healey JH, Gorlick R. Polymorphisms and methylation of the reduced folate carrier in osteosarcoma. *Clin. Orthop. Relat. Res.* 2008; 466:2046–51.

[10]   Shafran A, Ifergan I, Bram E, Jansen G, Kathmann I, Peters GJ, Robey RW, Bates SE, Assaraf YG. ABCG2 harboring the Gly482 mutation confers high-level resistance to various hydrophilic antifolates. *Cancer Res.* 2005; 65:8414–22.

[11]   Assaraf YG. Molecular basis of antifolate resistance. *Cancer Metastasis Rev.* 2007; 26:153-81.

[12]   Bleyer WA. Methotrexate: clinical pharmacology, current status and therapeutic guidelines. *Cancer Treat. Rev.* 1977; 4:87.

[13]   Bannwarth B, Péhourcq F, Schaeverbeke T, Dehais J. Clinical pharmockinetics of low-dose pulse methotrexate in rheumatoid arthiritis. *Clin. Pharmacokinet.* 1996; 30:194-210.

[14]   Jolivet J, Cowan KH, Curt GA, Clendeninn NJ, Chabner BA. The pharmacology and clinical use of methotrexate. *N. Engl. J. Med.* 1983; 309:1094–1104.

[15]   Leeb BF, Smolen JS. Low dose methotrexate therapy in chronic polyarthritis--an update. *Acta Med. Austriaca* 1996; 23:114-9.

[16]   Silverman E, Mouy R, Spiegel L, Jung LK, Saurenmann RK, Lahdenne P et al. Leflunomide or Methotrexate for Juvenile Rheumatoid Arthritis. *N. Engl. J. Med.* 2005; 352:1655-66.

[17]   Giannini EH, Brewer EJ, Kuzmina N, Shaikov A, Maximov A, Vorontsov I, Fink CW, Newman AJ, Cassidy JT, Zemel LS. Methotrexate in resistant juvenile rheumatoid arthritis. Results of the U.S.A.-U.S.S.R. double-blind, placebo-controlled trial. The

Pediatric Rheumatology Collaborative Study Group and The Cooperative Children's Study Group. *N. Engl. J. Med.* 1992; 326:1043-9.

[18]   Kuhn A, Ruland V, Patsinakidis N, Luger TA. Use of methotrexate in patients with psoriasis. *Clin. Exp. Rheumatol.* 2010; Sep-Oct; 28:S138-44.Epub 2010 Nov 2.

[19]   Ceponis A, Kavanaugh A.Use of methotrexate in patients with psoriatic arthritis. *Clin. Exp. Rheumatol.* 2010 Sep-Oct; 28:S132-7.Epub 2010 Oct 28.

[20]   Pigatto PD, Gibelli E, Ranza R, Rossetti A. Methotrexate in psoriatic polyarthritis. *Acta Derm. Venereol. Suppl.* (Stockh) 1994; 186:114-5.

[21]   Binder V, Hendriksen C, Kreiner S. Prognosis in Crohn's disease--based on results from a regional patient group from the county of Copenhagen.*Gut.*1985; 26:146-50.

[22]   Alfadhli AA, McDonald JW, Feagan BG. Methotrexate for induction of remission in refractory Crohn's disease. *Cochrane Database Syst. Rev.* 2005;(1): CD003459.

[23]   Weiss B, Lerner A, Shapiro R, Broide E, Levine A, Fradkin A, Bujanover Y. Methotrexate treatment in pediatric Crohn disease patients intolerant or resistant to purine analogues. *J. Pediatr. Gastroenterol. Nutr.* 2009; 48:526-30.

[24]   De Groot K, Rasmussen N, Bacon PA, Cohen Tervaert JW, Feighery C, Gregorini G, et al. Randomized trial of cyclophosphamide versus methotrexate for induction of remission in early systemic antineutrophil cytoplasmic antibody–associated vasculitis. *Arthritis Rheum.* 2005; 52:2461–9.

[25]   Gold R, Schneider-Gold C. Current and future standards in treatment of myasthenia gravis. *Neurotherapeutics.* 2008; 5:535-41.

[26]   Sathasivam S. Steroids and immunosuppressant drugs in myasthenia gravis. *Nat. Clin. Pract. Neurol.* 2008; 4:317-27.

[27]   Tranchant C. [Therapeutic strategy in myasthenia gravis]. *Rev. neurol.* (Paris) 2009; 165: 149-54.

[28]   Kjellman P, Eriksson H, Berg P. A retrospective analysis of patients with bullous pemphigoid treated with methotrexate. *Arch. Dermatol.* 2008; 144:612-6.

[29]   Dahlman-Ghozlan K, Ortonne J-P, Bahadoran P, Spadafora A, Stephansson E. Low-dose Oral Methotrexate Induces Apoptosis of Tissue Eosinophils in Bullous Pemphigoid. *Acta Derm. Venereol.* 2008; 88:219–22.

[30]   Spies CM, Burmester GR, Buttgereit F. Methotrexate treatment in large vessel vasculitis and polymyalgia rheumatica. *Clin. Exp. Rheumatol.* 2010 Sep-Oct; 28:S172-7. Epub 2010 Oct 28.

[31]   Mitsunaka H, Tokuda M, Hiraishi T, Dobashi H, Takahara J. Combined use of cyclosporine A and methotrexate in refractory polymyositis. *Scand. J. Rheumatol.* 2000; 29:192-4.

[32]   Baughman RP, Costabel U, du Bois RM. Treatment of sarcoidosis. *Clin. Chest Med.* 2008; 29:533-48.

[33]   Gedalia A, Molina JF, Ellis GS Jr, Galen W, Moore C, Espinoza LR. Low-dose methotrexate therapy for childhood sarcoidosis. *J. Pediatr.* 1997; 130:25-9.

[34]   Aaron SD, Dales RE, and Pham B. Management of steroid-dependent asthma with methotrexate: a meta-analysis of randomized clinical trials. *Respir. Med.* 1998; 92:1059-65.

[35]   Yao M, Tulandi T. Current status of surgical and nonsurgical management of ectopic pregnancy. *Fertil. Steril.* 1997; 67:421-33. Comment in Fertil Steril 1997; 68:945-7.

[36] Barnhart KT, Gosman G, Ashby R, Sammel M. The medical management of ectopic pregnancy: a meta-analysis comparing "single dose" and "multidose" regimens. *Obstet. Gynecol.* 2003; 101:778-84.

[37] Mori T, Aisa Y, Nakazato T, Yamazaki R, Shimizu T, Mihara A, et al. Tacrolimus and methotrexate for the prophylaxis of graft-versus-host disease after unrelated donor cord blood transplantation for adult patients with hematologic malignancies. *Transplant. Proc.* 2007; 39:1615-9.

[38] Nishida T, Murayama T, Hirai H, Okamoto S, Sao H, Hara M, et al. Phase II study of tacrolimus and methotrexate for prophylaxis of acute graft-versus-host disease after HLA-A, B, and DRB1 genotypically mismatched unrelated bone marrow transplantation among Japanese patients. *Int. J. Hematol.* 2009; 89:98-105.

[39] Sorda J, Findor J. Methotrexate therapy in primary biliary cirrhosis. *Acta Gastroenterol. Latinoam.* 2000; 30:221-5.

[40] Swamy BN, McCluskey P, Nemet A, Crouch R, Martin P, Benger R, et al. Idiopathic orbital inflammatory syndrome: clinical features and treatment outcomes. *Br. J. Ophthalmol.* 2007; 91:1667-70.

[41] Hayden A, Wilson DJ, Rosenbaum JT. Management of orbital xanthogranuloma with methotrexate. *Br. J. Ophthalmol.* 2007; 91:434-6.

[42] Soper JT, Clarke-Pearson DL, Berchuck A, Rodriguez G, Hammond CB. 5-day methotrexate for women with metastatic gestational trophoblastic disease. *Gynecol. Oncol.* Jul 1994; 54:76-9.

[43] Foulmann K, Guastalla JP, Caminet N, Trillet-Lenoir V, Raudrant D, Golfier F et al. What is the best protocol of single-agent methotrexate chemotherapy in nonmetastatic or low-risk metastatic gestational trophoblastic tumors? A review of the evidence. *Gynecol. Oncol.* Jul 2006; 102:103-10.

[44] Roberts JP, Lurain JR. Treatment of low-risk metastatic gestational trophoblastic tumors with single-agent chemotherapy. *Am. J. Obstet. Gynecol.* Jun 1996; 174:1917-23; discussion 1923-4.

[45] Ngan HY, Odicino F, Maisonneuve P, Creasman WT, Beller U, Quinn MA, et al. Gestational trophoblastic neoplasia. FIGO 6th Annual Report on the Results of Treatment in Gynecological Cancer. *Int. J. Gynaecol. Obstet.* Nov 2006; 95 Suppl 1:S193-203.

[46] Escobar PF, Lurain JR, Singh DK, Bozorgi K, Fishman DA. Treatment of high-risk gestational trophoblastic neoplasia with etoposide, methotrexate, actinomycin D, cyclophosphamide, and vincristine chemotherapy. *Gynecol. Oncol.* Dec 2003; 91:552-7.

[47] Dubertret L. Retinoids, methotrexate and cyclosporine. Curr Probl Dermatol. 2009; 38:79-94.

[48] [Pincus T. Furer V, Sokka T. Underestimation of the efficacy, effectiveness, tolerability, and safety of weekly low-dose methotrexate in information presented to physicians and patients. *Clin. Exp. Rheumatol.* 2010; 28:S68-S79.

[49] Foulmann K, Guastalla JP, Caminet N, Trillet-Lenoir V, Raudrant D, Golfier F, et al. What is the best protocol of single-agent methotrexate chemotherapy in nonmetastatic or low-risk metastatic gestational trophoblastic tumors? A review of the evidence. Gynecol. Oncol. 2006; 102:103-10.

[50] Shiroky JB, Neville C, Esdaile JM, Choquette D, Zummer M, Hazeltine M et al. Low-dose methotrexate with LV (folinic acid) in the management of rheumatoid arthritis. Results of a multicenter randomized, double-blind, placebo-controlled trial. *Arthritis Rheum.* 1993; 36:795-803.

[51] Govert, J. Patton S, Fine RL. Pancytopenia from using trimethoprim and methotrexate. *Ann. Intern. Med.* 1992; 117: 877-78.

[52] Berkowitz RS, Goldstein DP, Bernstein MR Ten year's experience with methotrexate and folinic acid as primary therapy for gestational trophoblastic disease. *Gynecol. Oncol.* 1986; 23:111-8.

[53] Prey S, Paul C. Effect of folic or folinic acid supplementation on methotrexate-associated safety and efficacy in inflammatory disease: a systematic review. *Br. J. Dermatol.* 2009; 160:622-8.

[54] Kawatani T, Suou T, Tajima F, Ishiga K, Omura H, Endo A et al. Incidence of hepatitis virus infection and severe liver dysfunction in patients receiving chemotherapy for hematologic malignancies. *Eur. J. Haematol.* 2001; 67:45-50.

[55] Kremer JM, Alarcon GS, Lightfoot RW, Willkens RF, Furst DE, Williams HJ, et al. Methotrexatefor rheumatoid arthritis. Suggested guidelines for monitoring liver toxicity. American College of Rheumatology. *Arthritis Rheum.* 1994; 37:316-28.

[56] Hsu P, Lan JL, Hsieh TY, Jan YJ, Huang WN. Methotrexate pneumonitis in a patient with rheumatoid arthritis. *J. Microbiol. Immunol. Infect.* 2003; 36:137-40.

[57] Mornex JF, Cordier G, Pages J, Vergnon JM, Lefebvre R, Brune J et al. Activated lung lymphocytes in hypersensitivity pneumonitis. *J. Allergy Clin. Immunol.* 1984;74:719-27.

[58] KimYJ, Song M, Ryu JC. Inflammation in methotrexate-induced pulmonary toxicity occurs via the p38 MAPK pathway. *Toxicology* 2009; 256:183-90.

[59] Fujimori Y, Kataoka M, Tada S, Takehara H, Matsuo K, Miyake T, et al. The role of Interleukin-8 in interstitial pneumonia. *Respirology* 2003; 8:33-40.

[60] RobbinsRA, Jinkins PA, Bryan TW, Prado SC, Milligan SA. Methotrexate inhibition of inducible nitric oxide synthase in murine lung epithelial cells in vitro. *Am. J. Respir. Cell Mol. Biol.* 1998; 18:853-59.

[61] Schnabel A, Gross W. Low-dose methotrexate in rheumatic diseases—efficacy, side effects, and risk factors for side effects, *Semin. Arthritis Rheum.* 1994; 5:310–27.

[62] Berthelot JM, Maugars Y, Hamidou M, Chiffoleau A, Barrier J, Grolleau JY, et al. Pancytopenia and severe cytopenia induced by low-dose methotrexate. Eight case-reports and a review of one hundred cases from the literature (with twenty-four deaths), *Rev. Rhum. Engl. Ed.* 1995; 62:477–86.

[63] Kamen B. Folate and antifolate pharmacology. *Semin. Oncol.* 1997; 24: S18-30-S18-39.

[64] Matherly LH, Barlowe CK, Goldman ID. Antifolate polyglutamylation and competitive drug displacement at dihydrofolate reductase as important elements in LV rescue in L1210 cells. *Cancer Res.* 1986; 46:588-93.

[65] Ackland SP, Schilsky RL. High-dose methotrexate: a critical reappraisal. *J. Clin. Oncol.* 1987; 5:2017-31.

[66] Abelson HT, Fosburg MT, Beardsley GP, Goorin AM, Gorka C, Link M, et al. Methotrexate-induced renal impairment: clinical studies and rescue from systemic toxicity with high-dose LV and thymidine. *J. Clin. Oncol.* 1983;1:208–16.

[67] Widemann BC, Adamson PC. Understanding and managing methotrexate nephrotoxicity. *Oncologist* 2006;11:694-703.

[68] Relling MV, Fairclough D, Ayers D, Crom WR, Rodman JH, Pui CH, et al. Patient characteristics associated with high-risk methotrexate concentrations and toxicity. *J. Clin. Oncol.* 1994;12:1667–72.

[69] BleyerWA. Methotrexate clinical pharmacology, current status and therapeutic guidelines. *Cancer Treat Rev.* 1977; 4:87–101.

[70] Alarcon G. Methotrexate: its use for the treatment of rheumatoid arthritis and other rheumatic disorders. In: W. Koopman, Editor, Arthritis and allied conditions. A textbook of rheumatology (13th ed.), Williams and Wilkins, London 1997, p 679–698.

[71] McKendry RJ. The remarkable spectrum of methotrexate toxicities, *Rheum. Dis. Clin. North Am.* 1997; 4:939–54.

[72] Kalantzis A, Marshman Z, Falconer DT, Morgan PR, Odell EW. Oral effects of low-dose methotrexate treatment. *Oral Surgery, Oral Medicine, Oral Pathology, Oral Radiology, and Endontology* 2005;100:52-62.

[73] *Ortiz Z, Shea B, Suarez-Almazor ME, Moher D, Wells GA, Tugwell P.* The efficacy of folic acid and folinic acid in reducing methotrexate induced gastrointestinal toxicity in rheumatoid arthritis. A metaanalysis of randomized controlled trials. *J. Rheumatol.* 1998; 25:36-43.

[74] Van Ede AE, Laan RF, Rood MJ, Huizinga TW, Van De Laar MA, Van Denderen CJ et al. Effect of folic or folinic acid supplementation on the toxicity and efficacy of methotrexate in rheumatoid arthritis: a forty-eight week, multicenter, randomized, double-blind, placebo-controlled study. *Arthritis Rheum.* 2001; 44:1515-24.

[75] *Edelman J,* Biggs DF, JamaliF, Russell AS. Low-dose methotrexate kinetics in arthritis. *Clin. Pharmacol. Ther.* 1984; 35:382-6.

[76] *Herman* RA, Van Pedersen P, Hoffman J, Furst DE. *Pharmacokinetics of low dose methotrexate in rheumatoid arthritis patients. J. Pharm. Sci. 1989; 78:165-71.*

[77] Hendel J, Nyfors A. Nonlinear renal elimination kinetics of methotrexate due to saturation of renal tubular reabsorption. *Eur. J. Clin. Pharmacol.* 1984; 6:121-4.

[78] Hendel J, Brodthagen H. Enterohepatic cycling of methotrexate estimated by the use of the D-isomer as a reference marker. *Eur. J. Clin. Pharmacol.* 1984; 26:103-7.

[79] Ertmann R, Landbeck G. Effect of oral cholestyramine on elimination of high-dose methotrexate. *J. Cancer Res. Oncol.* 1985; 110:48-50.

[80] Lilly MB, Omura GA. Clinical pharmacology of oral intermediate-dose methotrexate with or without probenecid. *Cancer Chemo. Pharmacol.* 1985; 15:220-2.

[81] Frenia ML, Long KS. Methotrexate and nonsteroidal anti-inflammatory drug interactions. *Ann. Pharmacother.* 1992;26:234-7.

[82] Cha SH, Sekine T, Fukushima JI, Kanai Y, Kobayashi Y, Goya T, Endou H. Identification and characterization of human organic anion transporter 3 expressing predominantly in the kidney. *Mol. Pharmacol.* 2001; 59:1277–86.

[83] Tracy TS, Krohn K, Jones DR, Bradley JD, Hall SD, Brater DC. The effects of salicylate, ibuprofen, and naproxen on the disposition of methotrexate in patients with rheumatoid arthritis. *Eur. J. Clin. Pharmacol.* 1992; 42:121-5.

[84] Ellison NM, Servi RJ. Acute renal failure and sudden death following sequential intermediate-dose methotrexate and 5-FU:a possible adverse effect due to concomitant indomethacin administration. *Cancer Treat. Rep.* 1985;69:342–43.

[85] Anaya JM, Fabre D, Bressolle F, Bologna C, Alric R, Cocciglio M, Dropsy R, Sany J. Effect of etodolac on methotrexate pharmacokinetics in patients with rheumatoid arthritis. J. Rheumatol. 1994; 21:203-8.

[86] Johnson AG, Seidemann P, Day RO. NSAID-related adverse drug interactions with clinical relevance. An update. *Int. J. Clin. Pharmacol. Ther.* 1994; 32:509-32.

[87] Ng HW, Macfarlane AW, Graham RM, Verbov JL. Near fatal drug interactions with methotrexate given for psoriasis (letter). *Br. Med. J.* 1987; 295:752-3.

[88] Morgan SL, Baggott JE, Alarcon GS. Methotrexate and sulfasalazine combination therapy: is it worth the risk? *Arthritis Rheum.* 1993; 36:281-2.

In: Methotrexate
Editors: V. S. Castillo and L. A. Moyano

ISBN: 978-1-62100-596-4
© 2012 Nova Science Publishers, Inc.

Chapter V

Low Dose Methotrexate: Pharmacology, Clinical Uses and Adverse Effects[*]

A. N. Patel,[1] D. P. Hawley[2,†] and S. Rangaraj[1]

[1]Nottingham University Hospitals NHS Trust, Derby Road,
Nottingham, United Kingdom
[2]Sheffield Children's NHS Foundation Trust, Western Bank,
Sheffield, United Kingdom

Abstract

In the late 1940's methotrexate was developed for use primarily in haematological malignancies. Used at much lower doses, it has subsequently become an established treatment for a range of autoimmune conditions including: rheumatoid arthritis [1], psoriasis and psoriatic arthropathy [2], Crohn's disease [3], connective tissue disease [4] and Felty's syndrome [5].

Methotrexate is a structural analogue of folic acid. It competitively inhibits binding of dihydrofolic acid to the enzyme dihydrofolate reductase. The amount of intracellular folinic acid (the active metabolite of dihydrofolic acid) is thereby decreased, and intracellular metabolic pathways dependent on folinic acid affected. Purine and pyrimadine metabolism are two such pathways. Whilst these pathways are considered important, the exact mechanism of action by which methotrexate exerts clinical effect remains elusive [6].

[*] All authors had: (1) No financial support for the submitted work from anyone other than their employer; (2) No financial relationships with commercial entities that might have an interest in the submitted work; (3) No spouses, partners, or children with relationships with commercial entities that might have an interest in the submitted work; (4) No Non-financial interests that may be relevant to the submitted work."

[†] Corresponding author: Dr Daniel P Hawley BMBS, BmedSci, MRCPCH. E-mail: dhawley@doctors.org.uk.
The Corresponding Author has the right to grant on behalf of all authors and does grant on behalf of all authors, an exclusive licence, to permit this article (if accepted) to be published.

Low dose methotrexate has been shown to cause aplastic marrow failure [7], pulmonary fibrosis [8] and liver toxicity, including cirrhosis [9]. Hence strict monitoring and review becomes necessary. In 1982, the dermatology community released guidelines recommending regular liver biopsy once a critical cumulative dose (1.5g) was reached [10]. These guidelines were initially applied to patients with rheumatoid arthritis treated with low dose methotrexate [11]. Subsequent research revealed a good correlation between liver enzymes and histological changes on liver biopsy, and regular blood test monitoring has since been widely practiced as a screening tool for early liver disease [12, 13]. Low dose methotrexate can also cause nausea and vomiting and a significant minority of patients become intolerant due to these troublesome adverse effects.

Methotrexate is contraindicated in certain situations namely pregnancy, localised or systemic infection, renal impairment and unexplained cytopenia associated with marrow failure. Several drug interactions are also associated with its use.

Despite these problems, methotrexate has remained the first line agent in many diseases for many years. It is generally well tolerated and displays good efficacy.

We provide an overview of the use of low dose methotrexate in autoimmune conditions with respect to pharmacology, clinical uses, adverse effects and monitoring schedules.

References

[1] Kremer JM. Historical overview of the treatment of Rheumatoid arthritis with an emphasis on methotrexate. *J. Rheumatol.* 1996;23(Suppl 44):34–7.

[2] Saporito FC, Menter MA. Methotrexate and psoriasis in the era of new biologic agents. *J. Am. Acad. Dermatol.* 2004;50:301–9.

[3] Feagan BG, Rochon J, Fedorak RN et al. Methotrexate for the treatment of Crohn's disease. *N. Engl. J. Med.* 1995;332:292–7.

[4] Williams HC, Pembroke AC. Methotrexate in the treatment of vasculitic cutaneous ulcerations in rheumatoid arthritis. *J. R. Soc. Med.* 1989;82:763.

[5] Wassenberg S, Herborn G, Rau R. Methotrexate treatment in Felty's syndrome. *Br. J. Rheumatol.* 1998;37:908–11.

[6] Rajagopalan, P. T. Ravi; Zhang, Zhiquan; McCourt, Lynn; Dwyer, Mary; Benkovic, Stephen J.; Hammes, Gordon G. (2002). "Interaction of dihydrofolate reductase with methotrexate: Ensemble and single-molecule kinetics". *Proceedings of the National Academy of Sciences* 99 (21): 13481–6.

[7] Gutierrez-Ureña S, Molina JF, García CO, Cuéllar ML, Espinoza LR. Pancytopenia secondary to methotrexate therapy in rheumatoid arthritis. *Arthritis Rheum.* 1996;39(2): 272-6.

[8] Lateef O, Shakoor N, Balk RA. Methotrexate pulmonary toxicity. *Expert Opin. Drug Saf.* 2005 Jul;4(4):723-30.

[9] Roenigk HH Jr, Auerbach R, Maibach HI, Weinstein GD. Methotrexate guidelines: Revised. *J. Am. Acad. Dermatol.* 1982;6(2):145-55.

[10] Furst DE, Kremer JM. Methotrexate in rheumatoid arthritis. *Arthritis Rheum.* 1988; 31(3):305-14.

[11] Kremer JM, Kaye GI, Kaye NW, Ishak KG, Axiotis CA. Light and electron microscopic analysis of sequential liver biopsy samples from rheumatoid arthritis patients receiving long-term methotrexate therapy. Follow up over long treatment

intervals and correlation with clinical and laboratory variables. *Arthritis Rheum.* 1995; 38(9):1194-203.

[12] Kremer JM, Furst DE, Weinblatt ME, Blotner SD. Significant changes in serum AST across hepatic histological biopsy grades: prospective analysis of 3 cohorts receiving methotrexate therapy for rheumatoid arthritis. *J. Rheumatol.* 1996;23(3):459-61.

[13] Chalmers RJG, Kirby B, Smith A et al. Replacement of routine liver biopsy by procollagen III aminopeptide for monitoring patients with psoriasis receiving long-term methotrexate: a multicentre audit and health economic analysis. *Br. J. Dermatol.* 2005; 152:444–50.

Introduction

Methotrexate has been used since the late 1940's [1] It was previously known as amethopterin and is an antimetabolite and antifolate drug used in the treatment of inflammatory conditions as well as cancer, autoimmune conditions and medical abortions. Methotrexate was initially developed as an anti-cancer drug (for haematological malignancies) and received Food and Drug Administration (FDA) approval in 1953. It was first used to treat rheumatoid arthritis (RA) in 1951 [2]. Soon afterward it was noted that methotrexate effectively controlled psoriasis and in 1967 an abstract was published in Archives of Dermatology explaining its efficacy [3]. By 1971 methotrexate had received FDA approval for psoriasis. Methotrexate became widely used in the British Isles during the 1990s, when its beneficial role in Crohn's disease was also documented, following trials confirming efficacy over placebo and acceptable side effect profile [4]. Although not licensed for use in childhood its use is based on evidence from clinical trials and it is currently accepted in specialist practice as the first line systemic medication for juvenile idiopathic arthritis (JIA) [5] and psoriasis [6]. Methotrexate is effective in remission induction and maintenance in steroid-dependent Crohn's disease (CD), but is often considered to be a second-line immunosuppressive agent, to be used in cases of failure or intolerance to azathioprine (AZA) or 6-mercaptopurine (6-MP) [7].

It is essential that disease modifying anti-rheumatic drugs (DMARDs) are used in appropriate doses to achieve an optimal balance between benefit and risk. Methotrexate is known to cause aplastic marrow failure [8], pulmonary fibrosis [9] and liver toxicity, including cirrhosis [10]. In 1982 the dermatology community released guidelines suggesting regular liver biopsy once a critical cumulative dose (1.5g) of methotrexate was reached [10]. These guidelines were also initially applied to patients with RA treated with low dose methotrexate [11]. Subsequent research found a good correlation between elevation of liver enzymes and histological changes on liver biopsy, and regular blood test monitoring has since been widely practiced as a screening tool for early liver disease, avoiding the need for regular biopsy [12, 13].

Various monitoring guidelines have evolved over the past three decades. The American College of Rheumatology (ACR) published guidelines in 1994 when there was relatively little experience using methotrexate [14]. These guidelines were developed primarily for adult use, but were also widely used by paediatric rheumatologists. The British Society for Rheumatology (BSR) have also published guidelines [15] and more recently the British

Society for Paediatric and Adolescent Rheumatology (BSPAR) published specific paediatric guidelines in 2005 [5]. Anecdotal evidence suggests hospitals in the British Isles use local practice guidelines which are often adaptations of BSPAR, BSR, British Association of Dermatologists (BAD) or British Society of Gastroenterology (BSG) guidelines.

- BSR/BHPR guideline for disease modifying anti-rheumatic drug (DMARD) therapy in consultation with the British Association of Dermatologists 2008 [15]
- British Society for Paediatric and Adolescent Rheumatology (BSPAR)-Methotrexate use in Paediatric Rheumatology 2005 and 2010 [5, 16]
- Guidelines for the management of Inflammatory Bowel Disease in adults by the British Association of Gastroenterology 2010 [17]
- British Society for Rheumatology. National guidelines for the monitoring of second line drugs [18].

Currently there is varying opinion and practice regarding use and monitoring of low-dose methotrexate, which is at least partly explained by the relative paucity of evidence on which current guidelines are based.

The doses of methotrexate used in dermatology, rheumatology and gastroenterology are classed as 'low', reaching a maximum of 25mg per week. Doses used in the field of oncology can reach levels up to 2.5mg/kg daily, almost 100 times the doses used for RA, psoriasis, and inflammatory bowel disease (IBD). The high-dose use of methotrexate in oncology is beyond the scope of this book chapter.

Pharmacology

Folate antagonists were among the first anti-neoplastic agents to be developed. In 1948, aminopterin was used to induce remission in childhood acute lymphoblastic leukaemia (ALL), and the related agent methotrexate is still an important component of current treatment for ALL and a number of other hematologic malignancies [19]. Methotrexate was the first drug shown to cure a cancer when given as monotherapy, and as a single agent remains a cornerstone of treatment for malignant gestational trophoblastic disease [20]. The use of methotrexate in oncology patients who also had RA led to the discovery that methotrexate improves arthritis symptoms. Subsequent work revealed that the beneficial effects of methotrexate in treating arthritis could be gained using doses far lower than those used when treating cancer. The precise immunosuppressive actions of methotrexate are not fully understood however many proposed mechanisms exist:

- Methotrexate competitively inhibits dihydrofolate reductase (DHFR) - an enzyme involved in tetrahydrofolate synthesis [21].The affinity of methotrexate for DHFR is about one thousand-fold that of folate. DHFR catalyses the conversion of dihydrofolate to the active tetrahydrofolate. Folic acid is needed for the de novo synthesis of the nucleoside thymidine, in turn required for deoxyribonucleic acid (DNA), as well as for purine base synthesis. Methotrexate, therefore, inhibits the synthesis of DNA, Ribonucleic acid (RNA), thymidylates, and proteins.

- The structures of folic acid and methotrexate are similar, explaining how methotrexate acts as a competitive inhibitor. Methotrexate acts specifically during DNA and RNA synthesis, and thus it is cytotoxic during the S-phase of the cell cycle. The S phase starts when DNA synthesis commences; when it is complete, all of the chromosomes have been replicated. Thus, during this phase, the amount of DNA in the cell has effectively doubled. Rates of RNA transcription and protein synthesis are very low during this phase [22]. Methotrexate therefore has a greater toxic effect on rapidly dividing cells which replicate their DNA more frequently, thus inhibiting the growth and proliferation of these non-cancerous cells as well as causing the side effects listed below.

- In the use of methotrexate in RA, psoriasis and IBD the inhibition of DHFR is not thought to be the main mechanism, but rather the inhibition of enzymes involved in purine metabolism, leading to accumulation of adenosine, or the inhibition of T cell activation and suppression of intercellular adhesion [1].

- Methotrexate has also been found to reduce spontaneous and IL-15-induced tumour necrosis factor (TNF) production by splenic T-cells but not by macrophages from healthy mice in vitro in a dose-dependent manner [1]. In contrast, interferon-gamma (IFN-gamma) production was less strikingly reduced and IL-4 production was virtually unaffected.

The role of TNF in methotrexate-mediated effects on cytokine production was further underlined by the finding that methotrexate effects on IFN-gamma production were augmented in TNF-transgenic mice but abolished in mice in which the TNF-alpha gene had been inactivated (by homologous recombination). Thus, methotrexate specifically modulates spontaneous and IL-15-induced TNF-alpha production in mice. These data suggest that TNF production by T cells is an important target of methotrexate and may serve as a basis to understand and further analyse methotrexate-mediated mechanisms of immunosuppression in patients with RA [23].

Pharmacokinetics

Methotrexate is a weak acid (pKa ranges between 4.8 and 5.5), and thus it is mostly ionised at physiologic pH. It can be administered either orally or by injection (subcutaneous, intravenous or intramuscular). Oral absorption is saturable and therefore dose-dependent, with doses less than $40mg/m^2$ having 42% bioavailability and doses greater than $40mg/m^2$ only 18%. On a graph of bioavailability against dose, bioavailability drops off towards the upper end of the therapeutic window. Mean oral bioavailability is 33% (13-76% range), and there is no clear benefit to subdividing an oral dose. The non-oral routes of administration are not subject to this dose-dependent drop in bioavailability, and therefore may be preferable, particularly at higher doses.

Methotrexate is metabolised by intestinal bacteria to the inactive metabolite 4-amino-4-deoxy-N-methylpteroic acid which accounts for less than 5% loss of the oral dose.

Factors that decrease absorption include food, oral non-absorbable antibiotics (e.g. vancomycin, neomycin, and bacitracin) and more rapid transit through the gastrointestinal tract (GI) (eg. diarrhoea). Slower transit time in the GI tract (eg. constipation) increases absorption. Methotrexate can also be used for termination of pregnancy. It is administered into the placenta accreta, inhibiting the blood circulation to the target site [1].

Clinical Uses

Methotrexate has a relatively slow onset, taking weeks to months to produce a clinical response (typically two to three months) [15]. Patients need to be informed about the delayed action to aid compliance.

Licensed (UK) uses: RA [24] and psoriasis.

Unlicensed uses: Psoriatic arthritis [25], Crohn's disease [26], connective tissue disease [27], Felty's syndrome [28].

Dermatology

Systemic treatment of psoriasis with methotrexate was noted to be efficacious shortly after methotrexate gained FDA approval for cancer treatment in 1953. By the 1970's FDA approval was gained for treatment of psoriasis [29] and to this day remains first line systemic treatment in Europe for patients who cannot be controlled via topical agents or phototherapy.

Despite accumulating experience using methotrexate in dermatological conditions, controversy remains regarding optimal route of administration (subcutaneous vs oral), initial dosing, escalation to therapeutic doses, the role of folic acid supplementation and monitoring for toxicity.

These controversies remain largely due to a paucity of published data concerning methotrexate use in psoriasis. There are no published studies comparing different routes of administration of methotrexate in psoriasis. A recent systematic review of the literature [30] showed that clinical outcome in psoriasis appears to be dose dependant. In fact the primary end point, Psoriasis Area Severity Index 75% (PASI 75) response was achieved in 60% with a starting dose of 15mg/wk.

Patients start methotrexate orally at a dose of 5-10mg/week [15] and thereafter rapidly increase the dose (by 2.5-5mg) over four weeks up to a therapeutic target of 15-25mg/week depending on the condition. The maximum licensed dose is 25mg/week. If this dose is not effective, a non-oral route of administration should be considered. Lower doses should be considered for frail elderly patients with co-morbidities. A folic acid supplement is recommended based on expert evaluation at a dose of 5mg/day for one to three days starting 48 hours after methotrexate [31, 32, 33]. It should not be given on the same day as the methotrexate as this may reduce the anti-psoriatic effect of methotrexate [31].

Initial treatment should ideally be administered via the oral route. If there is not sufficient efficacy, or in case of poor absorption or GI intolerance, the subcutaneous or intramuscular route should be considered. If there is poor compliance then methotrexate can be administered parenterally [34].

Procollagen III peptide (PIIINP) testing is the gold standard guide to monitor for hepatic fibrosis. This should be tested at initiation and then every three to six months. Due to the excellent negative predicted value of this test liver biopsies can be deferred whilst procollagen III remains within normal limits [35, 36].

Methotrexate should be avoided in pregnancy, breast feeding, suspected local or systemic infection, bone marrow failure with unexplained anaemia and cytopenia and pre-existing liver disease.

Monitoring of methotrexate varies between different specialities. These differences are largely due to consensus-based opinion within the speciality.

Monitoring as per BAD [15] *(See Adverse Events)*

Pre-treatment assessment: Full Blood Count (FBC), Urea and Electrolytes (UandE), Liver Function Test (LFT), PIIINP and Chest X-Ray (CXR) (unless pre-existing CXR less than six months old). Lung function testing should be considered for selected patients.

White Blood Cells (WBC)<3.5×10^9/l	Withhold until discussed with specialist team.
Neutrophils<2.0×10^9/l	Withhold until discussed with specialist team.
Platelets<150×10^9/l	Withhold until discussed with specialist team.
Aspartate transaminase (AST), Alanine aminotransferase (ALT)>twice upper limit of reference range	Withhold until discussed with specialist team.
Albumin-unexplained fall (in absence of active disease)	Withhold until discussed with specialist team.
Rash or oral ulceration, nausea and vomiting, diarrhoea	Withhold until discussed with specialist team.
New or increasing dyspnoea or dry cough	Withhold until discussed with specialist team.
Mean Cell Volume (MCV)>105 fl	Withhold and check serum B12, Folate and TFT and discuss with specialist team if necessary
Mild to moderate renal Impairment	Withhold until discussed with specialist team
Severe sore throat abnormal bruising	Immediate FBC and withhold until the result of FBC is available

Monitoring: FBC, UandE, and LFT every week is considered essential to identify induced marrow failure, renal failure and hepatotoxicity. Gradually an increase in the interval between tests can be achieved, after which serological tests can be undertaken every two to three months. PIIINP testing can be undertaken every three to six months.

In suspected cases of methotrexate overdose, severe haematological toxicity, pre-renal or acute renal failure, consider treatment with folinic acid:

(a) Withold methotrexate.
(b) Give folinic acid rescue therapy:
(c) Consider immediate discussion with supervising specialist/team, medical on-call team or the local haematologist.

The initial dose of folinic acid should be at least 20mg, given intravenously. Subsequent doses of 15mg (which may be taken orally) should be given at six hourly intervals until the haematological abnormalities are improved (usually not more than two to eight doses).

Rheumatology

In the field of rheumatology methotrexate is used widely as a first-line DMARD for conditions including: RA, psoriatic arthropathy, JIA, connective tissue disorders and vasculitic disorders.

In adults, typical doses of methotrexate used range between 7.5-25mg once weekly. The starting dose may vary depending on the severity of disease and individual patient characteristics (eg. age, kidney function, other co-morbidities). The initial dose may be between 5-10mg once weekly, increasing by 2.5-5mg every two to six weeks until disease has stabilised [15, 37]. The maximum licensed dose in RA is 25mg per week. Lower doses should be used in frail elderly patients with poor renal function [15]. Although methotrexate is not licensed for use in children there is good evidence for its efficacy in various paediatric rheumatological conditions including JIA for which it is the first line DMARD. Methotrexate is usually started at a dose of 10-15mg once weekly in the paediatric population. Evidence for efficacy of doses of methotrexate above 25mg is lacking [38].

Formulation consists of 2.5mg and 10mg tablets, syrup and an injectable (subcutaneous, intravenous or intramuscular) liquid. It is good practice to prescribe single tablet strength to avoid patient confusion [39]. 10mg tablets are sometimes not available from community pharmacies following National Patient Safety Agency recommendations [16]. The oral suspension exists in varying concentrations predominantly for the paediatric population. If maximum oral dose is not effective or causes intolerance then alternate routes of administration (in particular subcutaneous injection) can be trialled. Whilst an intramuscular preparation is available, this route is much less preferable as it causes more discomfort with no added benefit in efficacy. A large study has shown the subcutaneous route of administration more clinically efficacious than the oral route in RA [34]. Prescribed dose does not vary according to route of administration although consideration should be given to the differences in bioavailability.

Folic acid may be given in combination with methotrexate. Folate is important as it reduces toxic effects of methotrexate in the GI tract and potentially improves continuation of therapy and compliance [40, 41]. There is little evidence regarding how folic acid should be given, however avoiding administration on the same day as methotrexate is thought to decrease GI intolerance and hepatotoxicity. The supplementing of folic acid in patients undergoing methotrexate treatment aims to give cells dividing less rapidly enough folate to maintain normal cell functions [40].

Whilst there is evidence for the use of folic acid to ameliorate adverse effects of methotrexate in adults, there is no supporting evidence for the paediatric population. Folic acid may be given, either when initiating methotrexate treatment, or in response to adverse effects (e.g. nausea, mouth ulcers). The usual dose is 5mg orally weekly (given on a different day to the weekly methotrexate dose) or 1mg orally daily [16].

It is recognised as good clinical practice that patients and carers receive comprehensive teaching about treatment with methotrexate including contra-indications, risks and side-effects. For home administration of subcutaneous methotrexate, a training plan ensuring clear understanding of the associated process and responsibilities is necessary. In the paediatric population a robust, risk-assessed system in which the paediatric rheumatology specialist nurse plays a key role is required to fulfil these requirements [42].

Monitoring as per BSR [15] *(See Adverse Events)*

Pre-treatment assessment: FBC, UandE, LFT and CXR (unless CXR performed within last six months)

Monitoring: FBC, UandE, LFT every two weeks, until the dose of methotrexate and monitoring results are stable for six weeks, after which monthly blood tests can be implemented [43] until the dose and disease are stable for one year. Thereafter monitoring can be reduced in frequency depending on physician's judgement taking into consideration risk factors (eg. age, co-morbidity, renal impairment).

Liver biopsy is not required in absence of pre-existing liver disease. Clinically significant liver damage is uncommon/rare [27].

Pulmonary Function Testing

Methotrexate is best avoided in established cases of Interstitial Lung Disease.

If the pre-treatment CXR is abnormal, consider performing a high resolution computerised tomography scan and pulmonary function tests. Transfer Factor of the Lung for Carbon Monoxide (TLCO) can be more sensitive than CXR [44, 45]

If evidence of bone marrow failure (anaemia, neutropenia and thrombocytopenia) is noted on blood test results, withhold methotrexate; if severe, discuss with a haematologist. Immediate admission for urgent folinic acid rescue may be needed [46].

Renal Failure or Severe Dehydration

Patients who develop dehydration, pre-renal or acute renal failure while on methotrexate should have methotrexate withheld and should be given folinic acid rescue [46]. Methotrexate elimination is predominantly by renal excretion. If patients develop worsening chronic renal failure UandE should be monitored closely and dose reduction considered.

Gastroenterology

Currently methotrexate is a second line immunosuppressive agent for the treatment of IBD (mainly CD). It is used in patients resistant to, or intolerant of, AZA or 6-MP. However it is currently unclear whether thiopurines (drugs that are purine antimetabolites) are any more effective than methotrexate for remission in IBD.

Efficacy in Crohn's Disease

Methotrexate is effective for the induction [47] and maintenance [48] of remission in CD and can induce mucosal healing [49, 50]. Evidence from a single large randomised controlled trial (RCT) of adult patients demonstrates that 25mg/week of intramuscular methotrexate is more effective than placebo at inducing steroid-free remission at 16 weeks [26]. In a subsequent study by Feagan et al, patients who responded to therapy at induction were randomised to 15mg/week of intramuscular methotrexate. 65% of patients in the treated group compared with 39% in the placebo group were in remission at 40 weeks [4].

Efficacy in Ulcerative Colitis

There have been no comparable trials that have addressed the role of methotrexate in the induction or maintenance of remission in ulcerative colitis. A single RCT did not show oral methotrexate (12.5mg weekly) to be beneficial at inducing or maintaining remission [51] and is the only study considered in a recent Cochrane review [52]. The low dose and oral administration may account for the disappointing response. Several retrospective series, using larger weekly doses, have reported more promising data with response or remission rates of up to 78% in patients with ulcerative colitis resistant or intolerant of AZA or 6-MP [53, 54, 55, 56].

Mode of Delivery

Parenteral administration (either subcutaneous or intramuscular) may be more effective than oral therapy and is recommended by the British Society of Gastroenterology for IBD, although oral dosing may be more convenient. Studies in RA indicate the bioavailability of intramuscular methotrexate is greater than oral administration and equivalent to subcutaneous dosing [57]. To date there are no comparable studies in IBD; however, small uncontrolled series indicate that parenteral may be superior to oral administration in maintaining remission [58, 59] and subcutaneous may be as effective as intramuscular dosing [60].

Monitoring as per BSG *(See Adverse Events)*

Measurement of FBC and LFT are advisable before and within four weeks of starting therapy, then monthly. One fairly common practice is to perform FBC every two to four weeks for two months and then every four to eight weeks. The rationale for this approach is that, of patients who develop myelotoxicity, approximately half will develop it within two months and nearly two thirds within four months [17, 61]. Patients should remain under specialist follow-up.

Duration of Therapy

There is a paucity of data regarding optimal duration of treatment. A recent meta-analysis of observational studies reports remission rates of 75%, 53% and 43% after one, two and three years of treatment respectively [62] This suggests a prolonged period of treatment makes relapse on stopping treatment less likely, in keeping with patterns seen in other conditions treated with low dose methotrexate.

Adverse Effects [15, 63, 64]

Adverse effects of methotrexate can be divided into two groups:

- Rare, severe side effects (eg. Hepatotoxicity)
- Less severe, common, troublesome intolerance (eg. Anticipatory nausea)

Adverse effects in either group can lead to drug cessation. Adverse effects are relatively common, reported in around 27-49% of patients and leading to drug cessation in 10-25%. Nausea, and in particular anticipatory nausea, commonly develops during treatment with methotrexate. Strategies to overcome this include addition of folic acid (if not already taking), altering the route of administration or addition of an antiemetic drug. Co-prescription of folic acid 5mg once a week limits GI side effects of nausea, vomiting, diarrhoea and stomatitis.

Other common side effects are mouth and nasal ulcers, fatigue, cutaneous reaction at injection site and flu-like symptoms. Less common side effects include arthralgia, facial flushing, eye irritation, dizziness, mild hair loss, loss of libido/impotence and decreased fertility (reversible on discontinuation of treatment), headache, acne, pruritis, photosensitivity, shortness of breath and numbness.

Hepatotoxicity, renal failure, pneumonitis, bone marrow suppression and opportunistic infections comprise the serious side effects which require close monitoring, for the duration an individual is being treated with methotrexate.

Liver: Hepatic fibrosis was first reported several decades ago. An accumulative dose of 1.5g of methotrexate might cause significant liver disease. Liver fibrosis may occur with normal liver enzymes and imaging findings [65]. Type-two diabetes, Hepatitis B and C, excessive alcohol consumption and obesity appear to be significant risk factors of developing hepatic fibrosis when on methotrexate [30]. Thus hepatotoxicity may be minimised by avoiding administration in these patients. Significant liver toxicity due to methotrexate is extremely rare in children [66].

Liver biopsy is not recommended as a routine but patients with persistent elevation of pre-treatment PIIINP above 8.0ug/l or abnormal PIIINP (>4.2g/l, in at least three samples over a 12 month period) should be considered. If there is pre-existing liver disease a baseline ultrasound guided biopsy should be carried out three to four months after starting the methotrexate [65]. Elevation of PIIINP above 10ug/l in at least three samples in a 12 month period should warrant discontinuation of methotrexate. PIIINP has not been shown to be a useful marker of liver toxicity in children and is not generally measured.

Elevation of alanine aminotransferase (ALT) levels occurs in about 10% and a two fold persistent elevation may necessitate a temporary withholding of methotrexate or a dose reduction. It is rarely necessary to permanently stop methotrexate. Sudden cessation should be avoided as this can lead to a flare in disease. A study of liver biopsies in patients with IBD taking methotrexate showed only mild histological abnormalities in most, despite cumulative doses of up to 5.410g. Surveillance liver biopsy is not warranted as there is no evidence that it is beneficial, but if ALT levels rise significantly it is sensible to withhold methotrexate until it returns to normal before a re-challenge.

Bone marrow: Methotrexate-induced bone marrow failure presents with significant fall in cell counts. It is more likely in the elderly and in patients with significant renal impairment or in patients with concomitant administration of anti-folate drugs. If there is a significant fall in cell count, this may suggest bone marrow failure (anaemia, neutropenia and thrombocytopenia). Methotrexate should be withdrawn and if severe, discussion with a haematologist should take place. Immediate admission for urgent folinic acid rescue may be needed [46].

Marrow suppression is usually dose dependent. A WCC of less than $3.5 \times 10^9/l$, a neutrophil count below $1.5 \times 10^9/l$ or platelets below $150 \times 10^9/l$ may indicate a need to discontinue methotrexate. Sore throat, bruising, ulceration or fever may indicate a leucopenia and need an urgent FBC.

Lung injury: Following treatment with methotrexate, lung injury is rare. If it does occur, methotrexate should be stopped. Methotrexate pneumonitis is a potentially life threatening hypersensitivity reaction and is less predictable than hepatic or haematological toxicity. It is thought to be more common in those with pre-existing lung disease and usually occurs within the first year of treatment [44, 45]. The prevalence of pneumonitis has been estimated to be two to three cases per 100 patient-years of exposure, but large series have not reported any cases. If the pre-treatment CXR if abnormal, further investigation (eg. pulmonary function testing, high resolution CT) should be considered before starting methotrexate. Whilst airway obstruction is not a contraindication to methotrexate therapy, interstitial lung disease is [67].

Infections

Methotrexate has a relatively low risk of infection associated with its use [68], however, serious infections are reported to occur more frequently. Thus vigilance is required to ensure infections are diagnosed at an early stage and systemic dissemination prevented. In certain cases methotrexate should be stopped immediately. If infection is associated with dehydration and pre-renal failure, cessation of methotrexate should occur and folinic acid rescue considered. Infections occurring in individuals taking methotrexate are caused by a range of organisms, from viral and bacterial to rare opportunistic infections. Significant mortality and morbidity has been reported in infections due to Herpes Zoster/Varicella [69].

Renal failure/Severe dehydration: Patients who develop dehydration, pre-renal or acute renal failure while taking methotrexate should have methotrexate withheld and should be given folinic acid rescue [46]. Methotrexate elimination is predominantly by renal excretion.

If patients develop worsening chronic renal failure FBC should be monitored closely and dose reduction considered.

Overdose: In suspected cases of methotrexate overdose, severe haematological toxicity, pre-renal or acute renal failure, consider treatment with folinic acid. The initial dose should be at least 20mg given intravenously. Subsequent doses can be given at a dose of 15mg orally at six hourly intervals until abnormalities improve [71].

Contraindications

Absolute

Active bacterial infection, active tuberculosis, active herpes-zoster infection, active life-threatening fungal infections, acute hepatitis B or C, planning (or in) pregnancy, breastfeeding.

Relative

Chronic hepatitis B or C, hepatic disease, renal disease, interstitial lung disease.

Vaccines

Prior to commencing methotrexate treatment, immunity status to varicella and measles should be checked. This is especially important in paediatric populations likely to be exposed frequently to chicken pox. If not immune these individuals should be vaccinated prior to commencing methotrexate treatment if possible. In patients receiving methotrexate exposed to chicken pox or shingles, immunity status should be checked. If the patient is not immune, passive immunisation should be given using Varicella Zoster Immunoglobulin (VZIG) or patients treated with aciclovir [16]. Patients developing clinical chickenpox or shingles should be treated with aciclovir. Patients receiving methotrexate must not receive live vaccines (eg. Measles Mumps, Rubella, Varicella, Bacille Calmette-Guérin known as the BCG, and Yellow Fever). If live vaccines are needed then methotrexate therapy should be postponed or withdrawn. Annual flu and pneumococcal vaccination is recommended.

Drug Interactions

Non steroidal anti-Inflammatory drugs (NSAIDs) and salicylates may reduce elimination of methotrexate and potentiate toxicity [72]. In practice NSAIDs and methotrexate are commonly co-administered. However patients and carers should be informed not to buy over the counter products containing NSAIDs or salicylates without speaking to their doctor or pharmacist. In these cases caution should be exercised regarding LFT and renal function, particularly in the elderly.

Co-trimoxazole and trimethoprim (antifolate effect of methotrexate is increased and significantly increases the risk of marrow aplasia), ciprofloxacin, tetracyclines, aminoglycosides, sulphonamides and penicillins all increase the risk of toxicity when given with methotrexate. Corticosteroids, ciclosporin and omeprazole may increase risk methotrexate toxicity. In practice however, toxicity is not generally seen when co-prescribing these medications.

Antibiotics: There is a risk of severe adverse reactions if penicillins or related antibiotics are used alongside methotrexate. There have been numerous case reports of possible decreased urinary excretion of methotrexate due to competition by some acidic drugs like beta-lactams (penicillins, cephalosporins, carbapenems, and monobactams) for secretion in the renal tubule, with toxicity resulting due to increased blood methotrexate concentration [24].

Other notable drug interactions include phenytoin (antifolate effect of methotrexate is increased), probenecid and tolbutamide (methotrexate concentration maybe increased in the serum) and co-trimoxazole.

Pregnancy, Fertility and Breast Feeding

Methotrexate is teratogenic, therefore pregnancy and breast feeding should be avoided during treatment [5, 73]. Methotrexate may damage sperm thus adequate contraception is essential for both men and women. It may persist in tissues for long periods, therefore conception should be avoided for three to six months after withdrawal of therapy [74]. Breast-feeding is not recommended as methotrexate passes into breast milk [75]. On stopping the drug fertility returns to pre-treatment levels.

Surgery

Recent studies suggest that continuation of methotrexate therapy does not increase the risk of infection or surgical complications [74, 75]. Vigilance for infection and complications is recommended [74]. Stopping methotrexate for surgery runs the risk of disease flare.

Alcohol

Alcohol should only be consumed moderately as methotrexate is metabolised by the liver. Generally speaking physicians would advise no more than one unit/day. Binge drinking is particularly advised against. Any patient suspected of alcohol abuse is usually unsuitable for methotrexate therapy [10].

References

[1] Methotrexate. Eds: Cronstein N, Bertino JR. ISBN 3-7643-5959-5, New York, Springer-Verlag, 2000, pp1-5.

[2] Gubner R, August S, Ginsberg V. Therapeutic suppression of tissue reactivity. II. Effect of aminopterin in rheumatoid arthritis and psoriasis. *Am. J. Med. Sci.* 1951;221(2):176-82.

[3] Rees RB, Bennett JH, Maibach HI et al. Methotrexate for Psoriasis. *Arch. Dermatol.* 1967;95(1):2-11.

[4] Feagan BG, Fedorak RN, Irvine EJ et al. A comparison of methotrexate with placebo for the maintenance of remission in Crohn's disease. North American Crohn's Study Group Investigators. *N. Engl. J. Med.* 2000;342(22):1627-32.

[5] BSPAR Guidelines on methotrexate use in paediatric rheumatology. Approved by the BSPAR executive committee in 2005. This guideline version no longer available via website but available from BSPAR upon request. http://www.bspar.org.uk Accessed July 2011.

[6] Warren RB, Chalmers RJ, Griffiths CE et al. Methotrexate for psoriasis in the era of biological therapy. *Clin. Exp. Dermatol.* 2008;33(5):551-4.

[7] Chande N, Ponich T, Gregor J. A survey of Canadian gastroenterologists about the use of methotrexate in patients with Crohn's disease. *Can. J. Gastroenterol.* 2005;19(9): 553-8.

[8] Gutierrez-Ureña S, Molina JF, García CO et al. Pancytopenia secondary to methotrexate therapy in rheumatoid arthritis. *Arthritis Rheum.* 1996;39(2):272-6.

[9] Lateef O, Shakoor N, Balk RA. Methotrexate pulmonary toxicity. *Expert Opin. Drug Saf.* 2005;4(4):723-30.

[10] Roenigk HH Jr, Auerbach R, Maibach HI et al. Methotrexate guidelines: Revised. *J. Am. Acad. Dermatol.* 1982;6(2):145-55.

[11] Furst DE, Kremer JM. Methotrexate in rheumatoid arthritis. *Arthritis Rheum.* 1988; 31(3):305-14.

[12] Kremer JM, Kaye GI, Kaye NW et al. Light and electron microscopic analysis of sequential liver biopsy samples from rheumatoid arthritis patients receiving long-term methotrexate therapy. Followup over long treatment intervals and correlation with clinical and laboratory variables. *Arthritis Rheum.* 1995;38(9):1194-203.

[13] Kremer JM, Furst DE, Weinblatt ME et al. Significant changes in serum AST across hepatic histological biopsy grades: prospective analysis of 3 cohorts receiving methotrexate therapy for rheumatoid arthritis. *J. Rheumatol.* 1996;23(3):459-61.

[14] Kremer JM, Alarcón GS, Lightfoot RW Jr et al. Methotrexate for rheumatoid arthritis: suggested guidelines for monitoring liver toxicity. American College of Rheumatology. *Arthritis Rheum.* 1994;37:316–28.

[15] Chakravarty K, McDonald H, Pullar T et al. BSR/BHPR guideline for disease-modifying anti-rheumatic drug (DMARD) therapy in consultation with the British Association of Dermatologists. Rheumatology. 2008;47(6):924-5. Published Online First: 28 August 2006. doi:10.1093/rheumatology/kel216a.

[16] Hawley DP, Rangaraj S, Heafield S. British Society for Paediatric and Adolescent Rheumatology (BSPAR) Guidelines on Methotrexate use in Paediatric Rheumatology

2010 (update). http://www.bspar.org.uk /pages/clinical_guidelines.asp Accessed July 2011.

[17] Mowat C, Cole A, Windsor A et al. Guidelines for the management of inflammatory bowel disease in adults. Gut. 2011;60(5):571-607 doi:10.1136/gut.2010.224154.

[18] British Society for Rheumatology. National guidelines for the monitoring of second line drugs, 2000. http://www.rheumatology.org.uk/includes/documents/cm_docs/2009/m/monitoring_second_line_drugs.pdf Accessed Jul 2011.

[19] Farber S, Diamond L, Mercer R et al. Temporary remission in ALL in children produced by folic acid antagonist aminopterin. *NEJM* 1948; 238:1787.

[20] Yarris JP, Hunter AJ. Roy Hertz MD (1909-2002): The cure of choriocarcinoma and its impact on the development of chemotherapy for cancer. *Gynecol. Oncol.* 2003;89(2): 193-8.

[21] Johnston A, Gudjonsson JE, Sigmundsdottir H et al. The anti-inflammatory action of methotrexate is not mediated by lymphocyte apoptosis, but by the suppression of activation and adhesion molecules. *Clin. Immunol.* 2005;114(2):154-63. doi:10.1016/j.clim.2004.09.001. PMID 15639649.

[22] Wu RS, Bonner WM. Separation of basal histone synthesis from S-phase histone synthesis in dividing cells. *Cell.* 1981 Dec;27(2 Pt 1):321-30. doi:10.1016/0092-8674(81)90415-3. PMID 7199388.

[23] Neurath MF, Hildner K, Becker C et al. Methotrexate specifically modulates cytokine production by T cells and macrophages in murine collagen-induced arthritis (CIA): a mechanism for methotrexate-mediated immunosuppression. *Clin. Exp. Immunol.* 1999; 115(1):42-55.

[24] Kremer JM. Historical overview of the treatment of Rheumatoid arthritis with an emphasis on methotrexate. *J. Rheumatol.* 1996;23(Suppl 44):34–7.

[25] Saporito FC, Menter MA. Methotrexate and psoriasis in the era of new biologic agents. *J. Am. Acad. Dermatol.* 2004;50:301–9.

[26] Feagan BG, Rochon J, Fedorak RN et al. Methotrexate for the treatment of Crohn's disease. *N. Engl. J. Med.* 1995;332:292–7.

[27] Williams HC, Pembroke AC. Methotrexate in the treatment of vasculitic cutaneous ulcerations in rheumatoid arthritis. *J. R. Soc. Med.* 1989;82:763.

[28] Wassenberg S, Herborn G, Rau R. Methotrexate treatment in Felty's syndrome. *Br. J. Rheumatol.* 1998;37:908–11.

[29] Weinstein GD. Methotrexate. *Ann. Intern. Med.* 1977;86(2):199-204.

[30] Montaudie H, Sbidian E, Paul C et al. Methotrexate in psoriasis: a systematic review of treatment modalities, incidence, risk factors and monitoring of liver toxicity. *J. Eur. Acad. Dermatol. Venereol.* 2011;25 (Suppl 2):12-8. doi: 10.1111/j.1468-3083.2011.03991.x.

[31] Chladek J, Simkova M, Vaneckova J et al. The effect of folic acid supplementation on the pharmacokinetics and pharmacodynamics of oral methotrexate during the remission-induction period of treatment of moderate to severe plaque psoriasis. *Eur. J. Clin. Pharmacol.* 2008; 64:347-55.

[32] Salim A, Tan E, Ilchyshyn A et al. Folic acid supplementation during treatment of psoriasis with methotrexate: a randomised double-blind placebo controlled trial *Br. J. Dermatol.* 2006;154:1169-74.

[33] Van Ede AE, Laan RF, Rood MJ et al. Effect of folic acid supplementation on the toxicity and efficacy of methotrexate in rheumatoid arthritis: a 48 week, multicentre, randomised, double-blind, placebo-controlled trial. *Arthrits Rheum.* 2001;44:1515-24.

[34] Braun J, Kastner P, Flaxenberg P et al. Comparison of clinical efficacy and safety of subcutaneous versus oral administration of methotrexate in patients with active rheumatoid arthritis: results of a six month, multicentre, randomised, double blind, controlled phase IV trial. *Arthrits Rheum.* 2008;58:73-81.

[35] Boffa MJ, Smith A, Chalmers RJ et al. Serum type III procollagen aminopeptide for assessing liver damage in methotrexate treated psoriatic patients. *Br. J. Dermatol.* 1996; 135:538-44.

[36] Zachariae H, Aslam HM, Bjerring P et al. Serum aminoterminal propeptide of type III procollagen in psoriasis and psoriatic arthritis: relation to liver fibrosis and arthritis. *J. Am. Acad. Dermatol.* 1991;25:50–3.

[37] Guidelines for monitoring drug therapy in rheumatoid arthritis. American College of Rheumatology Ad Hoc Committee on Clinical Guidelines. *Arthritis Rheum.* 1996;39: 723–31.

[38] Ruperto N, Murray KJ, Gerloni V et al. A randomized trial of parenteral methotrexate comparing an intermediate dose with a higher dose in children with juvenile idiopathic arthritis who failed to respond to standard doses of methotrexate. *Arthritis Rheum.* 2004;50(7):2191-201.

[39] Department of Health. 'Never Events List' for 2011-12. Feb 2011. http://www.dh.gov. uk/prod_consum_dh/groups/dh_digitalassets/documents/digitalasset/dh_124580.pdf Accessed July 2011.

[40] Ortiz Z, Shea B, Suarez-Almazor ME et al. The efficacy of folic acid and folinic acid in reducing methotrexate gastrointestinal toxicity in rheumatoid arthritis. A meta-analysis of randomised controlled trials. *J. Rheumatol.* 1998;25:36–43.

[41] Morgan SL, Baggott JE, Vaughn WH et al. Supplementation with folic acid during methotrexate therapy for rheumatoid arthritis: a double-blind placebo-controlled trial. *Ann. Intern. Med.* 1994;121:833–41.

[42] Oliver S, Livermore P. Administering subcutaneous methotrexate for inflammatory arthritis. RCN guidance for nurses. April 2004. http://www.rcn.org.uk/__data/assets/ pdf_file/0011/78608/002269.pdf Accessed July 2011.

[43] Whittle SL, Hughes RA. Folate supplementation and methotrexate treatment in rheumatoid arthritis: a review. *Rheumatology* 2004;43;267–71.

[44] Saravanan V, Kelly CA. Reducing the risk of methotrexate pneumonitis in rheumatoid arthritis. *Rheumatology* 2004;43:143–7.

[45] Imokawa S, Colby TV, Leslie KO, Helmers RA. Methotrexate Pneumonitis: review of the literature and histopathological findings in nine patients. *Eur. Respir. J.* 2000;15: 373–81.

[46] Strang A, Pullar T. Methotrexate toxicity induced by acute renal failure. *J. R. Soc. Med.* 2004;97:536–7.

[47] Alfadhli AA, McDonald JW, Feagan BG. Methotrexate for induction of remission in refractory Crohn's disease. *Cochrane Database Syst. Rev.* 2005;(1):CD003459.

[48] Patel V, Macdonald JK, McDonald JW et al. Methotrexate for maintenance of remission in Crohn's disease. *Cochrane Database Syst. Rev.* 2009;(4):CD006884.

[49] Kozarek RA, Patterson DJ, Gelfand MD et al. Methotrexate induces clinical and histologic remission in patients with refractory inflammatory bowel disease. *Ann. Intern. Med.* 1989;1;110(5):353-6.

[50] Manosa M, Naves JE, Leal C et al. Does methotrexate induce mucosal healing in Crohn's disease? *Inflamm. Bowel Dis.* 2010;16(3):377-8.

[51] Oren R, Arber N, Odes S, et al. Methotrexate in chronic active ulcerative colitis: a double-blind, randomized, Israeli multicenter trial. *Gastroenterology.* 1996;110(5): 1416-21.

[52] Ei-Matary W, Vandermeer B, Griffiths AM. Methotrexate for maintenance of remission in ulcerative colitis. *Cochrane Database Syst. Rev.* 2009;(3):CD007560.

[53] Fraser AG, Morton D, McGovern D et al. The efficacy of methotrexate for maintaining remission in inflammatory bowel disease. *Aliment Pharmacol. Ther.* 2002;16(4):693-7.

[54] Paoluzi OA, Pica R, Marcheggiano A et al. Azathioprine or methotrexate in the treatment of patients with steroid-dependent or steroid-resistant ulcerative colitis: results of an open-label study on efficacy and tolerability in inducing and maintaining remission. *Aliment Pharmacol. Ther.* 2002;16(10):1751-9.

[55] Cummings JR, Herrlinger KR, Travis SP et al. Oral methotrexate in ulcerative colitis. *Aliment Pharmacol. Ther.* 2005;21:385-9.

[56] Wahed M, Louis-Auguste JR, Baxter LM et al. Efficacy of methotrexate in Crohn's disease and ulcerative colitis patients unresponsive or intolerant to azathioprine /mercaptopurine. *Aliment Pharmacol. Ther.* 2009;30(6):614-20. Epub 2009 Jun 23.

[57] Jundt JW, Browne BA, Fiocco GP et al. A comparison of low dose methotrexate bioavailability: oral solution, oral tablet, subcutaneous and intramuscular dosing. *J. Rheumatol.* 1993;20:1845-9.

[58] Din S, Dahele A, Fennel J et al. Use of methotrexate in refractory Crohn's disease: the Edinburgh experience. *Inflamm. Bowel Dis.* 2008;14:756-62.

[59] Chong RY, Hanauer SB, Cohen RD. Efficacy of parenteral methotrexate in refractory Crohn's disease. *Aliment Pharmacol. Ther.* 2001;15:35-44.

[60] Nathan DM, Iser JH, Gibson PR. A single center experience of methotrexate in the treatment of Crohn's disease and ulcerative colitis: a case for subcutaneous administration. *J. Gastroenterol. Hepatol.* 2008;23:954-8.

[61] Colombel JF, Ferrari N, Debuysere H et al. Genotypic analysis of thiopurine S-methyltransferase in patients with Crohn's disease and severe myelosuppression during azathioprine therapy. *Gastroenterology.* 2000;118:1025-30.

[62] Hausmann J, Zabel K, Herrmann E et al. Methotrexate for maintenance of remission in chronic active Crohn's disease: Long-term single-center experience and meta-analysis of observational studies. *Inflamm. Bowel Dis.* 2010;16:1195-202.

[63] Fraser AG. Methotrexate: first-line or second-line immunomodulator? *Eur. J. Gastroenterol. Hepatol.* 2003;15:225-31.

[64] Te HS, Schiano TD, Kuan SF et al. Hepatic effects of long-term methotrexate use in the treatment of inflammatory bowel disease. *Am. J. Gastroenterol.* 2000;95:3150-6.

[65] Roenigk HH Jr, Auerbach R, Maibach H et al. Methotrexate in psoriasis: Consensus Conference. *J. Am. Acad. Dermatol.* 1998;38:478–85.

[66] Hawley DP, Camina N, Rangaraj S. British isles survey of methotrexate monitoring practice during treatment of juvenile idiopathic arthritis. Semin. Arthritis Rheum. 2011; 40(4):358-64.e1-2. Epub 2010 Sep 6.

[67] Schnabel A, Richter C, Bauerfeind S et al. Bronchoalveolar lavage cell profile in methotrexate induced pneumonitis. *Thorax.* 1997;52:377–9.

[68] Lovell DJ, Zaoutis TE, Sullivan K. Immunosuppressants, infection and inflammation. *Clin. Immunol.* 2004;113:137–9.

[69] Bernal I, Domènech E, García-Planella E et al. Opportunistic infections in patients with inflammatory bowel disease undergoing immunosuppressive therapy. *Gastroenterol. Hepatol.* 2003;26(1):19-22.

[70] Chalmers RJG, Boffa MJ. Current management of psoriasis: methotrexate. *J. Dermatol. Treat.* 1997;8:41–4.

[71] Ting TV, Hashkes PJ. Methotrexate/naproxen-associated severe hepatitis in a child with juvenile idiopathic arthritis. *Clin. Exp. Rheumatol.* 2007;25(6):928-9.

[72] Donnenfeld AE, Pastuszak A, Noah JS et al. Methotrexate exposure prior to and during pregnancy. *Teratology.* 1994;49:79–81.

[73] Mahadevan U, Kane S. American gastroenterological association institute technical review on the use of gastrointestinal medications in pregnancy. *Gastroenterology.* 2006;131:283-311.

[74] Bridges SL Jr, Lo´pez-Me´ndez A, Han KH et al. Should methotrexate be discontinued before elective orthopaedic surgery in patients with rheumatoid arthritis? *J. Rheumatol.* 1991;18:984–8.

[75] Grennan DM, Gray J, Loudon J et al. Methotrexate and early postoperative complications in patients with rheumatoid arthritis undergoing elective orthopaedic surgery. *Ann. Rheum. Dis.* 2001;60;214–7.

In: Methotrexate   ISBN: 978-1-62100-596-4
Editors: V. S. Castillo and L. A. Moyano   © 2012 Nova Science Publishers, Inc.

Chapter VI

Methotrexate: Update on Pharmacology, Clinical Applications and Warnings

Marcelo Derbli Schafranski, Alexandre Bueno Merlini,
Ewelyn Adriane Chaves de Araújo,
Natasha Lure Bueno de Camargo and Polliane Arruda
Department of Medicine, Universidade Estadual de Ponta Grossa (UEPG),
Ponta Grossa, Paraná, Brazil

1. Introduction

Methotrexate (MTX) is an antimetabolic agent that affects the metabolism of folic acid. The drug entered clinical medicine as an innovative antineoplastic drug in 1948, after the detection of its indirect effects on DNA synthesis. Although by a different mechanism, it resembled corticosteroid drugs by acting on the proliferation of connective tissue. The drug has thus been used in the treatment of psoriasis, psoriatic arthritis and rheumatoid arthritis (RA). Since then, studies have been carried out on the effectiveness, toxicity, doses and other features of methotrexate. It has also been compared more recently with different rheumatic drugs, such as corticosteroids and new immunosuppressive drugs, such as inhibitors of specific molecular components of inflammation. [1]

Increases in the number of patients treated with methotrexate and increases in doses are universal. [2] It is now commonly administered in combination with either biological agents or other small-molecule antirheumatic drugs. Combination therapies have been more effective than either monotherapy, without increasing toxicity. [3]

2. Pharmacology

2.1. Chemical Structure and Mechanisms of Action

Chemically, methotrexate is N - [4 - [[(2,4 – diamino – 6 - pteridinyl) methyl] methylamino] benzoyl] - L- glutamic acid.

Several pharmacological mechanisms of action have been suggested for it, including inhibition of purine and pyrimidine synthesis, suppression of transmethylation reactions with accumulation of polyamines, reduction of antigen-dependent T-cell proliferation, and promotion of adenosine release with adenosine-mediated suppression of inflammation [3,4]. It is possible that a combination of these mechanisms is responsible for the anti-inflammatory effects of methotrexate.

Pteroyl-glutamic acid was isolated in 1941 from leafy vegetables and named folic (foliage) acid. It has different coenzymatic functions depending on the position on the pteroyl ring at which a particular radical is attached. It differs structurally from folic acid at two sites: an amino is replaced by a hydroxyl at one site and a methyl group replaces an amino at another. The pharmaceutical pteroyl-glutamic acid is not an active co-enzyme. To become metabolically active, folic acid is reduced to dihydrofolate, and the dihydrofolate to tetrahydrofolate by enzyme dihydrofolate reductase. This happens before they can be utilized as carriers of one-carbon groups in the synthesis of purine nucleotides and thymidylate (at higher oncologic dosages). Other folate enzymes such as methylene tetrahydrofolate reductase (MTHFR) may be influenced.

Thus, it inhibits reductase and interferes with DNA repair, synthesis, and cellular replication. By inhibiting the generation of tetrahydrofolate, a donor of methyl groups required in a large number of biochemical reactions, methotrexate also inhibits transmethylation reactions required for inflammation. [5]

Actively proliferating tissues such as malignant cells, bone marrow, fetal cells, buccal and intestinal mucosa, and cells of the urinary bladder are in general more sensitive to its effect. When there is more cellular proliferation in malignant tissues than in normal tissues, methotrexate may impair malignant growth without irreversible damage to normal tissues.

It enters the cell via a saturable transporter, the reduced folate carrier 1 (RFC1), and is transformed into methotrexate polyglutamate (MTX_{Glu}) by the enzyme folypolyglutamate synthase (FPGS). There is an intracellular accumulation of MTX_{Glu} that inhibits aminoimidazole carboxamide ribonucleotide transformylase (AICAR T'ASE), a potent enzyme involved in *de novo* purine biosynthesis [6]. This inhibition leads to accumulation of AICAR intracellularly which, by competitively inhibiting AMP deaminase, leads to accumulation of AMP, which is released and converted extracellularly to adenosine, an endogenous purine nucleoside.

Its adenosine-mediated anti-inflammatory effect is still best supported by in vitro, in vivo, and clinical data. Methotrexate has previously been shown to induce adenosine release in animal models of inflammation, and in patients with RA and adenosine, by acting on its receptors, thus being a potent inhibitor of inflammation. [7]

Its mechanism of action on cell proliferation and apoptosis also depends on the alteration of the reactive oxygen species (ROS), in a time-concentration-dependent manner, by pathway enzymes. [8.9] Higher ROS levels are found in active lymphocytes and may induce apoptotic, whereas in monocytes an adaptive response of cell proliferation inhibition is found. The effects seem to be more profound in activated lymphocytes. [10]

It is an inhibitor of cytokine production, as well as inducing activation of T cells. It probably reduces the production of many cytokines, including IL-4, IL-13, TNF-α, IFNγ (interferon gamma) and GM-CSF (granulocyte-macrophage colony-stimulating factor), IL-6 in activated cells. Furthermore, it inhibits the upregulation of IL-15, IL-8, CD69, CD25 and IL-17. It has been suggested that this inhibition of cytokines is due to the *de novo* syntheses of purines and pyrimidines. However, there are only a few studies that have provided a molecular basis for these findings. [10,11]

Current results in RA patients suggest that it may reduce the expression of cellular adhesion molecules, but it is not clear whether this is a direct effect or an indirect one via the reduced expression of cytokines [10,12]. Through the action of IL-6, it also has a preventive effect on bone resorption by osteoclasts. [13]

Its clinical effects can therefore be attributed to multiple targets. Knowledge concerning the mechanism of this drug has been expanding in recent years, but more animal and patient studies are needed to reveal the precise interactions between drug, drug target and diseases.

2.2. Pharmacokinetics

Methotrexate is a weak dicarboxylic acid with pKa 4.8 and 5.5, and is thus mostly ionized at physiologic pH. It is metabolized by intestinal bacteria to the inactive metabolite 4-amino-4-deoxy-N-methylpteroic acid (DAMPA) and accounts for less than 5% loss of the oral dose. It can be taken orally or administered by injection (subcutaneous, intramuscular, intravenous or intrathecal). Its concentration in plasma and other biological fluids is measured, in order to study its pharmacokinetics as well as predict and prevent its toxicity when administered in high-dose intravenous infusions, by modifying the administration schedule of calcium folinate according to the plasma concentration. [14,15,16]

2.3. Absorption

Oral absorption in adults appears to be dose-dependent. Peak serum levels are reached within one to two hours. At doses of 30 mg/m^2 or less, it is generally well absorbed. The absorption of doses greater than 80 mg/m^2 is significantly less, possibly due to a saturation effect.

In leukemic pediatric patients, oral absorption of methotrexate appears to be as in adults, dose-dependent, and has been reported to vary widely (23% to 95%). A twenty-fold difference between highest and lowest peak levels (C_{max}: 0.11 to 2.3 μmol after a 20 mg/m^2 dose) has been reported. The absorption of doses greater than 40 mg/m^2 has been reported to be significantly less than that of lower doses. Food has been shown to delay absorption and reduce peak concentration. Methotrexate is generally completely absorbed from parenteral routes of injection. After intramuscular injection, peak serum concentrations occur in 30 to 60 minutes. As in leukemic pediatric patients, wide interindividual variability in the plasma concentrations of methotrexate has been reported in pediatric patients with JRA. Following oral administration of methotrexate in doses of 6.4 to 11.2 mg/m^2/week in pediatric patients with JRA, mean serum concentrations were 0.59 μmol (range, 0.03 to 1.40) at 1 hour, 0.44 μmol (range 0.01 to 1.00) at 2 hours, and 0.29 μmol (range 0.06 to 0.58) at 3 hours. In pediatric patients receiving methotrexate for acute lymphocytic leukemia (6.3 to 30 mg/m^2), or for JRA (3.75 to 26.2 mg/m^2), the terminal half-life has been reported to range from 0.7 to 5.8 hours or 0.9 to 2.3 hours, respectively. [18]

A study shows that food has no significant effect on its absorption or bioavailability. Patients may take it without regard to meals. When poor oral absorption is observed, it can be administered subcutaneously. [19]

2.4. Distribution

After intravenous administration, the initial volume of distribution is approximately 0.18 L/kg (18% of body weight) and steady-state volume of distribution is approximately 0.4 to 0.8 L/kg (40% to 80% of body weight). It competes with reduced folates for active transport across cell membranes by means of a single carrier-mediated active transport process. At serum concentrations greater than 100 μmol, passive diffusion becomes a major pathway by which effective intracellular concentrations can be achieved. Methotrexate in serum is approximately 50% protein-bound.

Methotrexate does not penetrate the blood-cerebrospinal fluid barrier in therapeutic amounts when given orally or parenterally. High CSF concentrations of the drug may be attained by intrathecal administration. [18]

2.5. Metabolism

After absorption, methotrexate undergoes hepatic and intracellular metabolism to polyglutamated forms which can be converted back to methotrexate by hydrolase enzymes. These polyglutamates act as inhibitors of dihydrofolate reductase and thymidylate synthetase. Small amounts of methotrexate polyglutamates may remain in tissues for extended periods. The retention and prolonged drug action of these active metabolites vary among different cells, tissues and tumors. A small amount of metabolism to 7-hydroxymethotrexate may occur at doses commonly prescribed. Accumulation of this metabolite may become significant at the high doses used in osteogenic sarcoma. The aqueous solubility of 7-hydroxymethotrexate is 3 to 5 times lower than the parent compound. It is partially metabolized by intestinal flora after oral administration. [18]

2.6. Excretion

Renal excretion is dependent upon dosage and route of administration. It is oxidised to 7-hydroxy-methotrexate by aldehyde reductase and primarily has renal excretion. Thus, its action is prolonged by renal failure. [4] About 40% of tritium-labeled methotrexate is excreted unchanged in the urine within 48 hours after intravenous administration. One to two percent per day is excreted for several weeks, largely as its cleavage products. [20]

There is limited biliary excretion amounting to 10% or less of the administered dose. Enterohepatic recirculation of methotrexate has been proposed. Renal excretion occurs by glomerular filtration and active tubular secretion. [18]

Its clearance rates vary widely and are generally decreased at higher doses. Its toxicity has been linked with delayed drug clearance, and has been identified as one of the major factors responsible for it. The normal tissues are more dependent upon the duration of exposure to the drug than to the peak level achieved. When a patient has delayed drug elimination due to compromised renal function, a third space effusion, or other causes, its serum concentrations may remain high for prolonged periods. [18]

2.7. Dosage and Administration

It is used at high doses, up to 5 to 24 g per adult per week (130-300 mg/kg) for several weeks for the treatment of cancer. This dose can yield serum concentrations of >1000 μM, a concentration range associated with its life-threatening toxicity.21 By contrast, a 1000-fold lower dose of methotrexate (LD-MTX) [0.1-0.4 mg/kg (7.5-30 mg per adult)] is used once weekly in the treatment of rheumatoid arthritis (RA), juvenile idiopathic arthritis (JIA) in children (including infants <one year old) and psoriasis. [22,23,24] This use of LD-MTX is relatively safe and well tolerated, children tolerating it better than adults. [24] Pharmacokinetic data indicate LD-MTX yields *in vivo* concentrations >250 nM, which can clear malaria parasites *in vivo* (MTX IC_{99} of 200-400 nM). [25,26,27] In addition, two small-scale clinical trials carried out in the 1970s indicated that LD-MTX, as low as 2.5 mg per dose per day, was safe and efficacious for treating *P. falciparum* and *Plasmodium vivax* in adults. [28,29]

Low-dose methotrexate (LDMTX), administered with folid acid, is commonly administered orally, intramuscularly or subcutaneously. It is used as a therapy for generalized and palmoplantar psoriasis resistant to tar, retinoids, psoralens and UVA-light, such as in the treatment of rheumatoid arthritis, sarcoidosis or Crohn's disease.

The most important aims in LDMTX therapy are, first, to induce remission of disease or at least to decrease its symptoms to an acceptable level, second to attain the lowest maintenance dose, and third to maintain remission over a long period without undue toxicity. [30]

A convenient regimen in adults is to start therapy with intermittent oral administration of 5–10 mg once a week. If, after 6–8 weeks, the response is not adequate and no adverse effects are present, the weekly dose can be gradually increased to 25 mg. [31]

2.8. Pharmacogenomics

In the enzymes associated with its metabolism, there is a prevalence of genetic variations (single-nucleotide polymorphisms (SNPs) which could be associated with clinical variations in patients receiving the drug.

There are many SNP pathways for folate enzymes. If these are known for certain in the patient it can lead to the correct form of treatment. [22]

The best studied enzyme is methylene tetrahydrofolate reductase (MTHFR), which is responsible for some side effects. It is a critical enzyme associated with the regeneration of 5-methyl-tetrahydrofolate from 5,10-methylene-tetrahydrofolate. The regenerated 5-methyl-tetrahydrofolate contributes a methyl group to homocysteine for regeneration of methionine, using B12 as a necessary cofactor. Thus, in the absence of adequate amounts of 5-methyl-tetrahydrofolate, more homocysteine accumulates and less methionine is regenerated. As methionine is a precursor in a wide range of downstream-1 carbon transfers, it is easy to see that a genetic defect in its regeneration can lead to the potential for toxicities associated with both hyperhomocysteinaemia and methionine deficiency. [33,34]

A severe deficiency is associated with neuropathy and encephalopathy as well as vasculopathy and coagulopathy. The neuropathy and encephalopathy toxicities are also seen with the neurotoxicity associated with B12 deficiency. The wild-type (CC) polymorphism in the C677T genotype is associated with normal activity, whereas the CT heterozygote, found in 40% of the population, is associated with a 40% decrease in the ability to regenerate 5-methyl-tetrahydrofolate. The homozygotic TT genotype is found in 8–12% of the population and is associated with a 70% decrease in the ability to regenerate 5-methyl-tetrahydrofolate. [35]

2.9. Drug Interactions

a) High serum concentration of methotrexate:
   - Penicilins (such as Ampicilin, Oxacilin, Dicloxacilin) – competitive inhibition in renal tube, reduced clearance of MTX;
   - NSAIDs (Ibuprofen, Diclofenac, Meloxicam) – increased risk of gastrointestinal side effects and serum concentration of MTX. Extreme increase of liver and renal toxicity;
   - Probenecid – inhibits renal elimination of MTX and increases effects and toxicity especially in high-dose patients;
   - Tetracycline – raises MTX concentration because it involves displacement of plasma proteins.
   - Steroids – increases toxicity (without raising liver enzymes) and bone marrow suppression.
   - Sulfonamides – high risk of liver and renal toxicity and bone marrow suppression
b) Decreased serum concentration of methotrexate:
   - azathioprine – inhibits hepatic metabolism
   - Its combination with potentially hepatotoxic drugs (acetaminophen, ACE inhibitors, interferons, thiazolidinediones, carbamazepine, valproic acid, fenofibrate, HMG-CoA redutase inhibitors) is not recommended. It is necessary to assess risks and benefits in individual cases.
c) Caffeine: above 180 mg/day can change its effects. The mechanism of interaction is not yet defined but includes adenoside receptors.
d) d) Alcohol: induces severe hepatotoxicity and potential renal damage. It is associated with hepatitis, chronic fibrosis and cirrhosis in long-term treatment. [64]

3. Clinical Uses

In medical practice, methotrexate is indicated for a plethora of clinical conditions. Its main uses can be divided into three groups:

- Autoimmune rheumatic conditions, such as *rheumatoid arthritis, systemic lupus erythematosus, psoriatic arthritis*, juvenile idiopathic arthritis, inflammatory myopathies, sarcoidosis, rheumatic polymyalgia, arthritis related to secondary amyloidosis and others;
- Other autoimmune conditions, such as Sjögren syndrome, inflammatory bowel disease, and vasculitis;
- Some types of neoplasms.

3.1. Rheumatoid Arthritis

Being a disease-modifying antirheumatic drug (DMARD), methotrexate reduces the rate of erosion of the joint spaces, and can change the progression of the disease by preventing irreversible damage. It is recommended that physicians should start administration of DMARD as soon as diagnosis of rheumatoid arthritis is established.

Because of its effectiveness, low price, and relatively propitious toxicity, methotrexate is the most commonly used and first choice DMARD as treatment.

The guidelines recommend a single oral dose of 7.5 mg weekly, or fractionally in three doses of 2.5 mg every 12 hours. The maximum dose ranges from 20 to 25 mg per week. [36]

3.2. Systemic Lupus Erythematosus

Studies showed that patients with systemic lupus erythematosus who received an average of 1.33 mg of methotrexate per day for twelve months obtained a cutback of 22% in the average-during-trial daily dosage of prednisone (an immunosuppressive drug). Its use is therefore beneficial for these patients, decreasing the adverse effects of immunosupression, such as Cushing's syndrome, steroid toxicity, greater predisposition to infectious and cardiovascular diseases, osteoporosis, hyperglycemic conditions and others. [37]

3.3. Psoriatic Arthritis

Psoriasis is a chronic autoimmune inflammatory disease which affects 1-3% of the global population. 5-40% of these patients suffer from psoriatic arthritis. As a possible treatment, methotrexate is administered in a single dosage of 10-25 mg, orally, intravenously or intramuscularly until the appropriate therapeutic aim is achieved; or fractionally in three doses of 2.5 mg every 12 hours. The maximum dosage is 30 mg per week. Since it has a great capacity for long-term toxicity and may not control the disease successfully, biological therapies are in different phases of pharmacological studies, as ways of substituting it. [38]

3.4. Juvenile Idiopathic Arthritis

A dosage of 10-15 mg/m^2 per week orally or parentally can be administered in children with juvenile idiopathic arthritis. With this dose, 60-70% of patients are benefited significantly 4 to 6 months after the outset of treatment. [39]

3.5. Dermatomyositis

Oral or subcutaneous methotrexate could be considered as a reference drug in the treatment of patients with dermatomyositis, depending on the progression of the disease. A mean dosage of 15 mg/m^2 weekly must be administered until four weeks after inception of the disease, reducing the predisposition to calcinosis and fractures. [40]

3.6. Sarcoidosis

Although its use in the treatment of sarcoidosis is not new – it has been administered for this condition for over 40 years – there are few studies to support its efficacy.

Schiff et al. claim that, as a cytotoxic agent, it may help patients who are not given corticosteroids. They mention its successful use in patients with acute and symptomatic pulmonary sarcoidosis, and stress that its use should be reserved for chronic cases.

Baughman et al. showed its action by the analysis of pulmonary vital capacity, % lymphocytes and % lymphocytes CD4 and CD8 in bronchoalveolar lavage and the production of TNF-α, which are reduced in patients with active pulmonary sarcoidosis. However, better results were obtained with prednisone, reinforcing its use in case of failure of corticosteroids.

The recommended dosage is 10-20 mg orally per week, and should be adjusted in accordance with toxicity. [42]

3.7. Rheumatic Polymyalgia

Corticoesteroids are the baseline treatment for rheumatic polymyalgia. However, an average of 50% of patients presents side-effects. In case of intolerance to them or failure to respond, methotrexate is an attractive therapeutic strategy, although its efficacy in this disease still remains a matter of debate. [41]

3.8. Arthritis Related to Secondary Amyloidosis

Fiter et al. found that a low dosage treatment of methotrexate in patients with amyloidosis secondary to rheumatoid arthritis resulted in a sharp decrease in proteinuria. [43]

3.9. Sjögren Syndrome

In a non-double-blind rheumatologic experimental study, methotrexate was administered to patients with Sjögren syndrome weekly in a dose of 0.2 mg/kg body weight for one year. There was improvement in some subjective symptoms, such as dry eyes and mouth, as well as increased frequency of hyperplasia of the parotid gland, purpura and cough. [37]

3.10. Inflammatory Bowel Disease

In a study by Burger et al., the authors found that a dose of 25 mg/week intramuscularly in steroid-dependent patients with Crohn's disease or ulcerative colitis could replace immunosuppressive therapy and lead to remission. [44]

3.11. Vasculitis

De Groof et al. carried out a randomized trial comparing methotrexate (20-25 mg/week) and cyclophosphamide (2 mg/kg/day) in the induction of remission in early systemic antineutophil cytoplasmatic antibody-associated vasculitis. With median time of remission as a criterion, cyclophosphamide proved to be more effective. Since the effect of methotrexate is reduced in extensive disease and pulmonary involvement, it can be used to substitute cyclophosphamide in the initial treatment of this disorder. [41]

3.12. Oncologic Conditions

Acute Lymphoblast Leukemia

- Induction: 3,3 mg/m^2/day orally or intramuscularly
- Maintenance: 15 mg/m^2 twice a week orally or intramuscularly
- Alternate remission dose: 2.5 mg/kg intravenously up to two weeks [45]

Choriocarcinoma and Trophoblastic Disease
Dosage of 15 to 30 mg/day orally or intramuscularly for five days. This dosage must be repeated three to five times, with an interval $\geq$ 1 week. 1 or 2 of these courses should be applied after βhCG normalization.

Lymphoma

- Stages I and II of Burkitt's lymphoma: 10 to 25/mg/day orally for 4-8 days;
- Stage III of a malignant lymphoma: 0,625 to 2.5 mg/day orally associated with chemotherapy.

In general, several courses of methotrexate must be considered at each different stage. [46]

Meningeal Leukemia

A dosage of 12 mg/m^2 intrathecally for up to 2-5 days is recommended for patients with meningeal leukemia. The treatment must be maintained until the cell count of cerebrospinal fluid returns to normal. If necessary, an additional dose may be applied. [47]

Osteosarcoma

The initial dosage is 12g/m^2 intravenously in an infusion that lasts 4 to 6 hours. A mean peak serum methotrexate threshold above 700-1000 μmol/L is necessary for effective therapy. If this target is not achieved, dosage must be raised to 15 mg/m^2. [49]

Neoplastic Disorders

The dosage ranges from 30-40 mg/m^2 to 100-12000 mg/m^2 intravenously, with the support of leucovorin (folinic acid). [48]

A sufficient interval between courses of methotrexate must be respected in each patient, enabling the minor risk of toxic symptoms to subside.

4. Adverse Effects

The majority of side effects are caused by its pharmacological effect, although they can be reverted when detected in their initial phase. More than half of patients present some type of adverse effect during treatment, and these are the main cause of abandonment of short-term treatment. In long-term treatment the opposite occurs, with methotrexate being relatively well tolerated among DMARD drugs. [50] Patients in treatment reported significantly more side effects than the placebo group [51], but they are generally self-limited or preventable. These differences can occur because of great variability in the bioavailability of oral methotrexate and another pathway. It should be recalled that low-dose methotrexate is considered safe for treatment of rheumatoid arthritis. [52]

These effects are proportional to dose, [53] time of use and initial dose. [54] For example: higher starting doses are more effective but induce more gastrointestinal toxicity, while a lower dose can achieve the same clinical effect without side effects. Reviews classify drug effects in four classes:

- Type A: dose dependent
- Type B: idiosyncratic
- Type C: result of long-term therapy based on drug exposure
- Type D: delayed effects (including those that occur after interruption of treatment)

As the majority of uses of MTX are long-term, it is clinically useful to know about type B, C and D effects. [55]

It is important to emphasize that blood monitoring, evaluation of normalized liver enzymes and renal function should be carried out quarterly.

4.1. Gastrointestinal System

These are the most common side effects [56] and can affect up to 70% of patients. They consist of an increase of liver enzymes (mostly above upper normal limit, especially during the initial stage of treatment); a reduction of liver enzymes in long-term treatments; nausea and vomiting (which can lead to the interruption of treatment) [57]; diarrhea; stomatitis (dose-dependent – it should disappear two or three weeks after cessation of drug); mucosal ulceration; anorexia; hematemesis; melena; dyspepsia and weight loss. Most cases can be solved by introducing antiemetic drugs and folate supplementation. Four studies showed significant reduction of GI effects with folic acid 7-35 mg/week, in contrast with two using 5 mg/week. [58,59] Moreover, the use of folate supplement can prevent or minimize anemia, neutropenia, stomatitis and oral ulcers; effects such as liver and pulmonary fibrosis and renal failure are not related to folate and do not affect its efficacy. [4]

4.2. Hepatic Toxicity

A high level of liver enzymes is the most common sign that associates methotrexate with hepatotoxicity, but this is associated with short-term treatments and normalizes after treatment ends. However, in long-term (more than 55 months) treatment liver fibrosis can occur. This may be caused by the cumulative effect of the drug or by high doses, and can be detected by liver biopsy. The correlation with cirrhosis is not defined yet, but it is rare for this to be caused by the drug alone. Some comorbidities can exacerbate liver degeneration, such as obesity, diabetes, viral hepatitis, and alcoholism (associated with adenosine A2 receptors). Liver enzymes should be constantly monitored and special cases should be treated with caution and biopsy. Interactions with drugs that use hepatic metabolism can accentuate degeneration; for this reason they are not recommended. [60]

4.3. Skin Disorders

Usually caused by high oncologic doses, they are now being reported as adverse effects of low doses. They are numerous but, in most cases, do not affect the therapeutic plan. They may take the form of acne, alopecia, anaphylactic reaction, ecchymosis, depigmentation or hyperpigmentation of skin, urticaria, rashes of several kinds, photosensitivity or exacerbation of photosensitivity lesions, skin dryness, skin ulceration or necrosis and vasculitis (both rare), and nodulosis (related to adenosine A1 receptor). Skin eruptions and toxic eruptions and Stevens-Johnson Syndrome have also been reported. [61,62]

4.4. Hematopoietic System

Bone marrow suppression is the most dangerous side effect that can be caused, so the blood cell count should be monitored. This normally manifests as aplastic anemia, anemia, leukopenia, thrombocytopenia – associated with hypoalbuminemia - and pancytopenia.

Pancytopenia seems to be uncommon and can appear at any time during treatment; it does not appear to be dose-dependent, and may occur through a cumulative process. Myelosuppression can be exacerbated by combinations of drugs (corticosteroids, cyclosporin, NSAID's, omeprazole, peniciline, tetracycline, retinoids among others). As already observed, supplements of folic acid reduce the incidence of cytopenias. [50]

4.5. Central Nervous System

These effects are mostly nonspecific, because of which they are poorly described. They can be caused by methotrexate or any other reason, and were not studied by clinical trials. They are induced by low doses and can appear at any time during treatment. The best documented effects are headache, drowsiness, dizziness, vertigo, a feeling of light-headedness, and mood changes - normally presented as depression, confusion, possibly including memory and cognitive alterations – insomnia and delirium. Rare cases of increased intracranial pressure and epilepsy have been reported. High doses of methotrexate intrathecally or intraventricularly are associated with severe cases of neurotoxicity in patients with craniospinal irradiation. The events are subacute neurotoxicity with encephalopathy presenting paresis or plegia, dementia or confusion, tremor, ataxia and in progressive cases these can be fatal. [53]

4.6. Respiratory System

Clinical findings include acute interstitial pneumonitis (the most common effect), followed by interstitial fibrosis, with pleuritis and pleural effusion, pulmonary nodules and lung edema being rare. These may be accompanied by dyspnea, dry cough, fever, headache, cyanosis, hypoxemia and possible respiratory failure. These effects are classified as inflammatory, infectious and neoplastic. Some cases can present broncho-alveolar infiltration of cells and inflammation, such as peripheral eosinophilia. Rapid evolution shows a restrictive pattern and treatment includes suspension of methotrexate. Some factors can increase pulmonary toxicity: age > 60 years, previous use of DMARD's, hypoalbuminemia, renal failure, diabetes, or concomitant use of medications that decrease its plasma concentration. Moreover creatinine clearance lower than 79mL/minute severely increases pulmonary toxicity. [3] Risk factors are not defined but may include smoking and use of NSAIDs. [53]

4.7. Renal System

Methotrexate presents renal toxicity, decreases creatinine clearance and glomerular filtration rate. These adverse effects occur mainly in patients who concomitantly use NSAIDs and who have previously used nephrotoxic drugs. The adverse effects combined with risk factors can lead to renal failure. Renal function exams are used to evaluate patients, as methotrexate is known to be excreted by kidney and metabolite 7-OH- methotrexate precipitates in the glomerulus. Other effects are cystitis, hematuria, dark urine or blood in urine. [50]

4.8. Immune System

Low doses usually do not increase the probability of opportunistic infections and do not seem to be related to serious infection, although some infections have been reported, including *Pneumocystis carinii* pneumonia – the most common - cytomegalovirus, arpergillosis, sepsis, nocardiosis, herpes zoster and simplex hepatitis. These occur because the immune system is impaired due to the blocking of the inflammatory response. There was also a higher rate of post-operative infections in this group. [53]

4.9. Reproductive System, Pregnancy and Breastfeeding

Teratogenic alterations resulting from folate deficit have long been known, which is why methotrexate is not recommended for pregnant woman. As a rule it should not be used for at least three months in men, and a year in women, before pregnancy begins, as it may cause defects or miscarriage. A pregnancy test is recommended before starting treatment. According to the Food and Drug Administration (FDA), it can cause teratogenicity or miscarriage. The most common congenital effects are: low ears, hypertelorism, different heart position, depressed nasal bridge, cleft palate, syndactyly with long fingers, and neural tube defects such as spina bifida, mental retardation, hydrocephalus, anencephaly, cleft palate and syndactyly, and teratogy of Fallot. Some theories claim that the drug may remain in the maternal tissue for a longer period of time, in comparison to non-pregnant women. In rare cases, when associated with chemotherapy or myelosupressions, congenital defects were not found, according to significant data. Data suggest that it is secreted in maternal milk in low concentrations, resulting in the possibility of accumulation of the drug in the child's tissues causing adverse effects and various potential problems. For this reason MTX is not recommended during breast-feeding.

There have been rare cases of male infertility when oncologic doses are used. [50,53]

4.10. Carcinogenesis

There is some evidence that methotrexate can be oncogenic, notably in lymphomas and leukemias. Nevertheless, there does not seem to be a relation between cumulative tissue concentration and hematologic diseases.

According to the FDA, the risk of developing lymphoma in patients treated with biological agents is not related to TNF, but with the higher risk of lymfoproliferative diseases when compared with the normal population, especially in psoriasis patients who used methotrexate and cyclosporine. RA patients also have an increased risk of lymphoma compared to the normal population, although there is no evidence that it is caused by methotrexate, because studies have not considered RA as a risk condition for lymphoma disease. It should be recalled that RA or Sjoören's syndrome are isolated risk factors for the deployment of non-Hodgkin's lymphoma. Reported cases have shown a relation between Epstein-Barr virus and lymphoproliferative diseases responsive to it. [53]

4.11. Cardiovascular System

The principal side effects reported are pericarditis, pericardial effusion, hypotension and thromboembolic events – including arterial, pulmonary and cerebral.

RA patients treated with methorexate have reduced cardiovascular mortality when compared to other DMARD drugs. Its use is not a risk factor for cardiovascular diseases and events. [50]

4.12. General Manifestation

General side effects are frequent and include fatigue, arthralgias and myalgias, classic cases of anaphylaxis; endocrinologic manifestation in RA patients include gynecomastia, conjunctivitis and visual changes. [53]

Conclusion

As can be seen from this review, methotrexate is one of the best studied drugs, for its complex mechanisms of actions and its range of clinical uses. Its effects are distinct in different patients and in different medical conditions.

Many immunological, biochemical, pharmacological and genetic aspects remain uncertain, leaving wide scope for research and discoveries, which will result in ways to boost its uses, to reduce its toxicity and adverse effects, thereby bringing numerous benefits, improvement of diseases and health quality in patients.

References

[1]   Benedek TG. Methotrexate: from its introduction to non-oncologic therapeutics to anti-TNF-α. *Clin. Exp. Rheumatol.* 2010; 5(61): 3-8.

[2]   Sokka T. Increases in use of methotrexate since the 1980s. *Clin. Exp. Rheumatol.* 2010; 5(61): 13-20.

[3]   Cronstein B. Low-dose methotrexate: a mainstay in the treatment of rheumatoid arthritis. *Pharmacol. Rev.* 2005; 57(2):163-72.

[4]   Tian H, Cronstein B. Understanding the mechanisms of action of methotrexate: implications for the treatment of rheumatoid arthritis. *Bull. NYU Hosp. Jt Dis.* 2007; 65(3): 168-73.

[5]   Cronstein B, How does methotrexate suppress inflammation? *Clin. Exp. Rheumatol.* 2010; 5(61): 21-23.

[6]   Baggott JE, Morgan SL, Vaughn WH. Differences in methotrexate and 7-hydroxymethotrexate inhibition of folate-dependent enzymes of purine nucleotide biosynthesis. *Biochem. J.* 1994; 300 (Pt 3): 627-9.

[7]   Riksen NP, Barrera P, van den Broek PH et al. Methotrexate modulates the kinetics of adenosine in humans in vivo. *Ann. Rheum. Dis.* 2006; 65: 465-70.

[8]   Herman S, Zurgil N, Langevitz P et al. The induction of apoptosis by methotrexate in activated lymphocytes as indicated by fluorescence hyperpolarization: a possible model for predicting methotrexate therapy for rheumatoid arthritis patients. *Cell Struct. Funct.* 2003; 28:113–22.

[9]   Herman S, Zurgil N, Deutsch M. Low dose methotrexate induces apoptosis with reactive oxygen species involvement in T lymphocytic cell lines to a greater extent than in monocytic lines. *Inflamm. Res.* 2005; 54:273–80.

[10]   Wessels JA, Huizinga TW, Guchelaar HJ. Recent insights in the pharmacological actions of methotrexate in the treatment of rheumatoid arthritis. *Rheumatology* 2008; 47:249–255.

[11]   Gerards AH, de Lathouder S, de Groot ER et al. Inhibition of cytokine production by methotrexate. Studies in healthy volunteers and patients with rheumatoid arthritis. *Rheumatology* 2003; 42:1189–96.

[12]   Johnston A, Gudjonsson JE, Sigmundsdottir H et al. The anti-inflammatory action of methotrexate is not mediated by lymphocyte apoptosis, but by the suppression of activation and adhesion molecules. *Clin. Immunol.* 2005; 114:154–63.

[13]   Yoshida M, Kanno Y, Ishisaki A et al. Methotrexate suppresses inflammatory agonist induced interleukin 6 syntheses in osteoblasts. *J. Rheumatol.* 2005; 32:787–95.

[14]   Boyd JR. (1992) (Ed) *Drugs Facts and Comparisons*, JP Lippincot Company, St. Louis, 653-654.

[15]   Fleisher M.(1993) Antifolate analogs: mechanism of actions, analytical methodology, and clinical efficacy, *Ther. Drug Monit.* 15,521-529.

[16]   Dollery C. (Ed) (1991).*Therapeutic Drugs.* Vol. 2, Churchill Livingston, London M101-M110.

[17]   Wyeth TM. METHOTREXATE - Methotrexate Tablets USP - Methotrexate Injection USP, Antimetabolite. PRODUCT MONOGRAPH. April 1, 2003. Pfizer Canada Inc.

[18]   Hamilton RA, Kremer JM. The effects of food on methotrexate absorption. *J. Rheumatol.* 1995 Apr;22(4):630-2.

[19]   Johns DG, Hollingsworth JW, Cashmorear *et al.*: Methotrexate displacement in man. *J. Clin. Invest.* 1964; 43: 621-9.

[20]   Chabner BA, Amrein P, Drucker B, Michealson M, Mitsiades C, Goss P, Ryan D, Ramachandra S, Richardson P, Supko J, Wilson W. In: *The pharmacological basis of therapeutics 9/e.* Brunton L, editor. New York: McGrwa-Hill; 2006. Antineoplastic agents; pp. 1315–1465.

[21]   Kalb RE, Strober B, Weinstein G, Lebwohl M. Methotrexate and psoriasis: 2009 National Psoriasis Foundation Consensus Conference. *J. Am. Acad. Dermatol.* 2009; 60:824–837. doi: 10.1016/j.jaad.2008.11.906.

[22]   Swierkot J, Szechinski J. Methotrexate in rheumatoid arthritis. *Pharmacol. Rep.* 2006;58:473–492.

[23] Niehues T, Lankisch P. Recommendations for the use of methotrexate in juvenile idiopathic arthritis. *Paediatric drugs.* 2006;8:347–356. doi: 10.2165/00148581-200608060-00003.

[24] Chladek J, Grim J, Martinkova J, Simkova M, Vaneckova J. Low-dose methotrexate pharmacokinetics and pharmacodynamics in the therapy of severe psoriasis. *Basic Clin. Pharmacol. Toxicol.* 2005;96:247–248. doi: 10.1111/j.1742-7843.2005.pto960318.x.

[25] Grim J, Chladek J, Martinkova J. Pharmacokinetics and pharmacodynamics of methotrexate in non-neoplastic diseases. *Clin. Pharmacokinet.* 2003;42:139–151. doi: 10.2165/00003088-200342020-00003.

[26] Chladek J, Grim J, Martinkova J, Simkova M, Vaniekova J, Koudelkova V, Noiekova M. Pharmacokinetics and pharmacodynamics of low-dose methotrexate in the treatment of psoriasis. *Br. J. Clin. Pharmacol.* 2002;54:147–156. doi: 10.1046/j.1365-2125.2002. 01621.x.

[27] Wildbolz A. Methotrexate in the therapy of malaria. *Ther. Umsch.* 1973;30:218–222.

[28] Sheehy TW, Dempsey H. Methotrexate therapy for *Plasmodium vivax* malaria. *Jama.* 1970;214:109–114. doi: 10.1001/jama.214.1.109.

[29] Hendel J, Nyfors A. Non-linear renal elimination kinetics of methotrexate due to saturation of renal tubular reabsorption. *Eur. J. Clin. Pharmacol.* 1984;26:121–124.

[30] Songsiridej N, Furst DE. Methotrexate – the therapy rapidly acting drug. *Baillieres Clin. Rheumatol.* 1990;4:575–593.

[31] JM Kremer Methotrexate pharmacogenomics, Observations of clinical effects of methotrexate will help in patient management decisions. *Ann. Rheum. Dis.* 2006;65: 1121-1123.

[32] Kim RJ, Becker RC. Association between factor V Leiden, prothrombin G20210A, and methylenetetrahydrofolate reductase C677T mutations and events of the arterial circulatory system: a meta-analysis of published studies. *Am. Heart J.* 2003;146:948–57.

[33] Gos M Jr, Szpecht-potocka A. Genetic basis of neural tube defects. II. Genes correlated with folate and methionine etabolism. *J. Appl. Genet.* 2002;43:511–24.

[34] Schwahn B, Rozen R. Polymorphisms in the methylenetetrahydrofolate reductase gene: clinical consequences. *Am. J. Pharmacogenomics* 2001:189–201.

[35] Beukelman, T, Patkar NM, Saag KG et al. 2011 American College of Rheumatology recommendations for the juvenile idiopathic arthritis: initiation and safety monitoring of therapeutic agents for the treatment of arthritis and systemic features. *Arthritis Care Res.* (Hoboken). 2011

[36] Wizer M, Aringer M. Use of methotrexate in patients with systemic lupus erythematosus and primary Sjögren's syndrome. *Clin. Exp. Rheumatol.* 2010

[37] Cantini F, Nicolli L, Nannini C et al. Psoriatic arthritis: a systematic review. *Int. J. Rheum. Dis.* 2010 Oct;13(4):300-17.

[38] Boros C, Whitehead B. Juvenile idiopathic arthritis. *Aust. Fam. Physician.* 2010 Sep;39(9):630-6.

[39] Rosa Neto NS, Goldenstein-Schainberg C. Juvenile dermatomyositis: review and update of the pathogenesis and treatment.

[40] Spies CM, Burmester GR, Buttgereit F. Methotrexate treatment in large vessel vasculitis and polymyalgia rheumatica. *Clin. Exp. Rheumatol.* 2010

[41] Kiltz U, Braun J. Use of methotrexate in patients with sarcoidosis. *Clin. Exp. Rheumatol.* 2010 Sep-Oct;28.

[42] Yasuda M. Secondary amyloidosis in patients with rheumatoid arthritis. *Nippon. Rinsho.* 2005.

[43] Carbonnel F. Methotrexate: a drug of the future in colitis ulcerative? *Curr. Drug Targets.* 2011.

[44] Pieters R. Acute lymphoblastic laukeamia in children and adolescents: chance of cure now higher than 80%. Ned Tijdschr Geneeskd. 2010;154:A1577.

[45] ten Kate-Booij MJ, Lok CA, Verheijen RH et al. Trophoblastic diseases. Ned Tijdschr Geneeskd. 2008 Oct 11;152(41):2219-24.

[46] Carrabba MG, Reni M, Foppoli M et al. Treatment approaches for primary CNS lymphomas. *Expert Opin. Pharmacother.* 2010 Jun;11(8):1263-76.

[47] Thomas X, Pavan L, Le QH. Adult acute lymphoblastic leukemia with central nervous system involvement: an overview. *Bull. Cancer.* 2008 Jul-Aug;95(7):707-15.

[48] Dalen E, van As J, Camargo B. Methotrexate for high-grade osteosarcoma in children and Young adults. *Cochrane Database Syst. Rev.* 2011 May 11;5.

[49] Neves C, Jorge R, Barcelos A. A Teia de Toxicidade do metotrexato. *Acta Reumatol. Port.* 2009:34:11-34.

[50] Kozuch P, Hanauer S. Treatment of inflammatory bowel disease: A review of medical therapy. *World J. Gastroenterol.* 2008 January 21; 14(3): 354-377

[51] Osaki S. ANCA - associated Vasculitis: Diagnostic and Therapeutic Strategy. *Allergology International.* 2007;56:87-96.

[52] Taraborelli M, Andreoli L, Archetti S et al. I polimorfismi della metilentetraidrofolatoreduttasi (MTHFR) nel trattamento con methotrexate di pazienti con artrite reumatoide. Revisione della letteratura ed esperienza personale. *Reumatismo,* 2009; 61 (2):98-106.

[53] Visser K, Katchamart W, Loza E et al. Multinacional evidence-based recommendations for the use of methotrexate in rheumatic disorders with a focus on rheumatoid arthritis: integrating systematic literature research and expert opinion of a broad international panel of rheumatologists in the 3E initiative.

[54] McKendry R. The remarkable spectrum of methotrexate toxicities. Rheumatic Disease Clinice Of North America. November 1997; 23: 939-954.

[55] Salliot C, Heijde D. Long-term safety of methotrexate monotherapy in patients with rheumatoid arthritis: a systematic literature research. *Ann. Rheum. Dis.* 2009; 68:1100-1104.

[56] Ricci M, DeMarco G, Desiati F et al. Sopravvivenza a lungo termine del trattamento con methotrexate nell'artrite psoriasica. *Reumatismo,* 2009;61(2):125-131.

[57] Canhão H, Santos M, Costa L et al. Recomendações Portuguesas para utilização de metotrexato no tratamento de doenças reumáticas. *Acta Reumatol.* Port 2009;34;78-95.

[58] Warren R, Smith R, Campalani E et al. Outcomes of methotrexate for psoriasis and relationship to genetic polymorphisms. *British Journal of Dermatology* 2009;160: 438-441.

[59] Jensen P, Skov P, Zacharie C. Systemic Combination Treatment for Psoriasis: A Review.

[60] Dogra S, Kaur I. Childhood psoriasis. *Pediatric dermatoses* 2010;76: 357-365.

[61] Methotrexate and a compilation of methotrexate skin eruptions. *Dermatology Online Journal* 12(7):15.

[62] Drugs Information Online. Accessed in 2011 July 1st. Available in http://www.drugs.com.

In: Methotrexate
Editors: V. S. Castillo and L. A. Moyano

ISBN: 978-1-62100-596-4
© 2012 Nova Science Publishers, Inc.

Chapter VII

Factors Predicting Clinical Adverse Events during High-Dose Methotrexate Therapy

Yuko Kanbayashi[1], and Masafumi Taniwaki[2]*

[1]Department of Hospital Pharmacy, University Hospital,
Kyoto Prefectural University of Medicine, Kyoto, Japan
[2]Molecular Hematology and Oncology, Kyoto Prefectural University of Medicine,
Graduate School of Medical Science, Kyoto, Japan

Abstract

Sustained elevation of serum methotrexate (MTX) concentrations (>1.0 μM) for 48 h (48-h value) has been found to have predictive significance for the development of toxicity. However, severe adverse events are sometimes encountered during high-dose (HD)-MTX therapy even if serum MTX concentrations comply with recommended values. We designed and conducted a retrospective study to identify predictors for the occurrence of adverse events, and examined whether the 48-h value alone offers a significant predictor of clinical adverse events during HD-MTX therapy. The results showed that 48-h value is not the only predictive value for clinical adverse events during HD-MTX therapy, identifying long infusion time as a significant predictor of general fatigue and neutropenia and higher doses and combination chemotherapy as predictors for stomatitis. This chapter discusses predictors for clinical adverse events during HD-MTX therapy based on our study (retrospective study, n=58 episodes) and further review of recent findings, including genetic factors.

* Corresponding Author: Yuko Kanbayashi, PhD. Department of Hospital Pharmacy, Kyoto Prefectural University of Medicine, Kawaramachi Hirokoji, Kamigyo-ku, Kyoto 602-8566, Japan. E-mail: ykokanba@koto.kpu-m.ac.jp, Tel: +81-75-251-5865, Fax: +81-75-251-5863.

Introduction

The high-dose methotrexate (HD-MTX) regimen (6-h infusion) was established in 1970 as an effective treatment for osteosarcoma, lymphoma and metastatic carcinoma. Recently, HD-MTX with 24-h continuous intravenous infusion (24-h C-IV) procedures, such as hyper-CVAD (cyclophosphamide, vincristine, doxorubicin, and dexamethasone) and HD-MTX/cytarabine regimens have been developed for the treatment of lymphoid malignancies [1-9]. Whether the recommended serum concentration of 1 μM after 48 h of administration (48-h value) represents the only suitable factor for preventing the occurrence of severe adverse events remains unclear, particularly when the 24-h C-IV method is used [7-9]. We designed and conducted a retrospective study to identify predictors for the occurrence of adverse events, and examined whether the 48-h value is the only significant predictor of clinical adverse events during HD-MTX therapy. As a result, we reported "Statistical examination to determine whether only 48-h value for serum concentration during HD-MTX therapy is a predictor for clinical adverse events using ordered logistic regression analysis" [10].

Our Findings: Predictors of Clinical Adverse Events during HD-MTX Therapy

Table 1 shows the clinical characteristics of patients and various factors that could potentially be related to the occurrence of adverse events. All adverse events were categorized according to the Common Terminology Criteria for Adverse Events version 3.0 (CTCAE v3.0). All adverse events categorized by differential grade are listed in Table 2. The ordered logistic regression analysis used in our study demonstrated 24-h C-IV (long infusion time) was a significant predictor for fatigue and neutropenia, and that higher dose and combination chemotherapy were predictors for stomatitis during HD-MTX therapy. Our findings offer evidence of long infusion time as a significant predictor for general fatigue and neutropenia, while higher dose and combination chemotherapy are predictors for stomatitis (Table 3) [10].

MTX Pharmacology

MTX is an antimetabolite and antifolate agent with antineoplastic and immunosuppressant activities. This agent blocks de novo nucleotide synthesis by depleting reduced tetrahydrofolates, mainly through inhibition of dihydrofolate reductase (DHFR) and thymidylate synthase (TS), and subsequent inhibition of DNA and RNA synthesis. MTX also exhibits potent immunosuppressive activity, although the mechanisms of action remain unclear [11].

Following administration of HD-MTX, two metabolites are observed in plasma: 7-hydroxy-methotrexate (7-OH-MTX); and 2,4-diamino-N10-methylpteroic acid (DAMPA), an inactive metabolite. Within 12-24 h of the start of HD-MTX infusion, the plasma concentration of 7-OH-MTX, formed by the action of the hepatic enzyme aldehyde oxidase, exceeds the concentration of MTX [12-15]. Intracellular polyglutamation of 7-OH-MTX results in prolonged retention and enhanced MTX-induced cytotoxicity [16]. MTX and MTX polyglutamates (MTX-PGs) block de novo nucleotide synthesis, primarily by depleting cells of reduced tetrahydrofolate cofactors through inhibition of DHFR [17]. MTX-PGs and dihydrofolates that accumulate as a result of DHFR inhibition also inhibit TS and other enzymes involved in the purine biosynthetic pathway [14, 18, 19]. DAMPA, a minor, inactive [20-22] metabolite of MTX accounting for <5% of the total dose of drug that is excreted in urine [20], is presumably formed from MTX that is excreted into the intestinal tract, hydrolyzed by bacterial carboxypeptidases, and then reabsorbed [14]. Both DAMPA and 7-OH-MTX are six- to ten-fold less soluble than MTX in urine [14, 15].

Low-dose oral and HD-MTX are associated with large interindividual variations in pharmacokinetics, primarily reflecting renal clearance of MTX. For HD-MTX, rapid clearance has been linked to reduced cure rates [15, 23], although not all studies have confirmed this [15, 24]. HD-MTX refers to doses that range from 0.5 to 33.6 g/m^2 or even higher [15, 25]. In general, the higher doses are given with a shorter infusion time.

Table 1. Factors potentially contributing to frequency of adverse events

	n (0/1) or median (range)
Female/Male	28/30
Age <60 years / ≥60 years	35/23
Infusion time (6H/24H)	27/31
Combination chemotherapy	13/45
48-h value (μM)	0.18 (0.02-8.63)
Dose (low/high)	30/28
Disease (leukemia/lymphoma)	13/45

Binary variables were female = 0 and male = 1 for sex, <60 years = 0 and ≥60 years = 1 for age, <3.5 g = 0 and ≥3.5 g = 1 for dose, leukemia = 0, lymphoma = 1 for disease, ≤6 h (6-h C-IV) = 0, 24-h C-IV = 1 for infusion time, and absent = 0, present = 1 for combination chemotherapy.
6H, 6-h or less continuous infusion therapy, *24H*, 24-h continuous infusion therapy.

Table 2. Number of subjects per grade of adverse events *n*=58 (6H, *n*=27; 24H, *n*=31)

	Grade				
	0 (6H/24H)	1 (6H/24H)	2 (6H/24H)	3 (6H/24H)	4 (6H/24H)
Fatigue	22(13/9)	22(13/9)	3(1/2)	11(0/11)	0
Stomatitis	33(16/17)	12(6/6)	3(1/2)	10(4/6)	0
Skin manifestation	53(25/28)	1(0/1)	1(1/0)	2(0/2)	1(1/0)
Nausea/vomiting	24(14/10)	20(10/10)	7(1/6)	7(2/5)	0
Neutropenia	2(2/0)	5(5/0)	9(6/3)	7(4/3)	35(10/25)
Bilirubin	37(16/21)	16(8/8)	5(3/2)	0	0
AST	17(8/9)	28(14/14)	6(1/5)	5(4/1)	2(0/2)
ALT	14(6/8)	19(9/10)	16(9/7)	8(3/5)	1(0/1)
Serum creatinine	48(21/27)	5(2/3)	4(3/1)	1(1/0)	0

6H, ≤6-h continuous infusion therapy; *24H*, 24-h continuous infusion therapy; *AST*, aspartate aminotransferase; *ALT*, alanine aminotransferase.

Table 3. Results of ordered logistic regression analysis for variables extracted by forward selection N=58 episodes

Variable	Estimated value	Standard error	χ^2 value	P	OR	CI of OR	
						Lower 95%	Upper 95%
Response Y = Fatigue (accuracy = 33/58)							
Sex	-0.430	0.292	2.17	0.1411	0.650	0.367	1.153
Age	-0.402	0.271	2.21	0.1375	0.669	0.393	1.137
Dose	0.557	0.298	3.49	0.0618	1.745	0.973	3.131
Infusion time	1.061	0.338	9.92	0.0016[*]	2.890	1.493	5.594
Response Y = Stomatitis (accuracy=37/58)							
Dose	0.825	0.292	7.97	0.0048[*]	2.282	1.287	4.046
Combination chemotherapy	0.778	0.368	4.47	0.0344[*]	2.177	1.059	4.477
Response Y = Neutropenia (accuracy=39/58)							
Sex	-0.563	0.372	2.29	0.1299	0.569	0.275	1.180
48hr-value	-0.692	0.401	2.98	0.0843	0.501	0.228	1.098
Dose	-0.431	0.317	1.84	0.1745	0.650	0.349	1.211
Infusion time	0.945	0.433	4.76	0.0291[*]	2.573	1.101	6.016

OR, odds ratio; CI, confidence interval.
[*]P < 0.05.

The goals of HD-MTX with leucovorin rescue are to increase MTX concentrations in pharmacological sanctuaries (e.g., central nervous system (CNS) and testes), to increase both passive and active cellular MTX uptake in resistant tumor cells, to overcome intracellular resistance mechanisms, and to take advantage of a supposed dose-response relationship with regard to the propensity for MTX polyglutamation, which is lower in certain subsets, such as T-lineage acute lymphoblastic leukemia (ALL) and non-Hodgkin lymphoma (NHL) [15, 26-28]. However, whether these advantages of HD-MTX lead to increased efficacy is debatable, not least since much of the pharmacokinetic/pharmacodynamic HD-MTX data come from non-randomized studies [15, 25, 29-31]. Thus, even though HD-MTX leads to higher MTX concentrations in the cerebrospinal fluid, a recent meta-analysis was unable to demonstrate any significant reduction in the risk of CNS relapse [15, 32].

Predictive Factors for Clinical Adverse Events

1. Long Infusion Time (24-h C-IV)

Our finding that long infusion time (24-h C-IV) offers a significant predictor for the occurrence of neutropenia [10] is supported by the pharmacological features of MTX, because the critical determinant of MTX cytotoxicity is not only drug concentration, but also duration of exposure. In other words, high concentrations of MTX may be well tolerated for short periods of time, whereas prolonged exposure to low concentrations can result in life-threatening toxicity. The type of MTX toxicity is concentration- and time-dependent, and thus directly associated with the pharmacological features of MTX. Previous studies have clarified that exposure to millimolar concentrations of MTX for minutes to hours may lead to acute renal, CNS, and liver toxicity, while exposure to MTX concentrations as low as 0.01 and 0.005 μM for >24 h may result in bone marrow and gastrointestinal epithelial toxicities [14,33].

The relationship between long infusion time and each adverse event based on the existing literature is described as follows.

Stomatitis (Oral Mucositis)

A previous study clarified that no significant relationship exists between the serum MTX concentration and oral mucositis. This in vitro study demonstrated that cell injury was related to the duration of MTX exposure rather than a high MTX concentration [34]. On the other hand, some studies have discussed the relationship between serum MTX concentration and toxicity of oral mucositis. One preliminary study supported the hypothesis that the risk of oral mucositis is associated with the plasma concentration of MTX at 66 h after starting MTX infusion and the level of nausea/vomiting [35]. Another study found high plasma MTX concentrations at 48 h after MTX infusion were not significantly related to MTX-induced toxicities other than mucositis [36]. Mucosal lesions occurred significantly more often and were more severe after intermediate-dose methotrexate (IDM) treatment in a randomized comparison of 36-h IDM versus 4-h HD-MTX infusions for induction of remission in relapsed childhood ALL. Both regimens produced the same remission rates. A tendency toward better antileukemic activity with IDM was accompanied by more severe side effects as a consequence of long-lasting cytotoxic MTX levels. Long-term infusion of IDM followed by low-dose leucovorin is thus an effective treatment for recurrent ALL [37].

Woessmann et al. clarified that the incidence of mucositis grade III/IV (National Cancer Institute-Common Toxicity Criteria (NCI-CTC)) was significantly lower with 4-h HD-MTX infusions in all risk groups. They concluded that 4-h MTX infusion was less toxic than 24-h MTX. In comparison, 4-h MTX infusion was non-inferior to 24-h MTX infusion for limited-stage B-cell non-Hodgkin lymphoma (B-NHL), but not for advanced disease. For limited disease, MTX at 1 g/m^2 is non-inferior to that at 5 g/m^2 [38].

Neutropenia

Joerger et al. clarified that area under the curve (AUC) for HD-MTX did not predict toxicity, with the exceptions of liver toxicity and neutropenia [39]. Their findings agree with ours in terms of neutropenia. Rituximab plus hyper-CVAD alternating with rituximab/MTX/cytarabine is an effective dose-intense chemo-immunotherapy program for untreated mantle cell lymphoma, Burkitt lymphoma, atypical Burkitt lymphoma, and B-ALL. Toxicity is mainly hematological and significant, but expected [40].

2. Higher Dose

Our findings suggest that higher dose is a predictor of stomatitis. The relationship between higher dose and each adverse event based on the literature is described as follows.

Very high dose was associated with significant toxicities, particularly neutropenia, transient hepatic dysfunction and sepsis [25]. Erythrocyte levels of the metabolites and cumulative doses of 6-mercaptopurine (6MP) and MTX do not predict histological liver disease in children treated for ALL [41].

3. Combination Chemotherapy

Our findings also suggest that combination chemotherapy is a predictor for stomatitis. The relationship between combination chemotherapy and each adverse event based on the literature is described as follows.

Through inhibition of de novo purine synthesis and enhancement of 6MP bioavailability, HD-MTX may increase the incorporation into DNA of 6-thioguanine nucleotides (6TGN), a cytotoxic metabolite of 6MP.

van Kooten et al. demonstrated that toxicity after HD-MTX can be influenced by coadministrated antimetabolites, and modifiable by alterations in 6MP dose. Prevention of toxicity-related withdrawals through 6MP dose reduction could be a method of increasing total dose intensity [42]. Schmiegelow et al. also indicated that reductions in the dose of concurrently administered oral 6MP could be one way of reducing the risk of significant myelotoxicity following HD-MTX during maintenance therapy for childhood ALL [43]. Nygaard et al. demonstrated that a reduction in 6MP dosage during HD-MTX can significantly reduce the risk of severe myelotoxicity and prevent treatment interruptions. They concluded that reducing the dose of 6MP from 2 weeks before to 2 weeks after HD-MTX represents one way to decrease bone-marrow toxicity and avoid treatment interruptions in patients who have previously developed significant myelotoxicity after HD-MTX/6MP [44].

The risk here may be even higher in patients with low-activity alleles for thiopurine methyltransferase (TPMT), probably because such patients have higher cytosol levels of 6TGN [44, 45]. As for genetic factors, these are discussed in a later section.

4. Other Factors Predicting Adverse Events

Renal Dysfunction

HD-MTX-induced renal dysfunction leads to delayed renal excretion of MTX and sustained elevation of plasma MTX concentrations that can markedly enhance the toxicities of MTX. Pharmacological interventions to treat this emergency include administration of high-dose leucovorin [46, 47], glucarpidase (carboxypeptidase-G2) [48-50], or thymidine [50,51].

Green et al. found that male patients over 50 years old are at greatest risk of renal dysfunction [52]. MTX-associated nephropathy is a rare complication in pediatric oncology, and a review of the literature suggests that exposure to nephrotoxic agents may be a significant but perhaps under-recognized risk factor for the development of this pathology [53].

Hyper-alkalinization appears to offer an efficient and reliable method to prevent the acute renal toxicity of HD-MTX and allows safe administration in the outpatient setting [54].

Santucci et al. reported an interesting paper about Cola beverages, which show a low pH due to the phosphoric acid content that is excreted renally. They recommend patients receiving HD-MTX abstain from any cola drink from 24 h before MTX administration until complete elimination of the drug [55]. Yarlagadda et al. reported that acute renal failure can occur during HD-MTX due to precipitation of MTX crystals in the kidney [56], and such compromised kidney function will significantly delay MTX clearance. To date, no useful approaches are available to predict the individual risk of acute renal failure prior to HD-MTX therapy.

However, early recognition of the problem is feasible, as such patients often demonstrate an early rise in serum creatinine levels. Skärby et al. thus described a rise of more than 50% within 24 h from the start of MTX infusion (5.0-8.0 $g/m^2/24$ h) offered 32% sensitivity and 99% specificity for predicting delayed MTX elimination [9]. Thus, in courses with normal MTX elimination, 99% had a rise in serum creatinine under 50% [9]. This early prediction allows intensification of hydration and alkalization to reduce MTX crystallization and improve MTX excretion [14].

Jahnke et al. evaluated HD-MTX as a safe treatment for patients with primary CNS lymphoma regardless of age, with adherence to dose reduction as determined by calculating the GFR before each treatment cycle [57].

Hepatotoxicity

In a multivariate analysis, factors associated with abnormal markers of liver fibrosis were body mass index over 28 kg/m^2 and high alcohol consumption. Neither long duration of MTX administration nor cumulative dose was associated with elevated Fibro Scan or Fibro Test results. Severe liver fibrosis is a rare event in patients treated with MTX and is probably unrelated to the total dose. Patients with other risk factors for liver disease should be closely monitored with non-invasive methods before and during MTX treatment [58]. Halonen et al. concluded that erythrocyte levels of metabolites or cumulative doses of 6MP and MTX do not predict histological liver disease in children treated for ALL [59].

5. Genetic Polymorphisms

Recent studies showing a correlation between MTX clearance and various single nucleotide polymorphisms (SNPs) are described as follows.

Methylenetetrahydrofolate Reductase

5,10-Methylene-tetrahydrofolate reductase (MTHFR) is central to folate metabolism and has two common functional polymorphisms: C677T and A1298G. MTX inhibits the synthesis of thymidylate monophosphate (dTMP) needed for DNA replication by blocking the conversion of 5,10-methylene-tetrahydrofolate(MTHF) to 5- MTHF by MTHFR. The MTHFR C677T polymorphism is a common mutation of the gene encoding the enzyme that catalyzes the reduction of 5,10-MTHF to 5-MTHF, a carbon donor in the metabolism of folate. Several reports have evaluated the MTHFR C677T variant allele and MTX toxicity. Reported toxicities include hepatotoxicity, gastrointestinal toxicity, therapy interruption and vomiting, bone marrow toxicity, neurotoxicity, mucositis and prolonged thrombocytopenia [15].

Ulrich et al. first described an association between the MTHFR C677T variant genotype and an increased oral mucositis index in 220 patients receiving MTX in allogeneic stem cell transplantation for chronic myelogenous leukemia. They concluded that patients with decreased MTHFR activity appear at risk of higher MTX toxicity. Given the high prevalence of the TT genotype, these results may have implications for MTX dosage [60]. Chiusolo et al. reported on a group of 61 patients, finding that those individuals heterozygous for the MTHFR C677T polymorphism showed an increased risk of treatment-related toxicity in four different adult ALL protocols with different doses and schedules of MTX administration. They concluded that the TT genotype may indicate a need to reduce the MTX dose during prolonged administration. Considering the high prevalence of homozygous individuals in the Italian population, pretreatment screening may be worthwhile [61].

Ongaro et al. found that hepatic toxicity increased in proportion to the number of 677T alleles present in the genotype of patients (32% CC, 47% CT and 73% TT). Patients with the TT genotype showed a 5.23-fold increased risk of developing hepatic toxicity (p=0.028) when compared to patients with the wild-type genotype (CC). Furthermore, TT patients also exhibited a 6.43-fold increase in the risk of leukopenia (p=0.019), although this was found only in univariate analysis [62]. Müller et al. hypothesized that MTX toxicity could be explained by the association between homozygosity of the MTHFR C677T polymorphism causing disturbances in folate status and thus enhanced vulnerability of the CNS to antimetabolites and prolonged MTX exposure due to delayed MTX clearance [63]. Faganel et al. clarified that a population pharmacokinetic model developed in their study implied only a limited influence of genetic factors on the systemic disposition of MTX. Clearance is moderately reduced in patients with the MTHFR 677TT genotype. In addition, genetic polymorphisms in the folate metabolic pathway and solute carrier (SLC) 19A1 and reduced folate carrier (RFC) genes were associated with HD-MTX toxicity. They concluded that the protective role of the MTHFR 1298A>C, TS 2R>3R and SLC19A1 80A>G polymorphisms in HD-MTX-associated toxicities was demonstrated and an increased risk for HD-MTX-associated mucositis was found with the MTHFR 677 C>T polymorphism [64].

Kantar et al. found that the A1298C gene, but not the C677T polymorphism, is associated with MTX-related toxicity [65]. Patiño-García et al. found that patients with osteosarcoma with severe hematological toxicity were more frequently TT than CT/CC for C677T/MTHFR (P = .023) and GG for A2756G/MTR. They concluded that the roles of C677T/MTHFR and A2756G/MTR in chemotherapy-induced toxicity should be further investigated for pediatric osteosarcomas receiving HD-MTX [66]. Gemmati et al. suggested that MTHFR gene variants play a critical role in NHL outcome, possibly by interfering with the action of MTX, with significant effects on toxicity and survival. Genotyping of the folate pathway gene variants might be useful to enable reductions in chemotherapy toxicity and/or to improve survival by indicating when dose adjustments or alternative treatments are necessary [67].

On the other hand, Kishi et al. found no association between the MTHFR C677T variant allele and either seizure or thrombosis risk among 53 pediatric patients receiving HD-MTX therapy for de novo ALL; other toxicity end points were not reported [68]. Aplenc et al. reported that they did not observe any association between MTX toxicity and MTHFR C677T variant allele [69]. Seidemann et al. found no association of MTHFR 677 genotype with clinical characteristics (sex, age, and tumor stage), outcomes, or therapy-related toxicities could be detected. They thus concluded that the MTHFR 677 C-->T polymorphism did not appear to influence outcomes or therapy-associated toxicities in pediatric patients with NHL treated in their multicenter trial with Berlin-Frankfurt-Münster (BFM) protocols [70]. Shimasaki et al. also found no significant differences in the development of other toxicities or in plasma MTX concentrations for the different MTHFR 677C>T orRFC1 80G>A polymorphisms. They suggested, but could not confirm, that the RFC1 80G>A polymorphism may contribute to interindividual variability in responses to high-dose MTX [71].

Polyglutamation

In contrast, low-activity SNPs in c-glutamyl hydrolase, such as GGH 452C>T, may increase intracellular MTX-PGs and MTX cytotoxicity against leukemic cells. These studies demonstrated a substrate-specific functional SNP (452C>T) in the human gamma-glutamyl hydrolase gene that is associated with lower catalytic activity and higher accumulation of long-chain MTX-PGs in leukemia cells of patients treated with HD-MTX [72].

Transport

RFC is involved in the transport of MTX across the cell membrane. The RFC gene (SLC19A1) is located on chromosome 21. Gregers et al. found the reduced folate carrier SLC19A1 80G>A polymorphism interacts with copy numbers of chromosome 21 and affects both efficacy and toxicity of MTX [73].

Rau et al. suggest a hitherto unknown gender-specific impact of the -24C>T ATP-binding cassette, sub-family C, number 2 (ABCC2) gene polymorphism on HD-MTX pharmacokinetics. While a nonfunctional multidrug resistance-related protein 2 (MRP2) variant has been described in a patient with severe impairment of MTX excretion, their study is the first study to suggest that a frequent ABCC2 polymorphism contributes to the variability of MTX kinetics [74].

Conclusion

Predictive factors for clinical adverse events were described based on our previous research. Our study was able to show that the 48-h value is not the only predictor of clinical adverse events during HD-MTX therapy. A major limitation of the study was the small number of subjects.

However, our findings suggest that long infusion time is a significant predictor for general fatigue and neutropenia, and that higher doses and combination chemotherapy are predictors for stomatitis. Risk factors for high-dose MTX-induced toxicity such as gene polymorphism have already been reported [60-74], but the interrelationship of pharmacokinetics and gene polymorphisms in particular will need to be verified in further investigations.

However, to ensure patient safety and satisfactory outcomes, a prospective study is needed to establish optimal therapeutic drug monitoring, particularly during long infusion of HD-MTX therapy.

References

[1]   Ritchie DS, Seymour JF, Grigg AP, Roberts AW, Hoyt R, Thompson S, Szer J, Prince HM. (2007). The hyper-CVAD-rituximab chemotherapy programme followed by high-dose busulfan, melphalan and autologous stem cell transplantation produces excellent event-free survival in patients with previously untreated mantle cell lymphoma. *Ann. Hematol.* 86: 101-5.

[2]   Romaguera JE, Fayad L, Rodriguez MA, Broglio KR, Hagemeister FB, Pro B, McLaughlin P, Younes A, Samaniego F, Goy A, Sarris AH, Dang NH, Wang M, Beasley V, Medeiros LJ, Katz RL, Gagneja H, Samuels BI, Smith TL, Cabanillas FF. (2005). High rate of durable remissions after treatment of newly diagnosed aggressive mantle-cell lymphoma with rituximab plus hyper-CVAD alternating with rituximab plus high-dose methotrexate and cytarabine. *J. Clin. Oncol.* 23: 7013-23.

[3]   Hagemeister FB. (2003). Mantle cell lymphoma: non-myeloablative versus dose-intensive therapy. *Leuk. Lymphoma* 44: S69-75.

[4]   Todeschini G, Tecchio C, Pasini F, Benedetti F, Cantini M, Crippa C, Draisci M, Pizzolo G. (2005). Hyperfractionated cyclophosphamide with high-doses of arabinosylcytosine and methotrexate (HyperCHiDAM Verona 897). *Cancer* 104: 555-60.

[5]   Khouri IF, Saliba RM, Okoroji GJ, Acholonu SA, Champlin RE. (2003). Long-term follow-up of autologous stem cell transplantation in patients with diffuse mantle cell lymphoma in first disease remission: the prognostic value of beta2-microglobulin and the tumor score. *Cancer* 98: 2630-5.

[6]   Romaguera JE, Khouri IF, Kantarjian HM, Hagemeister FB, Rodriguez MA, McLaughlin P, Sarris AH, Younes A, Rodriguez J, Cabanillas F. (2000). Untreated aggressive mantle cell lymphoma: results with intensive chemotherapy without stem cell transplant in elderly patients. *Leuk. Lymphoma* 39: 77-85.

[7]   Rask C, Albertioni F, Bentzen SM, Schroeder H, Peterson C. (1998). Clinical and pharmacokinetic risk factors for high-dose methotrexate-induced toxicity in children with acute lymphoblastic leukemia--a logistic regression analysis. *Acta Oncol.* 37: 277-284.

[8]   Joannon P, Oviedo I, Campbell M. (2004). High-dose methotrexate therapy of childhood acute lymphoblastic leukemia: lack of relation between serum methotrexate concentration and creatinine clearance. *Pediatr. Blood Cancer* 43: 17-22.

[9]   Skärby T, Jönsson P, Hjorth L, Behrentz M, Björk O, Forestier E, Jarfelt M, Lönnerholm G, Höglund P. (2003). High-dose methotrexate: on the relationship of methotrexate elimination time vs renal function and serum methotrexate levels in 1164 courses in 264 Swedish children with acute lymphoblastic leukaemia (ALL). *Cancer Chemother. Pharmacol.* 51: 311-20.

[10] Kanbayashi Y, Nomura K, Okamoto K, Matsumoto Y, Horiike S, Takagi T, Taniwaki M. (2010). Statistical examination to determine whether only 48-h value for serum concentration during high-dose methotrexate therapy is a predictor for clinical adverse events using ordered logistic regression analysis. *Ann. Hematol.* 89: 965-9.

[11] http://www.cancer.gov/drugdictionary?CdrID=41719

[12] Jacobs SA, Stoller RG, Chabner BA, Johns DG. (1976). 7-Hydroxymethotrexate as a urinary metabolite in human subjects and rhesus monkeys receiving high dose methotrexate. *J. Clin. Invest.* 57: 534-8.

[13] Lankelma J, van der Klein E, Ramaekers F. (1980). The role of 7-hydroxymethotrexate during methotrexate anti-cancer therapy. *Cancer Lett.* 9: 133-42.

[14] Widemann BC, Adamson PC. (2006). Understanding and managing methotrexate nephrotoxicity. *Oncologist* 11: 694-703.

[15] Schmiegelow K. (2009). Advances in individual prediction of methotrexate toxicity: a review. *Br. J. Haematol.* 146: 489-503.

[16] Sholar PW, Baram J, Seither R, Allegra CJ. (1988). Inhibition of folate-dependent enzymes by 7-OH-methotrexate. *Biochem. Pharmacol.* 37: 3531-4.

[17] Messmann R, Allegra C. Antifolates. In Chabner B, Longo D, eds. Cancer Chemotherapy and Biotherapy. Philadelphia: Lippincott Williams and Wilkins, 2001: 139-184.

[18] Chabner BA, Allegra CJ, Curt GA, Clendeninn NJ, Baram J, Koizumi S, Drake JC, Jolivet J. (1985). Polyglutamation of methotrexate: is methotrexate a prodrug? *J. Clin. Invest.* 76: 907-12.

[19] Allegra CJ, Chabner BA, Drake JC, Lutz R, Rodbard D, Jolivet J. (1985). Enhanced inhibition of thymidylate synthase by methotrexate polyglutamates. *J. Biol. Chem.* 260: 9720-6.

[20] Donehower RC, Hande KR, Drake JC, Chabner BA. (1979). Presence of 2,4-diamino-N10-methylpteroic acid after high-dose methotrexate. *Clin. Pharmacol. Ther.* 6: 63-72.

[21] Widemann BC, Sung E, Anderson L, Salzer WL, Balis FM, Monitjo KS, McCully C, Hawkins M, Adamson PC. (2000). Pharmacokinetics and metabolism of the methotrexate metabolite 2, 4-diamino-N(10)-methylpteroic acid. *J. Pharmacol. Exp. Ther.* 294: 894-901.

[22] Widemann BC, Balis FM, Adamson PC. (1999). Dihydrofolate reductase enzyme inhibition assay for plasma methotrexate determination using a 96-well microplate reader. *Clin. Chem.* 45: 223-8.

[23] Evans WE, Crom WR, Abromowitch M, Dodge R, Look AT, Bowman WP, George SL, Pui CH. (1986). Clinical pharmacodynamics of high-dose methotrexate in acute lymphocytic leukemia. Identification of a relation between concentration and effect. *N. Engl. J. Med.* 314:471-7.

[24] Skarby TV, Anderson H, Heldrup J, Kanerva JA, Seidel H, Schmiegelow K. (2006). High leucovorin doses during high-dose methotrexate treatment may reduce the cure rate in childhood acute lymphoblastic leukemia. *Leukemia* 20: 1955-62.

[25] Nathan PC, Whitcomb T, Wolters PL, Steinberg SM, Balis FM, Brouwers P, Hunsberger S, Feusner J, Sather H, Miser J, Odom LF, Poplack D, Reaman G, Bleyer WA. (2006). Very high-dose methotrexate (33.6 g/m^2) as central nervous system preventive therapy for childhood acute lymphoblastic leukemia: results of National Cancer Institute/Children's Cancer Group trials CCG-191P, CCG-134P and CCG-144P. *Leuk. Lymphoma* 47: 2488-504.

[26] Jolivet, J. (1987) Biochemical and pharmacologic rationale for high-dose methotrexate. *NCI Monographs* 5: 61-5.

[27] Barredo JC, Synold TW, Laver J, Relling MV, Pui CH, Priest DG, Evans WE. (1994). Differences in constitutive and post-methotrexate folylpolyglutamate synthetase activity in B-lineage and T-lineage leukemia. *Blood*, 84: 564-9.

[28] Galpin AJ, Schuetz JD, Masson E, Yanishevski Y, Synold TW, Barredo JC, Pui CH, Relling MV, Evans WE. (1997). Differences in folylpolyglutamate synthetase and dihydrofolate reductase expression in human B-lineage versus T-lineage leukemic lymphoblasts: mechanisms for lineage differences in methotrexate polyglutamylation and cytotoxicity. *Mol. Pharmacol.* 52: 155-63.

[29] Mantadakis E, Cole PD, Kamen BA. (2005). High-dose methotrexate in acute lymphoblastic leukemia: where is the evidence for its continued use? *Pharmacotherapy* 25: 748-55.

[30] Whitehead VM, Shuster JJ, Vuchich MJ, Mahoney DH Jr, Lauer SJ, Payment C, Koch PA, Cooley LD, Look AT, Pullen DJ, Camitta B. (2005). Accumulation of methotrexate and methotrexate polyglutamates in lymphoblasts and treatment outcome in children with B-progenitor-cell acute lymphoblastic leukemia: a Pediatric Oncology Group study. *Leukemia* 19: 533-6.

[31] Pui CH (2006). Central nervous system disease in acute lymphoblastic leukemia: prophylaxis and treatment. Hematology American Society of Hematology. *Education Program* 142-6.

[32] Clarke M, Gaynon P, Hann I, Harrison G, Masera G, Peto R, Richards S. (2003) CNS-directed therapy for childhood acute lymphoblastic leukemia: Childhood ALL Collaborative Group overview of 43 randomized trials. *Journal of Clinical Oncology* 21: 1798-809.

[33] Chabner BA, Young RC. (1973).Threshold methotrexate concentration for in vivo inhibition of DNA synthesis in normal and tumorous target tissues. *J. Clin. Invest.* 52: 1804-11.

[34] Maiguma T, Hayashi Y, Ueshima S, Kaji H, Egawa T, Chayama K, Morishima T, Kitamura Y, Sendo T, Gomita Y, Teshima D. (2008).Relationship between oral mucositis and high-dose methotrexate therapy in pediatric acute lymphoblastic leukemia. *Int. J. Clin. Pharmacol. Ther.* 46: 584-90.

[35] Cheng KK. (2008). Association of plasma methotrexate, neutropenia, hepatic dysfunction, nausea/vomiting and oral mucositis in children with cancer. *Eur. J. Cancer Care* (Engl). 17: 306-11.

[36] Shimasaki N, Mori T, Samejima H, Sato R, Shimada H, Yahagi N, Torii C, Yoshihara H, Tanigawara Y, Takahashi T, Kosaki K. (2006). Effects of methylenetetrahydrofolate reductase and reduced folate carrier 1 polymorphisms on high-dose methotrexate-induced toxicities in children with acute lymphoblastic leukemia or lymphoma. *J. Pediatr. Hematol. Oncol.* 28: 64-8.

[37] Wolfrom C, Hartmann R, Fengler R, Brühmüller S, Ingwersen A, Henze G. (1993). Randomized comparison of 36-hour intermediate-dose versus 4-hour high-dose methotrexate infusions for remission induction in relapsed childhood acute lymphoblastic leukemia. *J. Clin. Oncol.* 11: 827-33.

[38] Woessmann W, Seidemann K, Mann G, Zimmermann M, Burkhardt B, Oschlies I, Ludwig WD, Klingebiel T, Graf N, Gruhn B, Juergens H, Niggli F, Parwaresch R, Gadner H, Riehm H, Schrappe M, Reiter A; BFM Group. (2005). The impact of the methotrexate administration schedule and dose in the treatment of children and

adolescents with B-cell neoplasms: a report of the BFM Group Study NHL-BFM95. *Blood* 105: 948-58.

[39]   Joerger M, Huitema AD, Krähenbühl S, Schellens JH, Cerny T, Reni M, Zucca E, Cavalli F, Ferreri AJ. (2010). Methotrexate area under the curve is an important outcome predictor in patients with primary CNS lymphoma: a pharmacokinetic-pharmacodynamic analysis from the IELSG no. 20 trial. *Br. J. Cancer* 102: 673-7.

[40]   Fayad L, Thomas D, Romaguera J. (2007). Update of the M. D. Anderson Cancer Center experience with hyper-CVAD and rituximab for the treatment of mantle cell and Burkitt-type lymphomas. *Clin. Lymphoma Myeloma Suppl.* 2: S57-62.

[41]   Halonen P, Mattila J, Mäkipernaa A, Ruuska T, Schmiegelow K. (2006) Erythrocyte concentrations of metabolites or cumulative doses of 6-mercaptopurine and methotrexate do not predict liver changes in children treated for acute lymphoblastic leukemia. *Pediatr. Blood Cancer*, 46: 762-6.

[42]   van Kooten Niekerk PB, Schmiegelow K, Schroeder H. (2008). Influence of methylene tetrahydrofolate reductase polymorphisms and coadministration of antimetabolites on toxicity after high dose methotrexate. *Eur. J. Haematol.* 81: 391-8.

[43]   Schmiegelow K, Bretton-Meyer U. (2001). 6-mercaptopurine dosage and pharmacokinetics influence the degree of bone marrow toxicity following high-dose methotrexate in children with acute lymphoblastic leukemia. *Leukemia* 15: 74-9.

[44]   Nygaard U, Schmiegelow K. (2003). Dose reduction of coadministered 6-mercaptopurine decreases myelotoxicity following high-dose methotrexate in childhood leukemia. *Leukemia* 17: 1344-8.

[45]   Andersen, J.B, Szumlanski, C, Weinshilboum, R.M, Schmiegelow, K. (1998). Pharmacokinetics, dose adjustments, and 6-mercaptopurine/methotrexate drug interactions in two patients with thiopurine methyltransferase deficiency. *Acta Paediatrica* 87: 108-11.

[46]   Bleyer WA. (1977). Methotrexate: clinical pharmacology, current status and therapeutic guidelines. *Cancer Treat. Rev.* 4: 87-101.

[47]   Djerassi I. (1975). High-dose methotrexate (NSC-740) and citrovorum factor (NSC-3590) rescue: background and rationale. *Cancer Chemother. Rep.* 6: 3-6.

[48]   Buchen S, Ngampolo D, Melton RG, Hasan C, Zoubek A, Henze G, Bode U, Fleischhack G. (2005). Carboxypeptidase G2 rescue in patients with methotrexate intoxication and renal failure. *Br. J. Cancer* 92: 480-7.

[49]   Schwartz S, Borner K, Müller K, Martus P, Fischer L, Korfel A, Auton T, Thiel E. (2007). Glucarpidase (carboxypeptidase g2) intervention in adult and elderly cancer patients with renal dysfunction and delayed methotrexate elimination after high-dose methotrexate therapy. *Oncologist* 12:1299-308.

[50]   Widemann BC, Balis FM, Murphy RF, Sorensen JM, Montello MJ, O'Brien M, Adamson PC. (1997). Carboxypeptidase-G2, thymidine, and leucovorin rescue in cancer patients with methotrexate-induced renal dysfunction. *J. Clin. Oncol.* 15:2125-34.

[51]   Howell SB, Herbst K, Boss GR, Frei E 3rd. (1980). Thymidine requirements for the rescue of patients treated with high-dose methotrexate. *Cancer Res.* 40:1824-9.

[52]   Green MR, Chamberlain MC. (2009). Renal dysfunction during and after high-dose methotrexate. *Cancer Chemother. Pharmacol.* 63: 599-604.

[53] Fong CM, Lee AC. High-dose methotrexate-associated acute renal failure may be an avoidable complication. (2006). *Pediatr. Hematol. Oncol.* 23: 51-7.

[54] Mir O, Ropert S, Babinet A, Alexandre J, Larousserie F, Durand JP, Enkaoua E, Anract P, Goldwasser F. (2010). Hyper-alkalinization without hyper-hydration for the prevention of high-dose methotrexate acute nephrotoxicity in patients with osteosarcoma. *Cancer Chemother. Pharmacol.* 66: 1059-63.

[55] Santucci R, Levêque D, Herbrecht R. (2010). Cola beverage and delayed elimination of methotrexate. *Br. J. Clin. Pharmacol.* 70: 762-4.

[56] Yarlagadda SG, Perazella MA. (2008). Drug-induced crystal nephropathy: an update. *Expert Opinion on Drug Safety* 7: 147-58.

[57] Jahnke K, Korfel A, Martus P, Weller M, Herrlinger U, Schmittel A, Fischer L, Thiel E; German Primary Central Nervous System Lymphoma Study Group (G-PCNSL-SG). (2005). High-dose methotrexate toxicity in elderly patients with primary central nervous system lymphoma. *Ann. Oncol.* 16: 445-9.

[58] Laharie D, Seneschal J, Schaeverbeke T, Doutre MS, Longy-Boursier M, Pellegrin JL, Chabrun E, Villars S, Zerbib F, de Lédinghen V. (2010). Assessment of liver fibrosis with transient elastography and FibroTest in patients treated with methotrexate for chronic inflammatory diseases: a case-control study. *J. Hepatol.* 53: 1035-40.

[59] Halonen P, Mattila J, Mäkipernaa A, Ruuska T, Schmiegelow K. (2006). Erythrocyte concentrations of metabolites or cumulative doses of 6-mercaptopurine and methotrexate do not predict liver changes in children treated for acute lymphoblastic leukemia. *Pediatr. Blood Cancer* 46: 762-6.

[60] Ulrich CM, Yasui Y, Storb R, Schubert MM, Wagner JL, Bigler J, Ariail KS, Keener CL, Li S, Liu H, Farin FM, Potter JD. (2001). Pharmacogenetics of methotrexate: toxicity among marrow transplantation patients varies with the methylenetetrahydrofolate reductase C677T polymorphism. *Blood*, 98: 231-4.

[61] Chiusolo P, Reddiconto G, Casorelli I, Laurenti L, Sorà F, Mele L, Annino L, Leone G, Sica S. (2002). Preponderance of methylenetetrahydrofolate reductase C677T homozygosity among leukemia patients intolerant to methotrexate. *Ann. Oncol.* 13: 1915-8.

[62] Ongaro A, De Mattei M, Della Porta MG, Rigolin G, Ambrosio C, Di Raimondo F, Pellati A, Masieri FF, Caruso A, Catozzi L, Gemmati D. (2009). Gene polymorphisms in folate metabolizing enzymes in adult acute lymphoblastic leukemia: effects on methotrexate-related toxicity and survival. *Haematologica* 94: 1391-8.

[63] Müller J, Kralovánszky J, Adleff V, Pap E, Németh K, Komlósi V, Kovács G. (2008). Toxic encephalopathy and delayed MTX clearance after high-dose methotrexate therapy in a child homozygous for the MTHFR C677T polymorphism. *Anticancer Res.* 28(5B): 3051-4.

[64] Faganel Kotnik B, Grabnar I, Bohanec Grabar P, Dolžan V, Jazbec J. (2011). Association of genetic polymorphism in the folate metabolic pathway with methotrexate pharmacokinetics and toxicity in childhood acute lymphoblastic leukaemia and malignant lymphoma. *Eur. J. Clin. Pharmacol.* in press.

[65] Kantar M, Kosova B, Cetingul N, Gumus S, Toroslu E, Zafer N, Topcuoglu N, Aksoylar S, Cinar M, Tetik A, Eroglu Z. (2009). Methylenetetrahydrofolate reductase C677T and A1298C gene polymorphisms and therapy-related toxicity in children

treated for acute lymphoblastic leukemia and non-Hodgkin lymphoma. *Leuk. Lymphoma*, 50: 912-7.

[66] Patiño-García A, Zalacaín M, Marrodán L, San-Julián M, Sierrasesúmaga L. (2009). Methotrexate in pediatric osteosarcoma: response and toxicity in relation to genetic polymorphisms and dihydrofolate reductase and reduced folate carrier 1 expression. *J. Pediatr.* 154: 688-93.

[67] Gemmati D, Ongaro A, Tognazzo S, Catozzi L, Federici F, Mauro E, Della Porta M, Campioni D, Bardi A, Gilli G, Pellati A, Caruso A, Scapoli GL, De Mattei M. (2007). Methylenetetrahydrofolate reductase C677T and A1298C gene variants in adult non-Hodgkin's lymphoma patients: association with toxicity and survival. *Haematologica* 92: 478-85.

[68] Kishi S, Griener J, Cheng C, Das S, Cook EH, Pei D, Hudson M, Rubnitz J, Sandlund JT, Pui CH, Relling MV. (2003). Homocysteine, pharmacogenetics, and neurotoxicity in children with leukemia. *J. Clin. Oncol.* 21: 3084-91.

[69] Aplenc R, Thompson J, Han P, La M, Zhao H, Lange B, Rebbeck T. (2005). Methylenetetrahydrofolate reductase polymorphisms and therapy response in pediatric acute lymphoblastic leukemia. *Cancer Res.* 65: 2482-7.

[70] Seidemann K, Book M, Zimmermann M, Meyer U, Welte K, Stanulla M, Reiter A. (2006). MTHFR 677 (C->T) polymorphism is not relevant for prognosis or therapy-associated toxicity in pediatric NHL: results from 484 patients of multicenter trial NHL-BFM 95. *Ann. Hematol.* 85: 291-300.

[71] Shimasaki N, Mori T, Samejima H, Sato R, Shimada H, Yahagi N, Torii C, Yoshihara H, Tanigawara Y, Takahashi T, Kosaki K. (2006). Effects of methylenetetrahydrofolate reductase and reduced folate carrier 1 polymorphisms on high-dose methotrexate-induced toxicities in children with acute lymphoblastic leukemia or lymphoma. *J. Pediatr Hematol. Oncol.* 28: 64-8.

[72] Cheng Q, Wu B, Kager L, Panetta JC, Zheng J, Pui CH, Relling MV, Evans WE. (2004). A substrate specific functional polymorphism of human gamma-glutamyl hydrolase alters catalytic activity and methotrexate polyglutamate accumulation in acute lymphoblastic leukaemia cells. *Pharmacogenetics* 14: 557-67.

[73] Gregers J, Christensen IJ, Dalhoff K, Lausen B, Schroeder H, Rosthoej S, Carlsen N, Schmiegelow K, Peterson C. (2010). The association of reduced folate carrier 80G>A polymorphism to outcome in childhood acute lymphoblastic leukemia interacts with chromosome 21 copy number. *Blood* 115: 4671-7.

[74] Rau T, Erney B, Göres R, Eschenhagen T, Beck J, Langer T. (2006). High-dose methotrexate in pediatric acute lymphoblastic leukemia: impact of ABCC2 polymorphisms on plasma concentrations. *Clin. Pharmacol. Ther.* 80:468-76.

In: Methotrexate
Editors: V. S. Castillo and L. A. Moyano

ISBN: 978-1-62100-596-4
© 2012 Nova Science Publishers, Inc.

Chapter VIII

Animals Models of Cognitive Impairment Induced by Methotrexate

Laura Lyons, Geoff Bennett
and Peter Wigmore
School of Biomedical Sciences, University of Nottingham, UK

Abstract

Methotrexate is an antimetabolite commonly used in adjuvant combination chemotherapy treatments. Patients treated with methotrexate have frequently complained of cognitive impairment. This phenomenon encompasses problems with memory and concentration and is reported to occur in many cancer survivors for several years after treatment.

Attempts to quantify these effects by psychometric testing of patients has been confounded by factors, including multi drug treatments, patient stress and fatigue and the effect of the cancer itself.

This has led to the use of rodent models to study chemotherapy-induced cognitive impairment. These studies have allowed the investigation of single chemotherapy agents and are not compromised by the confounding factors associated with patient testing. Animal investigations have used a range of behavioural tests including the Morris water maze, novel object/location recognition tasks and conditioning to investigate the effects of methotrexate on behaviour.

These tests have shown that methotrexate can significantly impair a range of memory paradigms. Furthermore research in rodents has allowed the investigation of potential underlying mechanisms including the effects of methotrexate on the proliferation, survival and apoptosis of cells involved in adult hippocampal neurogenesis and the demyelination of white matter tracts. Herein, we review this research and discuss potential approaches for intervention.

An Introduction to Chemotherapy-Induced Cognitive Impairment

As treatment for cancer has continually improved, this has led to a reduced risk of reoccurrence and a higher survival rate for patients. Therefore, it is becoming increasingly important to research possible improvements for the quality of life of cancer survivors as well as cancer treatment. Chemotherapy is often given as adjuvant treatment against cancer, frequently administered in combination with surgery, radiation and hormonal therapy. Although this treatment is often effective, chemotherapy is notorious for its many side effects. One area of side effects, described by a substantial number of patients, is problems with cognition including working memory, concentration and general confusion [1]. These symptoms have been reported to occur from immediately after chemotherapy administration to ten years after completion of treatment [2]. Although, the cognitive deficits are usually subtle [1], they have been reported to affect the ability of cancer survivors to return to work and resume a normal life [3].

Methotrexate is a folate antagonist which is used as a chemotherapy agent as well as an anti-inflammatory and/or immunosuppressive treatment for autoimmune diseases [4]. When used to treat malignancies, it is often used in chemotherapy combinations which are associated with cognitive decline [5-11]. Although chemotherapy-induced cognitive impairment has been reported in patients who have received treatment for solid tumours including breast, lung, prostate and ovarian cancers [12], the majority of clinical studies are carried out on survivors of breast cancer [13].

Clinical studies which have investigated chemotherapy combinations containing methotrexate have found a mild to moderate effect on working, visual and verbal memory [5, 10, 11]. It has been difficult to evaluate the prevalence of the cognitive impairment and estimations suggest between 13% and 75% of patients who have received methotrexate chemotherapy treatment have some form of cognitive decline [8, 14]. One reason for the variation in these figures may be the confounding factors of clinical trials which could contribute to the cognitive deficit observed in patients. Such factors include the stress and fatigue cancer patients are likely to experience during the course of treatment, as well as the effect of the cancer itself. Many variables including the dose, type and administration of chemotherapy and patient individuality (eg. age, menopausal status) have proved difficult to control, thereby contributing to a reduced sample size. It is also difficult to find appropriate controls to compare with chemotherapy treated patients. For these reasons animal models have been utilised to investigate chemotherapy-induced cognitive impairment in order to elucidate specific causal links.

Rodent models have made it possible to examine the effects of individual chemotherapy agents on memory together with the possible causes, and have made it possible to develop interventions to counteract the cognitive side effects of chemotherapy. Different chemotherapy agents have been investigated as single agents or in combinations with particular emphasis on the antimetabolites methotrexate (see Table 1) and 5-fluorouracil [15-17]. The effects of other chemotherapies with different mechanisms of action have also been investigated such as cyclophosphamide [17-19] and doxorubicin [20-22].

Table 1. Summary of rodent models investigating the effect of methotrexate (MTX) either alone or in combination with 5-fluorouracil (5-FU) on cognition, listed in chronological order from most recent

Study	Animals	Dose and administration of MTX	Time post MTX	Cognitive assessment and outcome	Comments
Walker et al., 2011	Male Swiss-Webster mice (20-25g)	MTX: 3.2 or 32mg/kg 5-FU: 75mg/kg MTX+5-FU: 3.2/32+75mg/kg all i.p. weekly for 3 weeks	8 and 9 days	Impaired acquisition and retention response (autoshaping)	Effects of MTX and 5-FU were potentiated in combination Impaired acquisition and retention response (autoshaping) with chronic tamoxifen treatment
Yang et al., 2011	Male C57BL/6 mice (8-9 weeks old)	40mg/kg, single i.p. injection	1 and 7 days	Impaired in NOR	Dose dependant reduction in proliferation of hippocampal cells Increased depression–like behaviour
Lyons et al., 2011	Male Lister-hooded rats (150-200g)	75 mg/kg, 2 i.p. weekly injections followed by LCV rescue	1 month	Impaired in NLR	Reduced proliferation and survival of hippocampal cells MTX impairments reversed by fluoxetine (10mg/kg/day)
Fardell et al., 2010	Male Wistar rats (303-460g)	250mg/kg, single i.p. injection followed by LCV rescue	11, 95 and 255 days	Impaired in NOR at all time points Impaired in MWM at 95 days	
Li et al., 2010b	Acute: Male Long-Evans rats (12 weeks old) Chronic: Male and female Long-Evans rats (2 weeks old)	Acute: 250mg/kg, single i.p. injection Chronic: 1mg/kg, 10 i.p. injections. 2 weekly for 2 weeks then weekly for 6 weeks	3-7 days	Acute and chronic: Impaired in NLR Unimpaired in NOR	Acute and chronic: No impairment in activity or motor coordination Reduced folate levels in both CSF and serum and decreased ratio of CSF S-adenosylmethionine to S-adenosylhomocysteine
Li et al., 2010a	Male Long-Evans rats (12 weeks old)	0.5mg/kg, intrathecal over 1min	3-7 days	Impaired in NOR and NLR	Reduced folate levels in both CSF and serum and increased CSF homocysteine No effect on locomotor, exploratory and anxiety-like behaviour
Seigers et al., 2009	Male Wistar rats (3 months old)	250mg/kg, single i.v. injection followed by LCV rescue	MWM: 1 week CFC: 1 month	Impaired in MWM and CFC	Reduced proliferation of hippocampal cells at 7 days, but not 1 day Reduced white matter density at 1 day and 1 and 3 weeks No reduction in apoptosis of hippocampal cells

Table 1. (Continued)

Study	Animals	Dose and administration of MTX	Time post MTX	Cognitive assessment and outcome	Comments
Foley et al., 2008	Male Swiss-Webster mice (20-35g)	MTX: 1-32mg/kg MTX+5-FU: 3.2+75mg/kg All single ip injections	1 and 2 days	MTX did not reduce operant conditioning either day MTX+5-FU reduced operant conditioning on both days	Enhanced effects with combined drugs
Gandal et al., 2008	Male C57BL/6Hsd mice (7-8 weeks old)	MTX+5-FU: 19+37.5mg/kg 37.5+75mg/kg 4 i.p. weekly injections	6-7 weeks	Unimpaired in NOR and CFC	Impaired gating of auditory stimuli (electrophysiology)
Seigers et al., 2008	Male Wistar rats (3 months old)	250mg/kg, single i.v. injection followed by LCV rescue	3-4 weeks	Impaired in MWM and NOR	Dose dependant reduction proliferation of hippocampal cells
Winocur et al., 2006	Female BALB/C mice (2 months old)	MTX+5-FU: 37.5+75mg/kg, single i.p. injection	1 month	Impaired in spatial MWM, NMTS and dNMTS Unimpaired in cue memory and discrimination learning	
Madhyastha et al., 2002	Male Wistar rats (4 months old)	1.5 or 2mg/kg, cannula into lateral ventrical, 3 doses, every other day	7 days	Impaired in conditioned aviodance learning and memory	Reduced concentrations of brain neurotransmitters (noradrenalin, dopamine, and serotonin) and 5-hydroxyindoleacetic acid No effect on anxiety-like behaviour
Sieklucka-Dziuba et al., 1998	Male and female Albino Swiss mice (20-25g)	10 mg/kg, single i.p. injection	24 h, 7 days and 14 days	Impaired passive avoidance at 14 days Unimpaired passive avoidance at 24 h and 7 days	Decreased GABA in brain tissue Increased susceptibility to seizures
Stock et al., 1994	Male and female Sprague-Dawley rats (17 days old)	0.005mg/kg, single i.p. injection	10 weeks	Unimpaired in taste aversive conditioning	
Yanovskiet al., 1989	Male and female Lewis-inbred rats (16-17 days old)	0.005mg/kg, single i.p. injection	10 weeks	Impaired in CER and taste aversive conditioning	

Abbreviations; MWM: Morris water maze, NOR: novel object recognition, NLR: novel location recognition, NMTS: non-matching to sample, dNMTS: delayed non-matching to sample, CFC: contextual fear conditioning, CSF: cerebrospinal fluid.

A number of behavioural tests have been used to investigate different areas of cognition (reviewed by Siegers and Fardell, 2011) and the majority of studies report that chemotherapy has a negative effect on cognition [15, 16, 18, 20-22]. In contrast, some studies found no effect on certain cognitive tasks [17, 19, 23] and one study curiously observed an improvement in spatial learning after treatment [17]. Variance of cognitive outcome is likely to be due to the different behavioural tests used, different dosing regimens and the particular chemotherapy agent used.

This chapter provides an overview of rodent studies investigating the effects of methotrexate on cognition and the possible underlying causes of the memory deficits it produces. Furthermore, potential pharmacological and behavioural methods of treatment to counteract cognitive decline are reviewed.

Animal Models of Cognitive Impairment and Neurobiological Changes Induced by Methotrexate

The recent use of *in vivo* animal models has provided a faster and more detailed method to research chemotherapy-induced cognitive impairment. In addition, they have enabled the investigation of the underlying mechanisms and neuropathological changes to discover the underlying basis for cognitive dysfunction. Existing models have used a number of cytostatic drugs, investigating the effects of both single agents and drugs used in combination [24]. Methotrexate is by far the most commonly investigated antimetabolite and studies to date are summarised in Table 1. The first study investigating the effect of methotrexate on cognition was in 1989 [25], although the majority have been carried out in the past 5 years using a range of behavioural tasks to explore different learning and memory paradigms (Table 1). In a number of these studies, the neurobiological changes and possible anatomical loci for the cognitive impairments have also been investigated.

Effects of Methotrexate in the Novel Object Recognition (NOR) Task in Rodent Models

An array of cognitive tests can be used to investigate different types of memory in rodents. In the literature, the behavioural test most frequently used to detect the cognitive effects of methotrexate, is the novel object recognition (NOR) task (Table 1). This task was first developed by Ennaceur and Delacour [26] and is a two trial recognition task used to assess working memory. During the task, an animal is allowed to explore two identical objects in an arena before being removed from the arena for a defined period of time (familiarisation trial). The animal is then returned to the arena with one of the objects replaced with a new object and exploration time of each object is again recorded (choice trial). If the animal has an unimpaired working memory, it will normally explore the novel object for longer during the choice trial due to an innate preference to explore novelty. This test is appropriate for investigating chemotherapy-induced cognitive impairment as working memory deficit has been described in chemotherapy patients [27, 28]. Results from using this test have however been contradictory with some reporting that methotrexate impairs performance in the NOR task indicating a deficit in working memory lasting from 1 to 255 days after treatment [29-32] while other studies using methotrexate, or a combination of methotrexate and 5-fluorouracil, found no effect on the performance of this task [23, 33].

Effects of Methotrexate in the Novel Location Recognition (NLR) and Morris Water Maze (MWM) Tasks in Rodent Models

Tasks which have been demonstrated to involve spatial working memory such as the novel location recognition (NLR) and Morris water maze (MWM) tasks have also been utilized to investigate cognitive effects of methotrexate in rodent models. The NLR task, developed by Dix and Aggleton [34], is a spatial variant of the NOR task which requires animals to remember the positions of two identical objects in an arena, rather than the objects themselves as in the NOR task. The MWM tests an animal's ability to remember the position of a hidden platform in a circular pool full of opaque water over a defined period of time. Ability in both of these tasks is impaired by hippocampal damage [35-37], consistent with the hippocampal association with spatial tasks.

Along with working memory, spatial memory has also been described as a cognitive deficit for patients who have received chemotherapy [38]. This also appears to be the case in animal models, as rodents which have received methotrexate treatment have been reported to be impaired in the NLR task from 3 days to a month after treatment [29, 33, 39] and the MWM task, with animals making a larger number of errors to find the submerged platform, for up to 255 days after treatment [31, 32, 40]. Brain regions involved with chemotherapy induced cognitive impairment are further discussed below.

Effects of Methotrexate in the Contextual Fear Conditioning (CFC), Conditioned Emotional Response (CER) and Other Tasks in Rodent Models

The contextual fear conditioning (CFC) task has been used in two methotrexate studies in rodents. It shows the ability of an animal to predict aversive footshocks, by measuring its freezing time when placed in a chamber where it previously received shocks. One study showed that drug-treated rats' ability was reduced in this task [40], indicating impaired contextual memory whilst another found that methotrexate had no effect [23]. The conditioned emotion response (CER) task is similar to the CFC but an auditory tone is given as a signal for a footshock rather than the animal being placed in a familiar environment. In the first study investigating methotrexate on cognition, rats which received a very low dose of methotrexate (0.005mg/kg) were impaired in this test 10 weeks after treatment [25]. Fear conditioning is a complex process reliant on a number of brain regions including the amygdala and cingulate gyrus, with the hippocampus more involved in CFC compared to CER [41-43]. Rodents' ability to perform other tasks including conditioned and passive avoidance has also been shown to be impaired by methotrexate [44, 45]. Two groups also looked at the effects of the chemotherapy drug on taste aversion, with one finding methotrexate impaired ability on this task [25] whilst the other study did not see an effect [46] after the same 10 week time period. Methotrexate induced effects on CFC and CER implicate various brain regions other than the hippocampus as discussed below.

Effects of Methotrexate and 5-Fluorouracil in Combination in Rodent Models

Clinically, methotrexate is often administered to cancer patients with other chemotherapy agents, including 5-fluorouracil. Two studies in rodents have investigated the effects of this combination on cognition. One found that treatment impaired the ability of mice in the MWM and in non-match to sample tasks but not in cue memory and discrimination learning [47]. A subsequent investigation did not find any effect of a methotrexate and 5-flourouracil combination on the NOR or CFC tasks [23]. Interestingly, in another study, methotrexate alone did not reduce operant conditioning in mice, but potentiated the effects of 5-fluoruacil Foley et al. [48]. Furthermore a dose dependant potentiating effect was seen in impaired acquisition and retention response (autoshaping) when methotrexate was co-administered with 5-fluorouracil [49]. These results suggest that combination chemotherapy may produce larger cognitive deficits than monotherapy with single agents. Studies investigating the effects of 5-fluorouracil alone have also associated 5-fluorouracil treatment with a cognitive deficit [15, 16].

Dose, Timing and Administration of Methotrexate in Rodent Models

In the studies described above, the dose and route of administration methotrexate varied widely with doses from 0.005mg/kg [25] to 250mg/kg [31-33, 40] showing cognitive decline. As very high doses of methotrexate can be toxic to patients and animals, a number of studies have co-administered [31, 32, 39, 40] calcium folinate (leucovorin/LCV) to replenish folate pools depleted by methotrexate [4]. However LCV alone has no effect on cognition in rodents [50].

When chemotherapy is administered to cancer patients, it is rarely given as a single dose. To model this, many of the studies in rodents have used chronic or sub-chronic dosing of methotrexate (Table 1), from 2 [39] to 10 [33] injections. Although, it is difficult to make direct comparisons between separate studies, it does not appear that chronic dosing increases any cognitive impairment observed (Table 1). For instance Li et al. [33] found that a series of 10 low dose injections of methotrexate had a similar effect to a single high dose injection, both protocols impairing the performance of rats in the NLR, but not the NOR task.

Another factor that has varied across the studies presented in Table 1 is the amount of time between the final methotrexate injection and the behavioural testing. One study found that cognition in mice was impaired in the NOR, 1 day after a single injection [30], whereas in a different behavioural test (operant conditioning), no impairment was seen at this time [48]. Different time points have also been investigated in single studies, demonstrating that the ability of mice in the passive avoidance task was impaired at 14 days, but not at 7 and 24 days after a single methotrexate injection [44]. In addition rats were impaired in the NOR task at 11, 95 and 255 days after a single high dose (250mg/kg) methotrexate injection, although these animals were only impaired in the MWM at the 95 day time point [31]. This highlights the importance of the time period between treatment and testing when comparing between individual studies.

Neurobiological Effects of Methotrexate and Potential Underlying Mechanisms of Chemotherapy Induced Cognitive Impairment

Brain Regions Associated with Chemotherapy-Induced Cognitive Impairment

It is probable that several brain regions are involved in chemotherapy induced cognitive impairment. A number of the tasks in which the animals' ability was impaired by methotrexate involve the hippocampus, an area associated with learning and memory consolidation [51]. Lesions in the hippocampus have been shown to impair performance in spatial memory tests such as the NLR, MWM and CFC tasks [35, 42, 43, 52]. More specifically, it has been reported that dentate gyrus lesions reduce rats' ability in the NLR task [53].

Methotrexate-treated animals are also impaired in behavioural tests involving fear conditioning, including the CFC and CER tasks. These tasks involve associating an unpleasant stimulus such as a footshock with a contextual or audio cue such as a familiar chamber or tone respectively. Learning this association requires the cingulate gyrus and the amygdala [41, 54]. Although the hippocampus is thought to be involved in the CFC, it is not required for the CER task [42, 43]. Therefore, it appears that numerous brain areas may be affected by methotrexate and it is not the effect of the chemotherapy on a single region of the brain which causes cognitive decline.

Effects of Methotrexate on Hippocampal Neurogenesis

Many studies have looked at structural changes in the brains of rodents after testing for the cognitive effects of methotrexate. In particular the impact of methotrexate on adult hippocampal neurogenesis which requires the continued proliferation of new cells in the dentate gyrus (see Table 1). The dentate gyrus is one of the few brain regions which continue to produce new neurones throughout adulthood and this neurogenic process is thought to be required for learning and memory [51]. Numerous studies in rodents have observed correlations between hippocampal neurogenesis and cognition, extensively reviewed by Zhao et al. [55]. These investigations have shown that environmental factors which increase hippocampal proliferation also have a positive effect on hippocampal dependant learning. This association is further strengthened by the finding that transgenic mice in which cell proliferation is decreased, are also impaired in memory tasks [55]. As methotrexate is a cytostatic agent, targeting proliferating cancerous cells, it is likely that it is also toxic to neural stem cells proliferating in the hippocampus, which could be one explanation for the cognitive deficit seen.

To date, all the studies in rodents have found that treatment with methotrexate reduces the number of proliferating neural progenitors in the hippocampus [30, 32, 39, 40]. This reduction in the production of the cells required for hippocampal neurogenesis has been shown to be dose dependant [30, 32] and to last for at least a month [39] after administration. The effect of methotrexate on cell proliferation may in fact increase with time after the completion of drug treatment and appears to be independent of apoptosis [40]. The long term survival of newly generated hippocampal cells has also been found to be reduced in animals which received methotrexate [39]. The significant and persistent effects of methotrexate on hippocampal neurogenesis provide one explanation for the long term effects on memory described by patients who have been given methotrexate chemotherapy.

Effects of Methotrexate on Levels of Neurotransmitters

The levels of several neurotransmitters have been shown to be affected by methotrexate. Concentrations of noradrenalin, dopamine, serotonin and its metabolite 5-hydroxyindoleacetic acid were all lower in the brains of rats treated with methotrexate and these animals were also cognitively impaired in conditioned avoidance testing [45]. Another study observed that methotrexate reduced levels of GABA in brain tissue of mice [44]. Such neurotransmitters are implicated in behavioural performance and in particular serotonin and dopamine modulate learning and memory [56], suggesting that a reduction of brain neurotransmitter function may be a mechanism by which methotrexate causes cognitive impairment.

Effects of Methotrexate on White Matter

Studies have demonstrated using MRI that adjuvant chemotherapy affects the white matter tracts of the CNS in patients with breast cancer [57]. The effects of high doses of methotrexate were investigated in rats and shown to induce white matter necrosis [58] and decreased white matter density in the corpus callosum [40]. White matter is important for neuronal signalling and damage to it could contribute to the delay in cognitive processing.

Effects of Cancer on Cognitive Impairment

It has been questioned whether the cancer itself could cause some of the cognitive deficits seen in cancer patients [59]. As the animals used to model the cognitive effects of chemotherapy in general do not have cancer this question has until recently not been addressed. However, one study has shown that the presence of a tumour in rats did cause some reduction in cell proliferation in the hippocampus. The presence of the tumour was however much less than the impact of methotrexate and the combination of tumour load and methotrexate showed no additive effect [60]. This could suggest that the cancer itself may contribute to cognitive impairment and may explain why some patients are found to have cognitive deficits prior to the start to treatment. This should be taken into account when considering memory deficits in cancer patients and tested during interludes between chemotherapy where possible.

Potential Methods of Intervention for Chemotherapy-Induced Cognitive Impairment

Despite the growing evidence of the negative effects of methotrexate on the brain and cognition, few studies have tested how to how to counteract these side effects. One difficulty is the variety of potential causes for cognitive impairments after chemotherapy, making it difficult to pin down a specific target. However, some preliminary potential methods of intervention have been investigated and suggested [15, 24, 39, 48].

As previously discussed, there is evidence to suggest that methotrexate targets proliferating neural precursors in the hippocampus which impacts on cognition. Fluoxetine, a selective serotonin reuptake inhibitor (SSRI) antidepressant, has been shown to up-regulate hippocampal neurogenesis [61-65].

Due to the correlation between fluoxetine and neurogenesis and neurogenesis and memory [51], it is reasonable to expect fluoxetine to enhance cognition. Although fluoxetine does not affect healthy subjects [66], several studies have found that fluoxetine improves cognition when it has been impaired. In clinical studies, fluoxetine has been reported to improve deficits in memory in patients suffering from moderate to severe depression [67-69], mild cognitive impairment [70], traumatic brain injury [71] and post traumatic stress disorder [72].

Effects of Fluoxetine on Methotrexate Induced Cognitive Decline

In addition, several experiments have been carried out to investigate the effects of fluoxetine on memory in rodents, reviewed by Monleon et al. [66]. Collectively these yield a range of results which could be due to the type of memory tested in the tasks or due to animals having no cognitive impairment before fluoxetine administration [66]. Positive effects of fluoxetine on cognition have also been reported in rodent models by counteraction of memory impairment caused from hypoxia [73], olfactory bulbectomy [74, 75], scopolamine and electroconvulsive shock [76].

Work within our laboratory in Nottingham has investigated the combined effects of fluoxetine and methotrexate in rat [39]. Rats sub-chronically treated with methotrexate alone (followed by leucovorin rescue) performed worse than the controls in the NLR spatial memory task compared to controls (Figure 1a). A separate group treated with both methotrexate and fluoxetine were unimpaired in this task, while animals treated with fluoxetine alone showed no cognitive enhancement compared to controls (Figure 1a). Methotrexate treated animals also had a lower number of proliferating cells in the subgranular zone of the dentate gyrus which was reversed by co-administration with fluoxetine (Figure 1b).

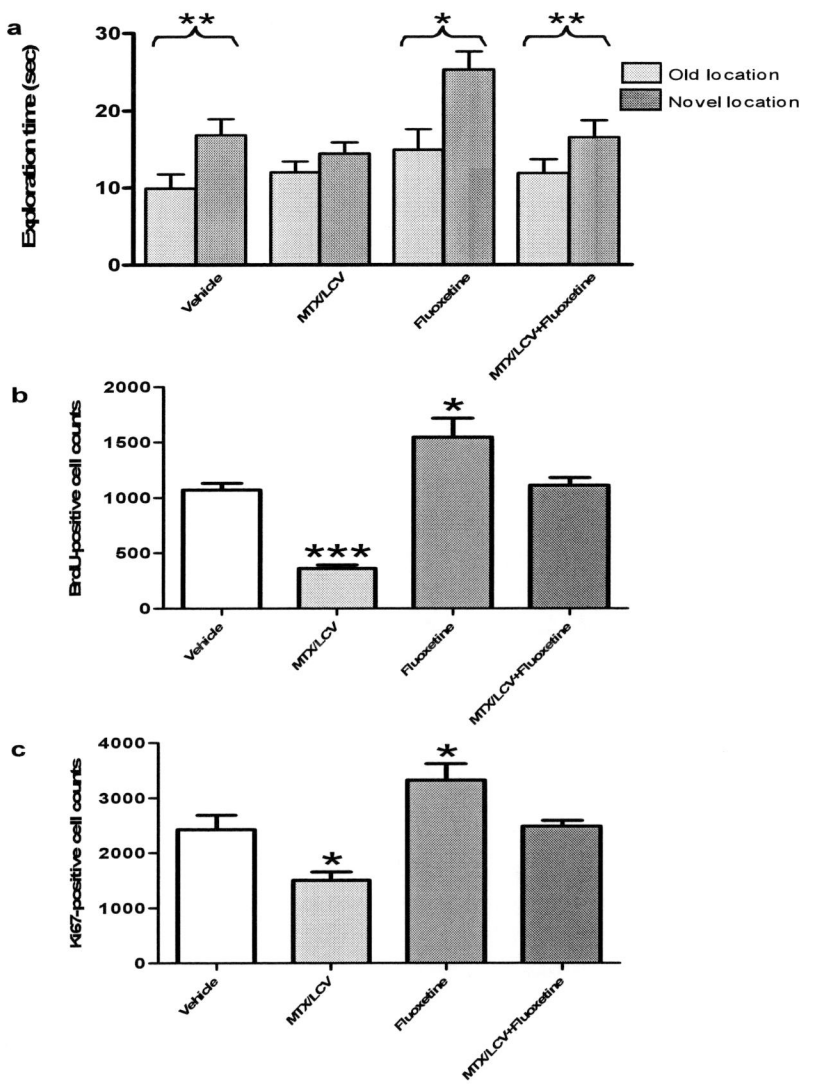

Figure 1. Effects of methotrexate (MTX; 75mg/kg, 2 weekly i.v. doses followed by leucovorin (LCV) rescue), selective serotonin reuptake inhibitor (SSRI) antidepressant, fluoxetine (10mg/kg/day) and both in combination in Lister-hooded rats (each group n=12). a) Exploration time in the test trial of the novel location recognition (NLR) task. Animals treated with MTX/LCV spent no significant difference in time exploring either object, indicating impairment in spatial working memory ($p > 0.05$, Student's paired t-test). All other groups spent longer exploring the object in the novel location memory (*$p < 0.05$, **$p < 0.01$, Student's paired t-tests), indicating that alone, fluoxetine has no effect on spatial working memory, but reverses the deficit caused by MTX. b) BrdU was administered with the first dose of MTX/LCV. The number of BrdU-positive cells in the dentate gyrus of the hippocampus was reduced in MTX/LCV (*$p < 0.05$, ***$p < 0.001$, one-way ANOVA) treated animals, and increased in animals which received fluoxetine. Animals treated with MTX/LCV and fluoxetine did not differ from the controls ($p > 0.05$). This suggests that MTX is toxic to newly proliferating hippocampal cells and the effect can be counteracted with co-administration of fluoxetine. c) The number of Ki67-positive cells in the dentate gyrus of the hippocampus was reduced in MTX/LCV (*$p < 0.05$, one-way ANOVA) treated animals, and increased in animals which received fluoxetine. Animals treated with MTX/LCV and fluoxetine did not differ from the controls (*$p > 0.05$) suggesting that fluoxetine is neuro-protective to proliferating hippocampal cells. Graphs all sourced from Lyons et al. 2011.

In addition, the survival of hippocampal cells which were dividing at the beginning of treatment which was reduced by methotrexate was similarly counteracted by administration of fluoxetine (Figure 1 c). This demonstrates that fluoxetine has neuro-protective properties and could offer a relatively simple method to alleviate the cognitive impairment produced by methotrexate [39]. It is likely that other antidepressants may have a similar effect, but at present have not been investigated as to their ability to reverse the effects of methotrexate.

External Factors Additional to Fluoxetine Treatment with Beneficial Reversal of Cognitive Decline

To the authors' knowledge there are no other animal models which successfully reverse the effects of cognitive impairment produced by methotrexate, although alternatives have been considered [24]. Physical activity is reported to have a beneficial influence on cognition and brain function in healthy subjects [77] and to improve cognitive performance in patients whose memory is impaired by bipolar disorder [78], Alzheimer's disease and aging [79]. Furthermore, exercise has been demonstrated to have a positive effect on neuronal mechanisms which are implicated in chemotherapy-induced cognitive impairment, such as hippocampal neurogenesis [80], neurotransmitter systems [81] and white matter integrity [82]. Therefore it would be practical to investigate the benefits of exercise in patients treated with methotrexate to see if it able to alleviate cognitive impairment.

A handful of clinical studies have been carried investigating possible interventions for chemotherapy-induced cognitive impairment. Administration of erythropoietin, a hormone which regulates the production of erythrocytes, along with adjuvant chemotherapy was shown to enhance cognitive function in breast cancer patients [83, 84]. In addition, the psychostimulant, modafinil, has been reported to improve cognitive performance in breast cancer patients, with the drug improving memory and attention skills [85]. Although not examined in these studies, it would be interesting to investigate the ability of these drugs to specifically counteract the effects of methotrexate.

Conclusion

Methotrexate is used in chemotherapy combinations which have been reported to cause memory deficits in cancer survivors. Although it is difficult to look directly at the cognitive and neurobiological effects of the drug in patients, there have been several investigations using rodents to model these effects, which avoid some of the confounding variables found in human patient trials. Results from these studies demonstrate that treatment with methotrexate can have a negative effect on cognition. However, this effect is highly dependent on different factors, including the dose of the drug, the behavioural test used and the time period between the two (Table 1). The use of rodent models has also enabled researchers to investigate the neurobiological changes of drug treatment, which have shown that methotrexate affects hippocampal neurogenesis, brain levels of a range of neurotransmitters and white matter tracts. Although further work is still necessary to fully understand the underlying neural mechanisms, literature is already emerging on potential strategies to counteract or reduce cognitive impairment induced by methotrexate.

References

[1]   Matsuda, T., et al., Mild cognitive impairment after adjuvant chemotherapy in breast cancer patients--evaluation of appropriate research design and methodology to measure symptoms. *Breast Cancer*, 2005. 12(4): p. 279-87.

[2]   Ahles, T.A. and A.J. Saykin, Breast cancer chemotherapy-related cognitive dysfunction. *Clin. Breast Cancer*, 2002. 3 Suppl 3: p. S84-90.

[3]   Boykoff, N., M. Moieni, and S. Subramanian, Confronting chemobrain: an in-depth look at survivors' reports of impact on work, social networks, and health care response. *Journal of Cancer Survivorship*, 2009. 3(4): p. 223-232.

[4]   Genestier, L., et al., Mechanisms of action of methotrexate. *Immunopharmacology*, 2000. 47(2-3): p. 247-257.

[5]   Kreukels, B.P., et al., Persistent neurocognitive problems after adjuvant chemotherapy for breast cancer. *Clin. Breast Cancer*, 2008. 8(1): p. 80-7.

[6]   Hurria, A., et al., Cognitive function of older patients receiving adjuvant chemotherapy for breast cancer: a pilot prospective longitudinal study. *J. Am. Geriatr. Soc*, 2006. 54: p. 925 - 931.

[7]   Donovan, K.A., et al., Cognitive functioning after adjuvant chemotherapy and/or radiotherapy for early-stage breast carcinoma. *Cancer*, 2005. 104(11): p. 2499-507.

[8]   Wieneke, M.H. and E.R. Dienst, Neuropsychological assessment of cognitive functioning following chemotherapy for breast cancer. *Psycho-oncology*, 1995. 4: p. 61-66.

[9]   Schagen, S.B., et al., Cognitive deficits after postoperative adjuvant chemotherapy for breast carcinoma. *Cancer*, 1999. 85(3): p. 640-50.

[10]   Brezden, C.B., et al., Cognitive function in breast cancer patients receiving adjuvant chemotherapy. *J. Clin. Oncol*, 2000. 18(14): p. 2695-701.

[11]   Shilling, V., et al., The effects of adjuvant chemotherapy on cognition in women with breast cancer--preliminary results of an observational longitudinal study. *Breast*, 2005. 14(2): p. 142-50.

[12]   Argyriou, A.A., et al., Either Called "Chemobrain" or "Chemofog," the Long-Term Chemotherapy-Induced Cognitive Decline in Cancer Survivors Is Real. *Journal of Pain and Symptom Management*, 2011. 41(1): p. 126-139.

[13]   Castellon, S.A., D.H. Silverman, and P.A. Ganz, Breast cancer treatment and cognitive functioning: current status and future challenges in assessment. *Breast Cancer Res. Treat*, 2005. 92(3): p. 199-206.

[14]   Schagen, S.B., et al., Late effects of adjuvant chemotherapy on cognitive function: a follow-up study in breast cancer patients. *Ann. Oncol*, 2002. 13(9): p. 1387-97.

[15]   ElBeltagy, M., et al., Fluoxetine improves the memory deficits caused by the chemotherapy agent 5-fluorouracil. *Behav. Brain Res*, 2010. 208(1): p. 112-117.

[16] Mustafa, S., et al., 5-Fluorouracil chemotherapy affects spatial working memory and newborn neurones in the adult rat hippocampus. *European Journal of Neuroscience*, 2008. 10(1111): p. 1460-9568.

[17] Lee, G.D., et al., Transient improvement in cognitive function and synaptic plasticity in rats following cancer chemotherapy. *Clin. Cancer Res*, 2006. 12(1): p. 198-205.

[18] Yang, M., et al., Cyclophosphamide impairs hippocampus-dependent learning and memory in adult mice: Possible involvement of hippocampal neurogenesis in chemotherapy-induced memory deficits. *Neurobiology of Learning and Memory*, 2010. 93(4): p. 487-494.

[19] Reiriz, A., Reolon, GK, Preissler, T, Rosado, JO, Henriques, JAP, Roesler, R, Schwartsmann, G, Cancer Chemotherapy and Cognitive Function in Rodent Models: Memory Impairment Induced by Cyclophosphamide in Mice Clinical Cancer Research Vol. 12, 5000-5001, August 15, 2006, 2006. 12: p. 5000-5001.

[20] Liedke, P.E.R., et al., Systemic administration of doxorubicin impairs aversively motivated memory in rats. *Pharmacology Biochemistry and Behavior*, 2009. 94(2): p. 239-243.

[21] Konat, G., et al., Cognitive dysfunction induced by chronic administration of common cancer chemotherapeutics in rats. *Metabolic Brain Disease*, 2008. 23(3): p. 325-333.

[22] MacLeod, J.E., et al., Cancer chemotherapy impairs contextual but not cue-specific fear memory. *Behavioural Brain Research*, 2007. 181(1): p. 168-172.

[23] Gandal, M.J., et al., A novel electrophysiological model of chemotherapy-induced cognitive impairments in mice. *Neuroscience*, 2008. 157(1): p. 95-104.

[24] Seigers, R. and J.E. Fardell, Neurobiological basis of chemotherapy-induced cognitive impairment: A review of rodent research. *Neuroscience and Biobehavioral Reviews*, 2011. 35(3): p. 729-741.

[25] Yanovski, J.A., et al., An animal model to detect the neuropsychological toxicity of anticancer agents. *Medical and Pediatric Oncology*, 1989. 17(3): p. 216-21.

[26] Ennaceur, A. and J. Delacour, A new one-trial test for neurobiological studies of memory in rats. 1: Behavioral data. *Behav. Brain Res*, 1988. 31(1): p. 47-59.

[27] Collins, B., et al., Cognitive effects of chemotherapy in post-menopausal breast cancer patients 1 year after treatment. *Psycho-oncology*, 2009. 18(2): p. 134-143.

[28] Jenkins, V., et al., A 3-year prospective study of the effects of adjuvant treatments on cognition in women with early stage breast cancer. *Br. J. Cancer*, 2006. 94(6): p. 828-34.

[29] Li, Y., et al., Intrathecal methotrexate induces focal cognitive deficits and increases cerebrospinal fluid homocysteine. *Pharmacology Biochemistry and Behavior*, 2010. 95(4): p. 428-433.

[30] Yang, M., et al., Neurotoxicity of methotrexate to hippocampal cells in vivo and in vitro. *Biochemical Pharmacology*, 2011. In Press, Corrected Proof.

[31] Fardell, J.E., et al., Single high dose treatment with methotrexate causes long-lasting cognitive dysfunction in laboratory rodents. *Pharmacology Biochemistry and Behavior*, 2010. 97(2): p. 333-339.

[32] Seigers, R., et al., Long-lasting suppression of hippocampal cell proliferation and impaired cognitive performance by methotrexate in the rat. *Behav. Brain Res*, 2008. 186: p. 168-175.

[33] Li, Y., et al., Systemic methotrexate induces spatial memory deficits and depletes cerebrospinal fluid folate in rats. *Pharmacology Biochemistry and Behavior*, 2010. 94(3): p. 454-463.

[34] Dix, S.L. and J.P. Aggleton, Extending the spontaneous preference test of recognition: evidence of object-location and object-context recognition. *Behav. Brain Res*, 1999. 99(2): p. 191-200.

[35] Mumby, D.G., et al., Hippocampal damage and exploratory preferences in rats: memory for objects, places, and contexts. *Learn Mem*, 2002. 9(2): p. 49-57.

[36] Clark, R.E., N.J. Broadbent, and L.R. Squire, The hippocampus and spatial memory: findings with a novel modification of the water maze. *J. Neurosci*, 2007. 27(25): p. 6647-54.

[37] D'Hooge, R. and P.P. De Deyn, Applications of the Morris water maze in the study of learning and memory. *Brain Research Reviews*, 2001. 36(1): p. 60-90.

[38] Tannock, I.F., et al., Cognitive impairment associated with chemotherapy for cancer: report of a workshop. *J. Clin. Oncol*, 2004. 22(11): p. 2233-9.

[39] Lyons, L., et al., Fluoxetine reverses the memory impairment and reduction in proliferation and survival of hippocampal cells caused by methotrexate chemotherapy. *Psychopharmacology*, 2011. 215(1): p. 105-115.

[40] Seigers, R., et al., Methotrexate decreases hippocampal cell proliferation and induces memory deficits in rats. *Behavioural Brain Research*, 2009. 201(2): p. 279-284.

[41] Ponnusamy, R., A.M. Poulos, and M.S. Fanselow, Amygdala-dependent and amygdala-independent pathways for contextual fear conditioning. *Neuroscience*, 2007. 147(4): p. 919-927.

[42] Radulovic, J. and N.C. Tronson, Molecular specificity of multiple hippocampal processes governing fear extinction. *Reviews in the Neurosciences*, 2010. 21(1): p. 1-17.

[43] Phillips, R.G. and J.E. LeDoux, Differential contribution of amygdala and hippocampus to cued and contextual fear conditioning. *Behavioral Neuroscience*, 1992. 106(2): p. 274-85.

[44] Sieklucka-Dziuba, M., et al., Central action of some cytostatics--methotrexate (MTX) and doxorubicin (DXR). I. Long-term influence on the pain sensitivity and activity of brain dopaminergic system in mice. *Ann. Univ. Mariae Curie Sklodowska Med*, 1998. 53: p. 71-9.

[45] Madhyastha, S., et al., Hippocampal brain amines in methotrexate-induced learning and memory deficit. *Canadian Journal of Physiology and Pharmacology*, 2002. 80(11): p. 1076-84.

[46] Stock, H.S., et al., Methotrexate does not interfere with an appetitive Pavlovian conditioning task in Sprague-Dawley rats. *Physiology and Behavior*, 1995. 58(5): p. 969-973.

[47] Winocur, G., et al., The effects of the anti-cancer drugs, methotrexate and 5-fluorouracil, on cognitive function in mice. *Pharmacology Biochemistry and Behavior*, 2006. 85(1): p. 66-75.

[48] Foley, J., R. Raffa, and E. Walker, Effects of chemotherapeutic agents 5-fluorouracil and methotrexate alone and combined in a mouse model of learning and memory. *Psychopharmacology* (Berl), 2008. 208(1): p. 112-7.

[49] Walker, E.A., Animal models. *Advances in Experimental Medicine and Biology*, 2010. 678: p. 138-46.

[50] Lalonde, R., C.C. Joyal, and M.I. Botez, Effects of folic acid and folinic acid on cognitive and motor behaviors in 20-month-old rats. *Pharmacology Biochemistry and Behavior*, 1993. 44(3): p. 703-707.

[51] Deng, W., J.B. Aimone, and F.H. Gage, New neurons and new memories: how does adult hippocampal neurogenesis affect learning and memory? *Nat. Rev. Neurosci*, 2010. 11(5): p. 339-350.

[52] Dere, E., J.P. Huston, and M.A. De Souza Silva, The pharmacology, neuroanatomy and neurogenetics of one-trial object recognition in rodents. *Neuroscience and Biobehavioral Reviews*, 2007. 31(5): p. 673-704.

[53] Lee, I., M.R. Hunsaker, and R.P. Kesner, The role of hippocampal subregions in detecting spatial novelty. *Behav. Neurosci*, 2005. 119(1): p. 145-53.

[54] Malin, E.L. and J.L. McGaugh, Differential involvement of the hippocampus, anterior cingulate cortex, and basolateral amygdala in memory for context and footshock. *Proceedings of the National Academy of Sciences of the United States of America*, 2006. 103(6): p. 1959-1963.

[55] Zhao, C., W. Deng, and F.H. Gage, Mechanisms and Functional Implications of Adult Neurogenesis. *Cell*, 2008. 132(4): p. 645-660.

[56] González-Burgos, I., et al., Serotonin/dopamine interaction in memory formation, in *Progress in Brain Research*. 2008, Elsevier. p. 603-623.

[57] Abraham, J., et al., Adjuvant chemotherapy for breast cancer: effects on cerebral white matter seen in diffusion tensor Imaging. *Clin. Breast Cancer*, 2008. 8: p. 88 - 91.

[58] Gregorios, J.B., et al., Morphologic alterations in rat brain following systemic and intraventricular methotrexate injection: light and electron microscopic studies. *Journal of Neuropathology and Experimental Neurology*, 1989. 48(1): p. 33-47.

[59] Shilling, V., V. Jenkins, and I.S. Trapala, The (mis)classification of chemo-fog - methodological inconsistencies in the investigation of cognitive impairment after chemotherapy. *Breast Cancer Res. Treat*, 2006. 95(2): p. 125-9.

[60] Seigers, R., et al., Inhibition of hippocampal cell proliferation by methotrexate in rats is not potentiated by the presence of a tumor. *Brain Research Bulletin*, 2010. 81(4-5): p. 472-476.

[61] Dranovsky, A. and R. Hen, Hippocampal Neurogenesis: Regulation by Stress and Antidepressants. *Biological Psychiatry*, 2006. 59(12): p. 1136-1143.

[62] Malberg, J.E., Implications of adult hippocampal neurogenesis in antidepressant action. *J. Psychiatry Neurosci*, 2004. 29(3): p. 196-205.

[63] Santarelli, L., et al., Requirement of hippocampal neurogenesis for the behavioral effects of antidepressants. *Science*, 2003. 301(5634): p. 805-9.

[64] Castrén, E. and T. Rantamäki, The role of BDNF and its receptors in depression and antidepressant drug action: Reactivation of developmental plasticity. *Developmental Neurobiology*, 2010. 70(5): p. 289-297.

[65] David, D.J., et al., Implications of the functional integration of adult-born hippocampal neurons in anxiety-depression disorders. *Neuroscientist*, 2010. 16(5): p. 578-91.

[66] Monleon, S., et al., Antidepressant drugs and memory: Insights from animal studies. *Eur. Neuropsychopharmacol.*, 2007.

[67] Vythilingam, M., et al., Hippocampal volume, memory, and cortisol status in major depressive disorder: effects of treatment. *Biological Psychiatry*, 2004. 56(2): p. 101-112.

[68] Gallassi, R., et al., Memory impairment in patients with late-onset major depression: The effect of antidepressant therapy. *Journal of Affective Disorders*, 2006. 91(2-3): p. 243-250.

[69] Levkovitz, Y., et al., The SSRIs drug Fluoxetine, but not the noradrenergic tricyclic drug Desipramine, improves memory performance during acute major depression. *Brain Research Bulletin*, 2002. 58(4): p. 345-350.

[70] Mowla, A.M.D., M.M.D. Mosavinasab, and A. Pani, Does Fluoxetine Have Any Effect on the Cognition of Patients With Mild Cognitive Impairment?: A Double-Blind, Placebo-Controlled, Clinical Trial. *Journal of Clinical Psychopharmacology*, 2007. 27(1): p. 67-70.

[71] Horsfield, S., et al., Fluoxetine's effects on cognitive performance in patients with traumatic brain injury. *Int. J. Psychiatry Med.*, 2002. 32(4): p. 337-44.

[72] Vermetten, E., et al., Long-term treatment with paroxetine increases verbal declarative memory and hippocampal volume in posttraumatic stress disorder. *Biol. Psychiatry*, 2003. 54(7): p. 693-702.

[73] Strek, K.F., K.R. Spencer, and V.J. DeNoble, Manipulation of serotonin protects against an hypoxia-induced deficit of a passive avoidance response in rats. *Pharmacology Biochemistry and Behavior*, 1989. 33(1): p. 241-244.

[74] Garrigou, D., C.L. Broekkamp, and K.G. Lloyd, Involvement of the amygdala in the effect of antidepressants on the passive avoidance deficit in bulbectomised rats. *Psychopharmacology*, 1981. 74(1): p. 66-70.

[75] Broekkamp, C.L., D. Garrigou, and K.G. Lloyd, Serotonin-mimetic and antidepressant drugs on passive avoidance learning by olfactory bulbectomised rats. *Pharmacology Biochemistry and Behavior*, 1980. 13(5): p. 643-646.

[76] Nowakowska, E., A. Chodera, and K. Kus, Anxiolytic and memory improving activity of fluoxetine. *Polish Journal of Pharmacology*, 1996. 48(3): p. 255-60.

[77] Hillman, C.H., K.I. Erickson, and A.F. Kramer, Be smart, exercise your heart: exercise effects on brain and cognition. *Nat. Rev. Neurosci*, 2008. 9(1): p. 58-65.

[78] Kucyi, A., et al., Aerobic physical exercise as a possible treatment for neurocognitive dysfunction in bipolar disorder. *Postgraduate Medicine*, 2010. 122(6): p. 107-16.

[79] van Uffelen, J.G., et al., The effects of exercise on cognition in older adults with and without cognitive decline: a systematic review. *Clinical Journal of Sport Medicine*, 2008. 18(6): p. 486-500.

[80] Lazarov, O., et al., When neurogenesis encounters aging and disease. *Trends in Neurosciences*, 2010. 33(12): p. 569-579.

[81] Cotman, C.W. and N.C. Berchtold, Exercise: a behavioral intervention to enhance brain health and plasticity. *Trends in Neurosciences*, 2002. 25(6): p. 295-301.

[82] Marks, B., et al., Aerobic fitness and obesity: relationship to cerebral white matter integrity in the brain of active and sedentary older adults. *British Journal of Sports Medicine*, 2011.

[83] Chang, J., et al., Weekly administration of epoetin alfa improves cognition and quality of life in patients with breast cancer receiving chemotherapy. *Support Cancer Ther*, 2004. 2(1): p. 52-8.

[84] Mar Fan, H.G., et al., The influence of erythropoietin on cognitive function in women following chemotherapy for breast cancer. *Psycho-Oncology*, 2009. 18(2): p. 156-161.

[85] Kohli, S., et al., The effect of modafinil on cognitive function in breast cancer survivors. *Cancer*, 2009. 115(12): p. 2605-2616.

In: Methotrexate
Editors: V. S. Castillo and L. A. Moyano

ISBN: 978-1-62100-596-4
© 2012 Nova Science Publishers, Inc.

Chapter IX

Damage and Recovery of the Bone and Bone Marrow Following Methotrexate Chemotherapy

Kristen R. Georgiou and Cory J. Xian[*]

Sansom Institute for Health Research, School of Pharmacy and Medical Sciences,
University of South Australia, Adelaide, SA, Australia

Abstract

The bone marrow microenvironment is home to mesenchymal and haematopoietic stem cells, and the interaction between these cell types and their respective progeny allows the maintenance of a steady-state functioning marrow, bone formation and turnover throughout life. Unfortunately, cancer chemotherapy, which commonly includes the anti-metabolite methotrexate (MTX), is a serious risk factor that disrupts homeostasis of the bone marrow and compromises bone formation, leading to myelosuppression and bone loss. MTX has been shown to cause significant damage to the bone marrow and reduce bone volume in both clinical and animal studies. Although the severity of damage to the bone marrow and the degree of ensuing recovery of marrow cell populations are dependent on the MTX dose and length of treatment, in order to re-establish the depleted marrow cavity, haematopoietic stem cells maintained at endosteal niche sites are induced to enter the cell cycle and differentiate down the appropriate lineage. Associated with damaged bone marrow stromal cells and a differentiation switch to adipogenesis at the expense of osteogenesis, are bone loss, increased marrow fat and fracture risk. This chapter will discuss mechanisms of how MTX chemotherapy causes myelosuppression, bone loss and marrow adiposity as reported in both clinical and animal studies, and will summarise changes in the relationship between cells of the mesenchymal and haematopoietic lineages in relation to MTX-induced damage and recovery of the bone and bone marrow.

[*] Correspondence to CJ Xian: cory.xian@unisa.edu.au.

Introduction

The bone marrow microenvironment houses mesenchymal and haematopoietic stem cells and their respective progeny (Figure 1). Regulation of the bone marrow stem cell niche and players involved in the maintenance of interactions between cells of the haematopoietic and mesenchymal lineages are becoming increasingly clear under both steady-state and damaged conditions. Under conditions of stress or injury, such as following cancer chemotherapy, homeostatic interactions are disrupted and early precursor cells held at the quiescent storage niche are induced to differentiate depending on environmental cues. These cells have the capacity to migrate and further differentiate in order to re-populate the depleted microenvironment, allowing tissue-specific regeneration. However, such damaging conditions also disrupt appropriate cell-cell signalling and environmental cues, altering appropriate regenerative mechanisms. This chapter aims to illustrate the damaging conditions that are induced within the bone marrow microenvironment by chemotherapy treatment with the commonly used anti-metabolite MTX and the subsequent intrinsic repair mechanisms that enable marrow recovery in both clinical and experimental animal studies.

Chemotherapy-Induced Damage to Bone Marrow Cell Populations

One of the myriad of undesirable side effects of intensive chemotherapy regimens is myelosuppression, characterized by depletion of cells of the haematopoietic lineage within the bone marrow (BM). Toxicity of chemotherapeutic agents to the BM depletes progenitor cell populations required for maintenance and establishment of the bone marrow microenvironment. Depending on severity of the illness, chemotherapeutic dosing regimen and patient capacity to re-establish the bone marrow, myelotoxicity may result in severe morbidity and in some cases mortality. However, the BM does appear to intrinsically recover, made possible by the conservation of undifferentiated quiescent stem cell pools (Das *et al.*, 2008), which allow release of quiescent stem cells enabling their differentiation in order to repopulate the depleted marrow cavity. In the clinic, myelotoxicity is measured by monitoring haemoglobin, white blood cell and absolute neutrophil counts, numbers of which fall substantially during MTX-inclusive treatments (de Wit *et al.*, 1996; Meropol *et al.*, 1992; Kiefer *et al.*, 2008; Nygaard and Schmiegelow, 2003). Conversely, depletion of marrow cells is used in patients suffering from haematological disorders as a method to re-engraft healthy or genetically advantaged haematopoietic stem cells (Belur *et al.*, 2005).

Steady-state interactions between cells of the haematopoietic and mesenchymal lineages maintain an optimally functioning bone marrow environment and appropriate haematopoiesis, bone turnover and homeostasis. Multipotent mesenchymal stem cells (MSC) have the capacity to differentiate into a number of cell types, namely osteoblasts, adipocytes and chondrocytes (Peled *et al.*, 1999), despite only representing a very small population of total marrow cells (0.001-0.01% of 1.077g/ml density gradient-isolated cells from a bone marrow aspirate) (Pittenger *et al.*, 1999; Fox *et al.*, 2007) (Figure 1). Along the bone cell differentiation lineage, MSCs are committed to highly proliferative osteoprogenitor cells, further differentiating into pre-osteoblasts and further still into mature osteoblasts (Long, 2001), initiated and regulated by transcription factors msh homeobox 2 (MSX2), runt-related transcription factor 2 (Runx2) and osterix (Osx) (Rodda and McMahon, 2006). These transcription factors allow target gene transcription of late stage differentiation-associated bone sialoprotein, type I collagen and osteocalcin (Kitazawa *et al.*, 2008). At this late stage, osteoblasts actively synthesise and mineralise the bone matrix, which acts as a scaffold for further bone formation and remodelling in order to maintain the trabecular bone structure (Chaudhary *et al.*, 2004). However, a characteristic phenotype observed in osteoporotic patients and following chemotherapy with glucocorticoid and other damaging treatments is an increase in marrow adiposity in parallel to reduced bone formation (Wittels, 1980; Brody *et al.*, 1985; Gerard *et al.*, 1992; Dalle Carbonare *et al.*, 2001). This is proposed to be due to a switch in favour of adipogenesis at the expense of osteogenic commitment and differentiation (Bennett *et al.*, 2005) (Figure 1). As with osteogenic commitment, adipogenesis is a highly regulated process in which transcription factors PPARγ and C/EBPα activate target gene transcription enabling commitment and differentiation to mature adipocytes (Scheideler *et al.*, 2008). Such terminal differentiation may be characterised by the induction of glycerol-3-phosphate dehydrogenase (GPDH), hormone-sensitive lipase (HSL), fatty acid synthase (FASN), fatty acid binding proteins (FABPs), perilipin (PLIN) and the secretion of adipokines such as leptin, adiponectin and adipsin (Scheideler, Elabd et al., 2008). However, the mechanisms by which such deregulated mesenchymal lineage determination is elicited remains to be clearly defined.

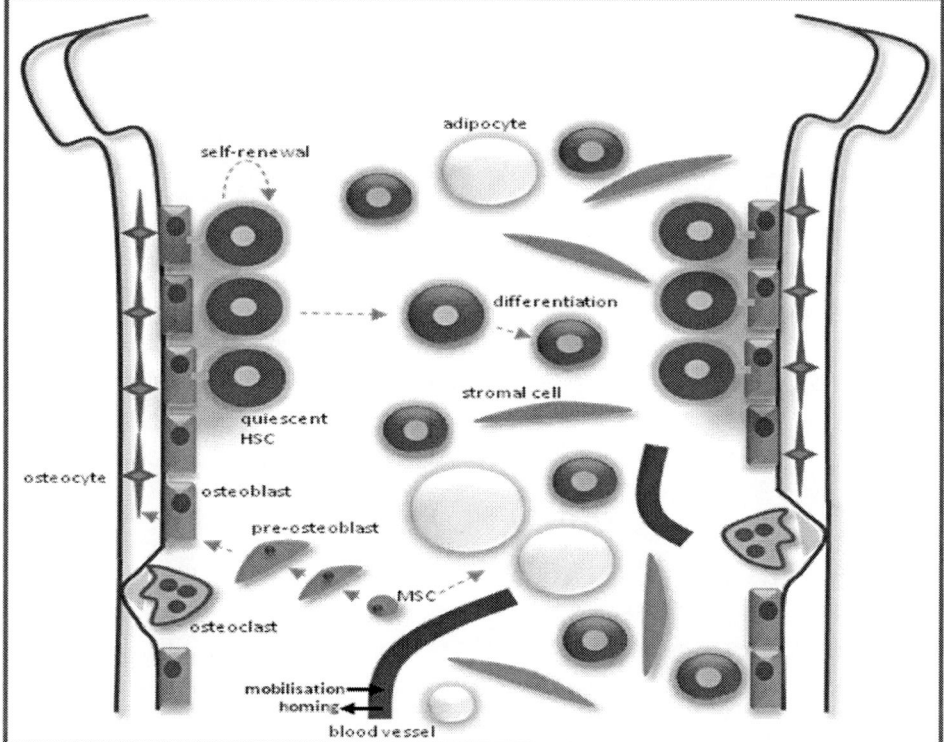

Figure 1. Representative diagram of the bone marrow microenvironment and the known locations of resident cell types.

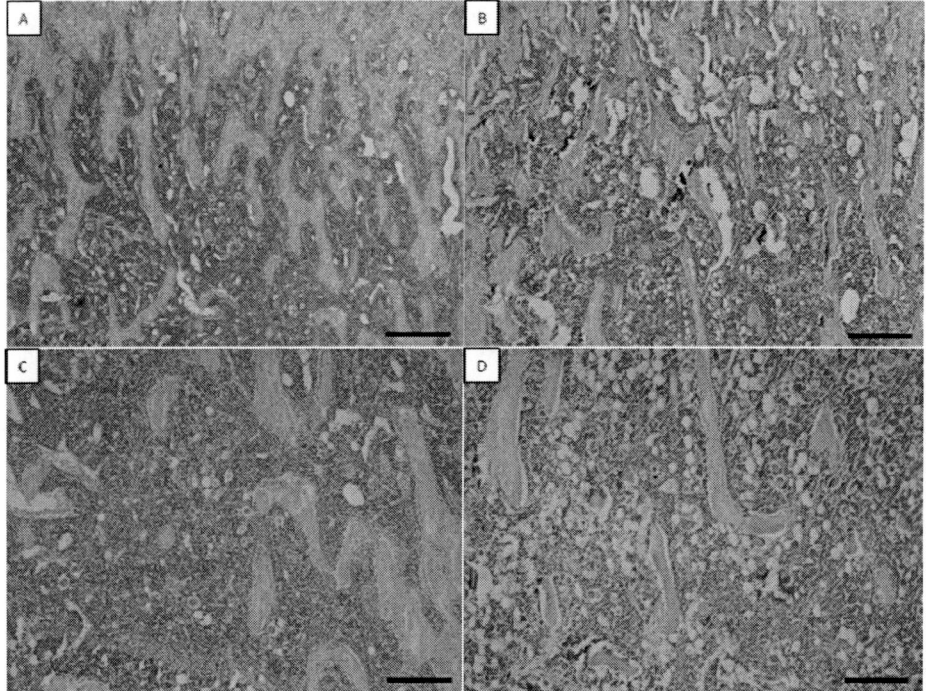

Figure 2. Bone marrow cavity of a control untreated rat (A, C) and a MTX-treated rat 24 hours after 5 consecutive daily doses of MTX (B, D), showing a reduced trabecular bone volume (A vs B) and an increased density of marrow adipocytes (C vs D) (scale bar A ,B 500µm; C, D 200µm).

Associated with the increased use of chemotherapy in cancer treatment regimens are long-term defects observed in bone such as osteopenia and osteoporosis which increase fracture risk (Schriock et al., 1991; Halton et al., 1996; Ahmed et al., 1997; Haddy et al., 2001). MSCs are also found to maintain an undifferentiated stem cell pool and upon depletion of the progenitor cell population these stem cells are triggered to differentiate, enabling marrow repopulation (Mueller et al., 2006) under conditions such as those induced following chemotherapy. Studies have suggested that while there is a reduction in more differentiated cell types in response to chemotherapy, the stem cell subset maintains a quiescent, unchanging precursor population (Li et al., 2004; Meng et al., 2003; Mueller, Luetzkendorf et al., 2006).

Methotrexate-Induced Damage and Recovery of the Bone and BM Microenvironment

The chemotherapeutic agent methotrexate (MTX) is an S-phase-specific antimetabolite, acting as a competitive inhibitor of dihydrofolate reductase. Methotrexate binds to the reduced folate receptor and upon entering the cell is polyglutamated by the enzyme folypolyglutamate synthase. MTX and its polyglutamates act to inhibit dihydrofolate reductase, in turn blocking the conversation of dihydrofolate to tetrahydrofolate. Depleted stores of tetrahydrofolate reduce the synthesis of thymidylate synthase, which is required for purine synthesis, ultimately affecting DNA and RNA synthesis and inducing cellular apoptosis (Chabner and Roberts, 2005). MTX is used in the treatment of osteosarcomas and acute lymphoblastic leukemia, also used in some breast cancer treatments, non-Hodgkin's lymphoma, and at lower doses in rheumatoid arthritis (Belur, James et al., 2005).

MTX in cancer treatment presents severe toxicity to the bone marrow (de Wit, Verweij et al., 1996; Meropol, Miller et al., 1992) and gastrointestinal tract (Xian, 2003; Xian *et al.*, 1999) and adversely affects bone, reducing bone turnover and formation (Friedlaender *et al.*, 1984; Wheeler *et al.*, 1995). There have also been recent studies in a rat model of acute short-term MTX treatment at a dose comparable to the induction phase of leukaemia treatment, as well as at a chronic low dose, which were found to induce significant effects on bone (Fan *et al.*, 2009; Xian *et al.*, 2007; Xian *et al.*, 2008). Such defects include reduced trabecular bone volume associated with a reduction in osteoblast number, reduced marrow stromal progenitor cell proliferation, decreased osteoprogenitor cell commitment but increased osteoclast progenitor cell numbers in the bone marrow and a higher density of osteoclasts on the bone surface (Fan, Cool et al., 2009; Xian, Cool et al., 2007; Xian, Cool et al., 2008). Furthermore, accompanying the decreased osteoprogenitor lineage commitment and osteogenesis after MTX treatment, a recent study has demonstrated that MTX chemotherapy causes an osteogenesis to adipogenesis switch in the MSC commitment, as clearly observed histologically by a fatty marrow cavity and reduced trabecular bone volume, increased *ex vivo* adipogenic potential but reduced osteogenic potential following MTX treatment *in vivo* (Georgiou *et al.*, 2011) (Figure 2).

When determining the effects of MTX treatment on a specific cell population, MTX *in vitro* caused suppression of cell proliferation and induced premature cell eath, particularly of osteoblast precursors (Davies *et al.*, 2002). However inconsistently, *ex vivo* MTX treatment did not induce apoptosis of BMSCs (Li, Law et al., 2004), nor did *in vivo* MTX treatment in a rat model induce obvious apoptosis among osteoblasts, pre-osteoblasts and bone stromal cells; however apoptosis was observed in the embedded osteocyte population (Fan, Cool et al., 2009; Xian, Cool et al., 2007; Xian, Cool et al., 2008). A clinical study showed that a single dose of MTX at 20mg/kg induced late apoptosis in the blood neutrophil population, as measured by uptake of both annexin V and propidium iodide (Cetiner *et al.*, 2005). Despite varied findings and an incomplete mechanistic understanding, previous studies have all demonstrated that MTX chemotherapy induces disruptions of steady-state bone and bone marrow cell regulation. Future investigations are required to determine the bone and bone marrow defects associated with long-term MTX treatment and potential signalling mechanisms underlying such deregulation, which would enable identification of potential therapeutic targets for the prevention or treatment of these defects.

Current Treatments for Enhancing Bone/Bone Marrow Regeneration after MTX Chemotherapy

As MTX acts as a folate inhibitor, concurrent treatment of folinic acid (Leucovorin) has become routine in the clinic to reduce MTX-induced toxicity to soft tissues, acting to replenish the depleted pool of intracellular folate. Adjustment of the length of folinic acid rescue according to the reduction of MTX plasma concentrations in the patient over the course of treatment has proven to be an effective method of managing MTX-induced toxicity and improved recovery in breast cancer (Monjanel-Mouterde *et al.*, 2002) and lymphoid malignancy patients (Faltaos *et al.*, 2006; Nygaard and Schmiegelow, 2003). Published clinical data have established that after haematological recovery 21-28 days after the induction phase of acute lymphoblastic leukemia treatment, $1.5g/m^2$ MTX is administered as 4-hour IV infusion followed by folinic acid rescue treatment commencing 18 hours after MTX infusion (Monjanel-Mouterde, Lejeune et al., 2002). In osteosarcoma patients, standard Leucovorin rescue is 15 mg/m^2 every 6 hours for 3 days, beginning 24 hours after the completion of MTX administration (Aquerreta *et al.*, 2004).

Methods of preventing damage to bone marrow stromal precursor cells and osteoblasts lining trabecular and endosteal bone regions are of great interest. Chemotherapy-induced damage to stromal precursors not only disrupts bone formation and maintenance, but alters haematopoietic cell preservation and differentiation as these cell lineages have a mutually dependent relationship at the endosteum (Figure 1). In experimental animal studies, folinic acid has been investigated as a protective therapy against toxicity to the bone following short- and long-term chemotherapy regimens (Faltaos, Hulot et al., 2006; Fan, Cool et al., 2009; Monjanel-Mouterde, Lejeune et al., 2002; Xian, Cool et al., 2008). In rats, supplementary folinic acid treatment appears to maintain the stromal cell pool, osteoblast number and bone mass during MTX chemotherapy (Fan, Cool et al., 2009; Xian, Cool et al., 2008). Interestingly, folinic acid treatment also prevented MTX chemotherapy-induced increased osteoclast precursor cell population and osteoclast density on bone surface, which may potentially have contributed to the overall preservation of bone mass during the MTX + folinic acid treatment (Fan, Cool et al., 2009; Xian, Cool et al., 2008). However despite these positive observations, further investigations are required to elucidate molecular regulators of bone marrow/bone homeostasis and molecules that can promote regeneration in order to reduce MTX-induced damage and promote recovery.

Conclusion

This chapter has outlined the effects of disrupting steady-state communication between stromal and haematopoietic cells of the bone marrow microenvironment and phenotypic outcomes of chemotherapy regimens, particularly MTX treatment. Preservation of bone marrow cell populations is not only required for optimal haematopoiesis and immune function, but also for bone formation and maintenance. As chemotherapy treatment disrupts the steady-state functioning of haematopoietic and stromal cell populations, and although the damage of a single exposure may be transient, repeated disruptions over time may lead to severe bone marrow toxicity and development of severe bone marrow and bone complications in later life. While folinic acid is currently used clinically to reduce marrow toxicity during MTX chemotherapy, further investigations into other potential safe and effective therapies are required in order to prevent or alleviate such detrimental defects in bone and bone marrow during or after MTX chemotherapy.

Acknowledgments

This book chapter has reviewed some of the authors' own work that had been funded in part by Bone Growth Foundation (Australia), Women's and Children's Hospital Foundation, Channel-7 Children's Research Foundation of South Australia, and NHMRC Australia. The authors thank valuable discussion with Drs Bruce Foster, Chiaming Fan, Tristan King, and Heather Tapp (Women's and Children's Hospital, South Australia).

References

Ahmed, S F, Wallace, W HKelnar, C J (1997) An anthropometric study of children during intensive chemotherapy for acute lymphoblastic leukaemia. *Horm. Res.* 48: 178-183.

Aquerreta, I, Aldaz, A, Giraldez, JSierrasesumaga, L (2004) Methotrexate pharmacokinetics and survival in osteosarcoma. *Pediatr. Blood Cancer* 42: 52-58.

Belur, L R, James, R I, May, C, Diers, M D, Swanson, D, Gunther, RMcIvor, R S (2005) Methotrexate preconditioning allows sufficient engraftment to confer drug resistance in mice transplanted with marrow expressing drug-resistant dihydrofolate reductase activity. *J. Pharmacol. Exp. Ther.* 314: 668-674.

Bennett, C N, Longo, K A, Wright, W S, Suva, L J, Lane, T F, Hankenson, K DMacDougald, O A (2005) Regulation of osteoblastogenesis and bone mass by Wnt10b. *Proc. Natl. Acad. Sci. USA* 102: 3324-3329.

Brody, J P, Krause, J RPenchansky, L (1985) Bone marrow response to chemotherapy in acute lymphocytic leukaemia and acute non-lymphocytic leukaemia. *Scand. J. Haematol.* 35: 240-245.

Cetiner, M, Sener, G, Sehirli, A O, Eksioglu-Demiralp, E, Ercan, F, Sirvanci, S, Gedik, N, Akpulat, S, Tecimer, TYegen, B C (2005) Taurine protects against methotrexate-induced toxicity and inhibits leukocyte death. *Toxicol. Appl. Pharmacol.* 209: 39-50.

Chabner, B ARoberts, T G, Jr. (2005) Timeline: Chemotherapy and the war on cancer. *Nat. Rev. Cancer* 5: 65-72.

Chaudhary, L, A., HHruska, K (2004) Differential growth factor control of bone formation through osteoprogenitor differentiation. *Bone* 34: 402-411.

Dalle Carbonare, L, Arlot, M E, Chavassieux, P M, Roux, J P, Portero, N RMeunier, P J (2001) Comparison of trabecular bone microarchitecture and remodeling in glucocorticoid-induced and postmenopausal osteoporosis. *J. Bone Miner. Res.* 16: 97-103.

Das, B, Antoon, R, Tsuchida, R, Lotfi, S, Morozova, O, Farhat, W, Malkin, D, Koren, G, Yeger, HBaruchel, S (2008) Squalene selectively protects mouse bone marrow progenitors against cisplatin and carboplatin-induced cytotoxicity in vivo without protecting tumor growth. *Neoplasia* 10: 1105-1119.

Davies, J, Evans, B, Jenney, MGregory, J (2002) In vitro effects of chemotherapeutic agents on human osteoblast-like cells. *Calcified Tissue International* 70: 408-415.

de Wit, R, Verweij, J, Bontenbal, M, Kruit, W H, Seynaeve, C, Schmitz, P IStoter, G (1996) Adverse effect on bone marrow protection of prechemotherapy granulocyte colony-stimulating factor support. *J. Natl. Cancer Inst* 88: 1393-1398.

Faltaos, D W, Hulot, J S, Urien, S, Morel, V, Kaloshi, G, Fernandez, C, Xuan, H, Leblond, VLechat, P (2006) Population pharmacokinetic study of methotrexate in patients with lymphoid malignancy. *Cancer Chemother. Pharmacol.* 58: 626-633.

Fan, C, Cool, J C, Scherer, M A, Foster, B K, Shandala, T, Tapp, HXian, C J (2009) Damaging effects of chronic low-dose methotrexate usage on primary bone formation in young rats and potential protective effects of folinic acid supplementary treatment. *Bone* 44: 61-70.

Fox, J M, Chamberlain, G, Ashton, B AMiddleton, J (2007) Recent advances into the understanding of mesenchymal stem cell trafficking. *Br J Haematol* 137: 491-502.

Friedlaender, G E, Tross, R B, Doganis, A C, Kirkwood, J MBaron, R (1984) Effects of chemotherapeutic agents on bone. I. Short-term methotrexate and doxorubicin (adriamycin) treatment in a rat model. *J. Bone Joint Surg. Am.* 66: 602-607.

Georgiou, K, Scherer, M, Fan, C, Cool, J, King, T, Foster, BXian, C (2011) Methotrexate chemotherapy reduces osteogenesis but increases adipogenic potential in the bone marrow. *Journal of Cellular Physiology* 2011 Apr 18. doi: 10.1002/jcp.22807.

Gerard, E L, Ferry, J A, Amrein, P C, Harmon, D C, McKinstry, R C, Hoppel, B ERosen, B R (1992) Compositional changes in vertebral bone marrow during treatment for acute leukemia: assessment with quantitative chemical shift imaging. *Radiology* 183: 39-46.

Haddy, T B, Mosher, R BReaman, G H (2001) Osteoporosis in survivors of acute lymphoblastic leukemia. *Oncologist* 6: 278-285.

Halton, J M, Atkinson, S A, Fraher, L, Webber, C, Gill, G J, Dawson, SBarr, R D (1996) Altered mineral metabolism and bone mass in children during treatment for acute lymphoblastic leukemia. *J. Bone Miner. Res.* 11: 1774-1783.

Kiefer, T, Kruger, W H, Montemurro, M, Schuler, F, Hirt, C, Pasold, R, Niederwieser, D, Schwenke, MDolken, G (2008) Mobilization of hemopoietic stem cells with high-dose methotrexate plus granulocyte-colony-stimulating factor in patients with primary central nervous system lymphoma. *Transfusion* 48: 2624-2628.

Kitazawa, R, Mori, K, Yamaguchi, A, Kondo, TKitazawa, S (2008) Modulation of mouse RANKL gene expression by Runx2 and vitamin D3. *J. Cell Biochem.* 105: 1289-1297.

Li, J, Law, H K, Lau, Y LChan, G C (2004) Differential damage and recovery of human mesenchymal stem cells after exposure to chemotherapeutic agents. *Br. J. Haematol.* 127: 326-334.

Long, M (2001) Osteogenesis and Bone-Marrow-Derived cells. *Blood cells, molecules and diseases* 27: 677-690.

Meng, A, Wang, Y, Brown, S A, Van Zant, GZhou, D (2003) Ionizing radiation and busulfan inhibit murine bone marrow cell hematopoietic function via apoptosis-dependent and -independent mechanisms. *Exp. Hematol.* 31: 1348-1356.

Meropol, N J, Miller, L L, Korn, E L, Braitman, L E, MacDermott, M LSchuchter, L M (1992) Severe myelosuppression resulting from concurrent administration of granulocyte colony-stimulating factor and cytotoxic chemotherapy. *J. Natl. Cancer Inst.* 84: 1201-1203.

Monjanel-Mouterde, S, Lejeune, C, Ciccolini, J, Merite, N, Hadjaj, D, Bonnier, P, Piana, PDurand, A (2002) Bayesian population model of methotrexate to guide dosage adjustments for folate rescue in patients with breast cancer. *J. Clin. Pharm. Ther.* 27: 189-195.

Mueller, L P, Luetzkendorf, J, Mueller, T, Reichelt, K, Simon, HSchmoll, H J (2006) Presence of mesenchymal stem cells in human bone marrow after exposure to chemotherapy: evidence of resistance to apoptosis induction. *Stem Cells* 24: 2753-2765.

Nygaard, USchmiegelow, K (2003) Dose reduction of coadministered 6-mercaptopurine decreases myelotoxicity following high-dose methotrexate in childhood leukemia. *Leukemia* 17: 1344-1348.

Peled, A, Petit, I, Kollet, O, Magid, M, Ponomaryov, T, Byk, T, Nagler, A, Ben-Hur, H, Many, A, Shultz, L, Lider, O, Alon, R, Zipori, DLapidot, T (1999) Dependence of human stem cell engraftment and repopulation of NOD/SCID mice on CXCR4. *Science* 283: 845-848.

Pittenger, M F, Mackay, A M, Beck, S C, Jaiswal, R K, Douglas, R, Mosca, J D, Moorman, M A, Simonetti, D W, Craig, SMarshak, D R (1999) Multilineage potential of adult human mesenchymal stem cells. *Science* 284: 143-147.

Rodda, S JMcMahon, A P (2006) Distinct roles for Hedgehog and canonical Wnt signaling in specification, differentiation and maintenance of osteoblast progenitors. *Development* 133: 3231-3244.

Scheideler, M, Elabd, C, Zaragosi, L E, Chiellini, C, Hackl, H, Sanchez-Cabo, F, Yadav, S, Duszka, K, Friedl, G, Papak, C, Prokesch, A, Windhager, R, Ailhaud, G, Dani, C, Amri, E ZTrajanoski, Z (2008) Comparative transcriptomics of human multipotent stem cells during adipogenesis and osteoblastogenesis. *BMC Genomics* 9: 340.

Schriock, E A, Schell, M J, Carter, M, Hustu, OOchs, J J (1991) Abnormal growth patterns and adult short stature in 115 long-term survivors of childhood leukemia. *J. Clin. Oncol.* 9: 400-405.

Wheeler, D, Vander Griend, R, Wronski, T, Miller, G, Keith, EGraves, J (1995) The short- and long-term effects of methotrexate on the rat skeleton. *Bone* 16: 215-221.

Wittels, B (1980) Bone marrow biopsy changes following chemotherapy for acute leukemia. *Am. J. Surg. Pathol.* 4: 135-142.

Xian, C, Cool, J, Scherer, M, Macsai, C, Fan, CFoster, B (2007) Suppression of endochondral bone formation by methotrexate chemotherapy and the protective effects of folinic acid supplementary treatment. *Bone* 40: S174.

Xian, C J (2003) Roles of growth factors in chemotherapy-induced intestinal mucosal damage repair. *Curr. Pharm. Biotechnol.* 4: 260-269.

Xian, C J, Cool, J C, Scherer, M A, Fan, CFoster, B K (2008) Folinic acid attenuates methotrexate chemotherapy-induced damages on bone growth mechanisms and pools of bone marrow stromal cells. *J. Cell Physiol.* 214: 777-785.

Xian, C J, Howarth, G S, Mardell, C E, Cool, J C, Familari, M, Read, L CGiraud, A S (1999) Temporal changes in TFF3 expression and jejunal morphology during methotrexate-induced damage and repair. *Am. J. Physiol.* 277: G785-795.

In: Methotrexate   ISBN: 978-1-62100-596-4
Editors: V. S. Castillo and L. A. Moyano   © 2012 Nova Science Publishers, Inc.

Chapter X

The Effects of β-Glucan Isolated from *Pleurotus Ostreatus* on Methotrexate Treatment in Rats with Adjuvant Arthritis[*]

Jozef Rovenský,[1,†] Mária Stančíková,[1] Karol Švík,[1]
Katarína Bauerová[2] and Jana Jurčovičová[3]
[1]National Institute of Rheumatic Diseases, Piešťany, Slovakia
[2]Institute of Experimental Pharmacology SAS, Bratislava, Slovakia
[3]Institute of Experimental Endocrinology SAS, Bratislava, Slovakia

Abstract

Objective. The purpose of this study was to evaluate the effect of Imunoglukan ® , β-(1,3/1,6)-D-glucan isolated from *Pleurotus ostreatus* (β-glucan-PO) on prophylactic treatment of adjuvant arthritis (AA) with methotrexate (MTX) in rats.

Methods. Groups of rats with AA were treated with methotrexate (1 mg/kg/week), β-glucan-PO (1 mg/kg every second day) or their combination for the period of 28 days from adjuvant application. Body mass, hind paw swelling, arthrogram scores and a level of serum albumin were measured as markers of inflammation and arthritis.

Results. Treatment with low dose of MTX significantly inhibited the markers of both inflammation and arthritis. MTX and its combination with β-glucan-PO significantly increased body mass of arthritic rats. β-glucan-PO administered alone significantly decreased both the hind paw swelling and arthritic score. In combination with MTX, β-glucan-PO markedly potentiated the beneficial effects of MTX, which resulted in a more significant reduction of hind paw swelling and arthritic scores. The concentration of

[*] This work was supported by APVV grant, number APVV-21-055205.
[†] Please address correspondence and reprint requests to: Prof. Jozef Rovenský, MD, DrSc, FRCP, National Institute of Rheumatic Diseases, Nábrežie I. Krasku 4, 921 01 Piešťany, Slovak Republic. Telephone: 004217 33 7969111, fax number: 004217 33 7721192. e-mail: rovensky.jozef@nurch.sk.

albumin in the serum of arthritic controls was significantly lower than in healthy controls. Both MTX alone and the combination treatment with MTX + β-glucan-PO significantly inhibited the decrease in serum albumin.

Conclusion. β-glucan-PO increased the treatment efficacy of basal treatment of AA with MTX.

Keywords: β-glucan, methotrexate, adjuvant arthritis

Introduction

Poly-branched β-1,3-(D)-glucans are naturally occurring polysaccharides, with or without β-1,6-(D)-glucose side chains, that are integral cell wall constituents in a number of bacteria, plants and yeasts. β-glucans from various sources are different in their structure, chemical, physical and biological properties [1]. Moreover, they represent the conserved structure - pathogen-associated molecular pattern (PAMP) and are effective biological response modifiers, non-specifically enhancing the host immune system by multiple interactions within innate and adaptive mechanisms [2]. The induction of cellular responses by β-glucans is likely to involve their specific interaction with several cell surface receptors, as complement receptor 3, lactosylceramide, selected scavenger receptors, and dectin-1 [3–5]. β-Glucans increase host immune defense by activating the complement system, enhancing the function of macrophages, leucocytes and natural killer cells. The use of β-glucans alone or as vaccine adjuvants for viral and bacterial antigens has been shown in animal models to increase resistance to a variety of bacterial, fungal, protozoan and viral infections [6-8]. β-Glucans also show anticarcinogenic activity. Its use as adjuvant to cancer chemotherapy and radiotherapy demonstrated the positive role in the restoration of hematopoiesis following bone marrow injury [9, 10, 11].

β-(1,3/1,6)-D-glucan is an insoluble polysaccharide isolated from the mushroom *Pleurotus ostreatus*. It is a safe and potent nutritional supplement with a profound systemic effect that can be described as nonspecific immune stimulation combined with antioxidant activity [11-13]. Recently, Smiderle et al. [14] described the antiinflammatory and analgesic activity of β-(1,3/1,6)-D-glucan isolated from *Pleorutus ostreatus* on the acetic acid-induced writhing reaction in mice, a typical model for quantifying inflammatory pain. The authors suggested that the glucan had potent anti-inflammatory and analgesic activities, possibly due to the inhibition of pro-inflammatory cytokines. In our previous studies with application of β-(1,3/1,6)-D-glucan isolated from *Pleurotus ostreatus* to rats with adjuvant arthritis we showed decreased activities of pro-inflammatory cytokine TNF-α, IL-1 and IL-6 in the serum of arthritic rats, decreased oxidative stress as well as the suppression of inflammatory and arthritic signs of arthritis [15, 16]. Protective antioxidant activity and anti-inflammatory activities of carboxylated (1-3)-beta-D-glucan isolated from *Saccharomyces cerevisiae* were reported in adjuvant arthritis in Lewis rats [17].

Methotrexate is an antifolate that is widely used in the treatment of rheumatic disorders and malignant tumors. The efficacy of methotrexate is often limited by severe side effects, which also includes the development of oxidative stress. Sener et al. [18] showed that β-glucan can ameliorate the methotrexate-induced oxidative organ injury (liver or kidney) in rats via its antioxidant and immunostimulatory effects.

Our previous results showed the beneficial effects of β-(1,3/1,6)-D-glucan in rat adjuvant arthritis, the aim of the present study was to evaluate its effect on methotrexate treatment of rats with adjuvant arthritis.

Materials and Methods

Materials. In this study methotrexate injection solution 10 mg/ml in sterile saline from Medac Company, Hamburg, Germany was used. ß-(1,3/1,6)-D-Glucan is insoluble micronized pure compound isolated from *Pleurotus ostreatus* (β-glucan-PO). ß-(1,3/1,6)-D-Glucan was obtained from Pleuran s.r.o. company (Bratislava, Slovakia). *Mycobacterium butyricum* was purchased from Difco Laboratories Co. Ltd. (Detroit, USA) and incomplete Freund's adjuvant from Sigma-Aldrich Chemie GmbH (Germany).

Animals. Male Lewis rats (160 - 180 g) obtained from Charles River Wiga, Germany were maintained during the experiment in standard animal facilities that comply with European Convention for the Protection of Vertebrate Animals Used for Experimental and Other Scientific Purposes. The animals were fed pelleted food (TOP DOVO, Dobrá Voda, Slovak Republic) and had free access to both food and water. The State Veterinary Committee of the Slovak Republic and the Ethics Committee for Control of Animals Experimentation at the National Institute of Rheumatic Diseases approved the experimental protocol and all procedures.

Induction of arthritis. The rats were injected with 0.1 ml suspension of heat killed *Mycobacterium butyricum* (12 mg/ml) in incomplete Freund's adjuvant intradermally at the base of the tail.

Treatment. MTX and β-glucan-PO were administered in corresponding doses from day 0 (the day of immunization) to day 28 of the study. MTX was prepared by dilution with sterile saline to yield the desired concentration of 0.5 mg in 0.1 ml saline, and applied twice a week *per os* (1 mg/kg in total per week). β-glucan-PO was administered orally as suspension in saline every second day in dose 1 mg/kg body mass. The untreated groups received the vehicle (sterile saline) in the same manner daily for 28 days.

The animals were divided into the following five groups of eight animals: group 1 - non-arthritic untreated healthy controls; group 2 - untreated rats with AA; group 3 - AA rats treated with β-glucan-PO; group 4 - AA rats treated with MTX; group 5 - AA rats treated with the combination of MTX + β-glucan-PO.

Evaluated Parameters

Body mass of rats was measured at the beginning of study and every week during the study.

Hindpaw swelling. The volume of the hind paw swelling was measured with an electronic water plethysmographically (UGO BASILE, Comerio-Varese, Italy) on days 14, 21 and 28.

Arthrogram score. The severity of arthritis was quantified by scoring each paw from 0 to 5, based on increasing levels of swelling and periarticular erythema. The sum of the scores for the limbs was calculated as the arthritic index, with a maximum possible score of 20 per rat. Arthrogram scores were evaluated on days 14, 21 and 28.

Serum albumin levels were measured on days 14, 21 and 28 in the rat serum by spectrophotometric method, using SYS 1 kit (BM/Hitachi, Boehringer Mannheim, Germany) on a Hitachi 911 automatic biochemical analyzer.

Statistical analysis of the results. One-way analysis of variance (ANOVA) was used for statistical analysis of the results, and $p < 0.05$ was considered as the significance limit for all comparisons.

Results

Body weight. In the first 7 days of the treatment, the increment in body weight was similar in all groups of rats (Table 1). However, on day 14, the body mass of arthritic control rats and rats treated with β-glucan-PO alone was significantly lower than that of the healthy controls and arthritic rats treated with MTX and with combination of MTX + β-glucan-PO. The loss of body mass in rats treated with combination MTX + β-glucan-PO was similar to that treated with MTX alone.

Hind paw swelling, arthrogram score. The clinical signs of arthritis reflect both inflammatory and arthritic changes occurring in rats with AA. The volume of the swollen hind paws in arthritic rats was significantly higher compared to healthy controls on days 14, 21 and 28, as supported by the mean value for two hind paws (Table 2). Statistically significant decreases of both hind paw swelling and arthrogram scores were observed in the arthritic rats treated with MTX on post-immunization days 14, 21 and 28 (Table 3). β-glucan-PO administered alone significantly decreased both the hind paw swelling and arthritic score on day 21 and 28. The combination treatment MTX + β-glucan-PO reduced these parameters statistically more significantly than MTX treatment alone (MTX vs. MTX+ β-glucan-PO, $P < 0.05$).

Table 1. The effect of MTX, β-glucan-PO,
and their combination on body mass of rats (g)

Groups of rats	Day 1	Day 7	Day 14	Day 21	Day 28
Healthy controls	167 ± 6	219 ± 13	224 ± 13 [**]	239 ± 14 [***]	250 ± 15 [***]
Untreated AA controls	170 ± 8	217 ± 12	186 ± 11	179 ± 18	199 ± 13
AA rats treated with:					
β-glucan-PO	171 ± 6	217 ± 7	193 ± 10	184 ± 9	212 ± 12
MTX	173 ± 6	227 ± 7	228 ± 17 [***]	236 ± 14 [***]	247 ± 15 [***]
MTX+β-glucan-PO	171 ± 6	228 ± 8	231 ± 18 [***]	230 ± 20 [***]	244 ± 24 [**]

Data represent mean value and standard deviation (mean value ± SD) for groups of 8 rats.
Significantly different from arthritic control rats: [**] $p < 0.01$, [***] $p < 0.001$.

Table 2. The effect of MTX, β-glucan-PO and their combination
on hind paws swelling (mL) in AA rats

Groups of rats	Day 14	Day 21	Day 28
Healthy controls	1.36 ± 0.04 ***	1.40 ± 0.02 ***	1.41 ± 0.05 ***
Untreated AA controls	2.25 ± 0.20	2.51 ± 0.18	2.34 ± 0.15
AA rats treated with:			
β-glucan-PO	2.05 ± 0.14	2.31 ± 0.09 *	2.16 ± 0.24 *
MTX	1.85 ± 0.23 **	2.16 ± 0.22 **	2.04 ± 0.30 **
MTX + β-glucan-PO	1.73 ± 0.22 ***	1.94 ± 0.37 ***†	1.88 ± 0.28 ***†

Data represent mean value and standard deviation (mean value ± SD) for groups of 8 rats.
Significantly different from arthritic control rats: *p<0.05, **p<0.01, ***p<0.001.
Significantly different from arthritic rats treated with MTX: †p<0.05.

Table 3. The effect of MTX, β-glucan-PO and their combination
on the arthrogram score in AA rats

Groups of rats	Day 14	Day 21	Day 28
Untreated AA controls	13.44 ± 1.81	17.22 ± 1.99	14.89 ± 2.26
AA rats treated with:			
β-glucan-PO	11.30 ± 1.46	14.25 ± 0.53 *	12.14 ± 2.10 *
MTX	8.50 ± 1.52 **	13.33 ± 3.44 **	11.00 ± 2.53 *
MTX+ β-glucan-PO	8.25 ± 2.25 ***	10.88 ± 2.85 ***†	9.88 ± 2.10 *** †

Data represent mean value and standard deviation (mean value ± SD) for groups of 8 rats.
Significantly different from arthritic control rats: *p<0.05, **p<0.01, *** p<0.001.
Significantly different from arthritic rats treated with MTX: †p<0.05.

Table 4. The effect of MTX, β-glucan-PO and their combination
on serum albumin concentrations (g/L) in AA rats

Groups of rats	Day 14	Day 21	Day 28
Healthy controls	42.00 ± 2.70 ***	39.92 ± 2.45 ***	42.15 ± 2.14 ***
Untreated AA controls	27.68 ± 1.08	30.91 ± 2.10	34.28 ± 1.22
AA rats treated with:			
β-glucan-PO	28.62 ± 1.26	30.66 ± 1.71	34.41 ± 2.04
MTX	32.01 ± 3.36 **	35.33 ± 1.79 ***	38.03 ± 2.19 **
MTX+ β-glucan-PO	36.01 ± 3.44 ***	36.33 ± 3.39 ***	37.84 ± 2.02 **

Data represent mean value and standard deviation (mean value ± SD) for groups of 8 rats.
Significantly different from arthritic control rats: * p<0.05, **p<0.01, *** p<0.001.

Serum albumin levels. Serum albumin acts as a negative acute phase reactant in both rat and human arthritis. Lower levels of serum albumin correspond to higher levels of inflammatory activity. The concentration of albumin in the serum of arthritic controls was significantly lower than in healthy controls (HC vs. AA rats, p< 0.001). Both MTX alone and the combination treatment with MTX + β-glucan-PO significantly inhibited the decrease in serum albumin (Table 4).

Discussion

This experiment was focused on the effect of β-(1,3/1,6)-D-glucan isolated from *Pleurotus ostreatus* on the inflammatory and arthritic markers in rats with AA during basal treatment with MTX. The treatment was prophylactic, which means that the animals were treated immediately after administration of the adjuvant.

The results of our investigation confirmed the previously reported effect of MTX treatment in rats with AA [19, 20]. Methotrexate at a dose of 1 mg/kg/week suppressed, but did not prevent, arthritis development. In our study, MTX significantly suppressed the hind paw swelling and decreased arthrogram scores. β-glucan-PO alone decreased both the hind paw swelling and the arthrogram on days 21 and 28. The remarkable finding was also that β-glucan-PO potentiated the beneficial effect of MTX; reduction of hind paw swelling and arthrogram scores on days 21 and 28 were more significant compared to the rats treated with MTX alone.

Serum albumin acts as a negative acute-phase reactant in rat arthritis. Decreased levels of serum albumin reflect the changes in synthesis of this protein in the liver secondary to the activation of hepatic cells by inflammatory cytokines, mainly interleukin-1 [20]. Our results correlate with the observation that MTX markedly prevents the albumin decrease in AA rats. The combination of MTX with β-glucan-PO had no additional effect compared to MTX alone (Table 4).

Systemic administration of β-glucan to rats and mice has been demonstrated to protect against various infections by activation of macrophages and attenuation of pro-inflammatory cytokine release [13, 21, 22, 23]. Hetland et al. [24] have showed that β-glucan reduced growth of *Mycobacterium tuberculosis* in macrophage cultures and had protective effect against *Mycobacterium bovis*, BCG infection in BALB/c mice [25]. Certain microbes, such as fungi and viruses led to generation and activation of autoimmune T cells resulting in a development of a particular autoimmune disease in genetically susceptible individuals. β-(1,3/1,6)-D-glucan, an effective activator of immune system may be beneficial also in humans in preventing or eliminating bacterial infections which are known to induce reactive arthritis.

In our study we tested the pure β-glucan isolated from *Pleurotus ostreatus*. This β-glucan decreased the arthritis development in rats and had additional beneficial effect to methotrexate treatment.

Acknowledgments

This work was supported by APVV Grant, number APVV-21-055205.

References

[1]   Akramiené D, Kondratos A, Didžiapetriené J, Kévelaitis E: Effects of ß-glucans on the immune system. *Medicina* (Kaunas) 2007; 43:597-606.

[2] Muta T: Molecular basis for invertebrate innate immune recognition of (1-->3)-beta-D-glucan as a pathogen-associated molecular pattern. *Curr. Pharm. Des.* 2006; 12: 4155-61.

[3] Ross G, Cain J, Myones B, Newman S, Lachmann P: Specificity of membrane complement receptor type 3 (CR3) for ß-glucans. *Complement* 1987; 4: 61–74.

[4] Brown GD, Tailor PR, Reid DM *et al.*: Dectin-1 is a major ß-glucan receptor on macrophages. *J. Exp. Med.* 2002; 196: 407-412.

[5] Brown GD, Gordon S: Immune recognition of fungal beta-glucans. *Cell Microbiol.* 2005; 7:471-9.

[6] Ben-Ami R, Lewis RE, Kontoyiannis DP: Immunocompromised hosts: immunopharmacology of modern antifungals. *Clin. Infect. Dis.* 2008; 47: 226-35.

[7] Kernodle DS, Gates H, Kaiser AB: Prophylactic anti-infective activity of poly-[1-6]-beta-D-glucopyranosyl-[1-3]-beta-D-glucopryanose glucan in a Guinea pig model of staphylococcal wound infection. *Antimicrob. Agents Chemother.* 1998; 42: 545-9.

[8] Vetvicka V, Vashishta A, Saraswat-Ohri S, Vetvickova J: Immunological effects of yeast- and mushroom-derived beta-glucans. *J. Med. Food* 2008; 11: 615-22.

[9] Weitberg AB: A phase I/II trial of beta-(1,3)/(1,6) D-glucan in the treatment of patients with advanced malignancies receiving chemotherapy. *J. Exp. Clin. Cancer Res.* 2008; 27: 40.

[10] Mantovani MS, Bellini MF, Angeli JP, Oliveira RJ, Silva AF, Ribeiro LR: Beta-Glucans in promoting health: prevention against mutation and cancer. *Mutat. Res.* 2008; 658:154-61.

[11] Bobek P, Galbavy S: Effect of pleuran (beta-glucan from *Pleurotus ostreatus*) on the antioxidant status of the organism and on dimethylhydrazine-induced precancerous lesions in rat colon. *Br. J. Biomed. Sci.* 2001; 58:164-8.

[12] Bobek P, Galbavy S, Ozdin L: Effect of oyster mushroom (Pleurotus ostreatus) on pathological changes in dimethylhydrazine-induced rat colon cancer. *Oncol. Rep.* 1998; 5:727-730.

[13] Nosál'ová V, Bobek P, Černá S, Galbavý S, Štvrtina S: Effects of pleuran (beta-glucan isolated from Pleurotus ostreatus) on experimental colitis in rats. *Physiol. Res.* 2001; 50: 575-81.

[14] Smiderle FR, Olsen LM, Carbonero ER *et al.*: Anti-inflammatory and analgesic properties in a rodent model of a (1-->3),(1-->6)-linked beta-glucan isolated from *Pleurotus pulmonarius*. *Eur. J. Pharmacol.* 2008; 597: 86-91.

[15] Bauerová K, Paulovičová E, Mihalová D, Švík K, Poništ S: Study of new ways of supplementary and combinatory therapy of rheumatoid arthritis with immunomodulators Glucomannan and Imunoglukán® in adjuvant arthritis. *Toxicol. Industrial Health* 2009; (in press).

[16] Stančíková M, Rovenský J, Švík K, Utěšený J, Bauerová K, Jurčovičová J: The effects of immunostimulatory drugs on rat adjuvant arthritis (in slovak). *Rheumatologia* 2008; 22: 9-11.

[17] *Kogan G, Staško A, Bauerová K et al.: Antioxidant properties of yeast (1→3)-β-d-glucan studied by electron paramagnetic resonance spectroscopy and its activity in the adjuvant arthritis.* Carbohydrate Polymers *(Elsevier). 2005; 61: 18–28.*

[18] Sener G, Ekşioglu-Demiralp E, Cetiner M, Ercan F, Yegen BC: Beta-glucan ameliorates methotrexate-induced oxidative organ injury via its antioxidant and immunomodulatory effects. *Eur. J. Pharmacol.* 2006; 542: 170-8.

[19] Welles WL, Silkworth J, Oronsky AL, Kerwar SS, Galivan J: Studies on the effect of low dose methotrexate in adjuvant arthritis. *J. Rheumatol.* 1985; 12: 904-6.

[20] Connolly KM, Stecher VJ, Danis E, Pruden DJ, LaBrie T. Alteration of interleukin-1 production and the acute phase response following medication of adjuvant arthritic rats with cyclosporin-A or methotrexate. *Int. J. Immunopharmacol.* 1988; 10: 717-28.

[21] Cleary JA, Kelly GE, Husband AJ: The effect of molecular weight and beta-1,6-linkages on priming of macrophage function in mice by (1,3)-beta-D-glucan. *Immunol. Cell Biol.* 1999; 77: 395-403.

[22] Onderdonk AB, Cisneros RL, Hinkson P, Ostroff G: Anti-infective effect of poly-beta-1-6-glucotriosyl-beta1-3-glucopyranose glucan *in vivo. Infect. Immun.* 1992; 60:1642-7.

[23] Bedirli A, Kerem M, Pasaoglu H *et al.*: Beta-glucan attenuates inflammatory cytokine release and prevents acute lung injury in an experimental model of sepsis. *Shock* 2007; 27: 397-401.

[24] Hetland G, Lovik M, Wiker HG: Protective effect of beta-glucan against mycobacterium bovis, BCG infection in BALB/c mice. *Scand. J. Immunol.* 1998; 47: 548-53.

[25] Hetland G, Sandven P: Beta-1,3-glucan reduces growth of *Mycobacterium tuberculosis* in macrophage cultures. *FEMS Immunol. Med. Microbiol.* 2002; 33: 41-5.

In: Methotrexate
Editors: V. S. Castillo and L. A. Moyano

ISBN: 978-1-62100-596-4
© 2012 Nova Science Publishers, Inc.

Chapter XI

Methotrexate: Pharmacology, Clinical Application and Adverse Effects

Chan-Mei Lv, Wen-Jing Zhao and Rui-Chen Guo[*]

Institute of Clinical Pharmacology,
Qilu Hospital of Shandong University, Jinan, Shandong, China

Abstract

Methotrexate (MTX) ($C_{20}H_{22}N_8O_5$) is an antimetabolite analogue of folic acid (4-amino-10-methylfolic acid) and is derived from N_{10} methylation of its precursor amethopterin. MTX is used as anti-inflammatory, antiproliferative and immunosuppressant agents for systemic treatments of plaque psoriasis, psoriatic erythroderma, generalized pustular psoriasis, nail psoriasis, palmoplantar psoriasis, and psoriatic arthritis. MTX is also used in combination with other medicine to increase the efficacy or reduce adverse effects. Contraindications and special precautions are supposed to be considered with care during MTX administration. MTX is absorbed and intracellularly accumulated as MTX-poly glutamates. It may induce liver toxicity with high doses in a long period. During MTX administration, liver enzymes increase, but only a few patients develop liver diseases. Hematologic toxicity and serious cytopenias were reported in patients with renal insufficiency or depleted folate storages without folic acid supplements. Different from the liver and the blood whose injury and toxicity are reversible, lung toxicosis may be fatal. Following MTX application, lung injury could happen at any time, even within a few weeks. Malignancies of MTX are considered co-carcinogenic, and malignant changes are elicited by synergistical effects with compounds. In addition, other side effects of MTX include carcinogenesis teratogenicity, direct potential mutagenic action, etc. MTX toxicities are numerous and involve almost any organ system.

[*] Corresponding Author: Rui-Chen Guo, No. 44, Wenhuaxi Road, Institute of Clinical Pharmacology, Qilu Hospital of Shandong University, Jinan 250012, Shandong, China. Ph: 86 531 82169636, Fax: 86 53186109975. Email: grc7636@126.com.

1. Introduction

Methotrexate (MTX) ($C_{20}H_{22}N_8O_5$) is an antimetabolite analogue of folic acid (4-amino-10-methylfolic acid) and derived from N_{10} methylation of the precursor, amethopterin. It is used in the treatment of certain neoplastic diseases, severe psoriasis, and adult rheumatoid arthritis. MTX competitively inhibits dihydrofolate reductase that catalyzes dihydrofolic acid (FH_2) to tetrahydrofolic acid (FH_4). Anti-metabolites prevent purine or pyrimidine, that are building blocks of DNA, from being incorporated into DNA during the "S" phase (of the cell cycle), resulting the block of its normal development and division.

MTX, is one of the most widely used anticancer agents for the treatment of various human malignancies. After entering cells, it potentially inhibit dihydrofolate reductase, or inhibit folate-dependent enzymes after conversion to MTX polyglutamates, reducing the availability of folate coenzymes that are required for synthesizing thymidylate, purines, methionine and serine. The influx of MTX into cells is an active transport system, and the intact membrane sulfhydryl groups were necessary for the protein carriers involved in the uptake.

2. Pharmacology

2.1. Folic Acid Reductase Inhibitor

MTX inhibits folic acid reductase, which is responsible for the conversion of folic acid to tetrahydrofolic acid. At two stages in the biosynthesis of purines and at one stage in the synthesis of pyrimidines, one-carbon transfer reactions occur which require specific coenzymes synthesized in the cell with tetrahydrofolic acid. Tetrahydrofolic acid itself is synthesized in the cell from folic acid with the help of folic acid reductase. MTX strongly binds to the enzyme and inhibits its activity to a large extent. Thus, DNA synthesis cannot proceed because no coenzymes that are used for one-carbon transfer reactions is produced duo to lack if tetrahydrofolic acid. MTX selectively affects the most rapidly dividing cells (neoplastic and psoriatic cells), therefore, it is also applied in severe, active, classical, and definite rheumatoid arthritis. MTX is used as anti-inflammatory, antiproliferative and immunosuppressant agents. It interferes the metabolic pathway of folic acid, competitively inhibits dihydrofolate reductase, resulting in activation folinic acid and blocking of deoxythymidylic acid synthesis, and then DNA synthesis is inhibited. MTX also partially inhibits forming purine ring of inosinic acid with less sensitivity, and inhibit protein synthesis with high doses.

2.2. Folate Antimetabolite

MTX is as antimetabolite, anionic cytostatic agent, and is commonly used in treating malignancies such as acute lymphoblastic leukemia, osteosarcoma, and head or neck tumors. In these indications, MTX is applied with high-dose regimen that may be associated with severe toxic reactions, particularly in patients with higher medicine plasma concentrations attained in a long period. MTX is indicated as a systemic treatment in moderate to severe plaque psoriasis, psoriatic erythroderma, generalized pustular psoriasis, nail psoriasis, palmoplantar psoriasis, and, especially, in psoriatic arthritis, which result from the inhibition of folic acid reductase, leading to inhibition of DNA synthesis and cellular replication. The mechanism involved in its activity against RA is unknown. MTX is a good therapeutic choice for psoriasis if it failed to topical therapies, acitretin, broadband and narrowband psoralen-UV-A (PUVA) and UV-B, or is rejected by patient. MTX is also used in combination with other systemic medicine to increase efficacy or to reduce the adverse effects. , MTX interferes with DNA synthesis, or repair, and cellular replication. Therefore, in general, MTX is sensitive to abnormally proliferating tissues, such as malignant cells, bone marrow, fetal cells, buccal and intestinal mucosa, and cells of the urinary bladder. When cellular proliferation in malignant tissues is greater than that in most normal tissues, MTX may impair malignant growth without irreversible damage to normal tissues. The mechanism of action in RA is unknown, but may affect the immune function of human body. It is reported MTX inhibition of DNA precursor following being uptaken by mononuclear cells in vitro, and spleen cell hyporesponses and suppressed IL 2 production by MTX in animal polyarthritis partial correction.

Further study is needed to clarify MTX effects on immune activity and the mechanism of rheumatoid immunopathogenesis.

3. Pharmacokinetics

3.1. Absorption

Oral absorption of MTX appears to be dose dependent in adults, and the peak serum levels are reached within 1-2 hours. MTX is well absorbed at dose of 30 mg·m^{-2} or less, with a mean bioavailability of about 60%, but significantly less absorbed at dose of larger than 80 mg·m^{-2} or larger , possibly due to a saturation effect.

In leukemic pediatric patients, oral absorption of MTX is also dose dependent and is reported to vary widely (23% to 95%). A twenty fold differences could happen for MTX plasma peak levels (C_{max}, 0.11 to 2.3 μmol) after an oral dose of 20 mg•m^{-2}. Significant inter-individual variability of time to peak concentration (T_{max}: 0.67 to 4 hrs after a 15 mg•m^{-2} dose) and fraction of dose absorbed is noted. The absorption fraction is significantly less at oral dose of 40 mg•m^{-2} than that at lower doses. Food delay absorption and reduce peak concentration. MTX is generally completely absorbed from parenteral routes of injection. The peak serum concentrations occur in 30 to 60 minutes after intramuscular injection. A wide inter-individual variability of MTX plasma concentrations is reported in pediatric patients with JRA. The mean MTX serum concentrations were 0.59 μmol (0.03 - 1.40) at 1 hour, 0.44 μmol (0.01 - 1.00) at 2 hours, and 0.29 μmol (0.06 - 0.58) at 3 hours following oral administration of MTX in doses of 6.4 to 11.2 mg•m^{-2}/week in pediatric patients with JRA. The terminal half-life ranges from 0.7 to 5.8 hours or 0.9 to 2.3 hours in pediatric patients receiving MTX for acute lymphocytic leukemia (6.3 to 30 mg•m^{-2}), or for JRA (3.75 to 26.2 mg•m^{-2}), respectively.

3.2. Distribution

The initial volume distribution of MTX is approximately 0.18 L·kg⁻(18% of body weight) and steady-state volume of distribution is approximately 0.4 to 0.8 L•kg⁻(40% to 80% of body weight) after intravenous administration. MTX competes with reduced folates and across cell membranes by means of a single carrier-mediated active transport process. At serum concentrations greater than 100 µmol, passive diffusion becomes a major pathway by which effective intracellular concentrations can be achieved. Approximately 50% of MTX in serum are bound with protein, and may be displaced from plasma albumin by various compounds including sulfonamides, salicylates, tetracyclines, chloramphenicol and phenytoin.

MTX does not penetrate the blood-cerebrospinal fluid barrier in therapeutic amounts when given orally or parenterally, and its high CSF concentrations may be attained by intrathecal administration.

3.3. Metabolism

MTX undergoes hepatic and intracellular metabolism to polyglutamated forms. Small amounts of MTX or polyglutamates may remain in tissues for longer. The retention and prolonged action of these active metabolites vary among cells, tissues and tumors. A small amount of 7-hydroxy MTX may occur at doses commonly prescribed, and its accumulation may become significant at the high doses used in osteogenic sarcoma. The aqueous solubility of 7-hydroxy MTX is 3 to 5 times lower than that of parent. MTX is partially metabolized by intestinal flora after oral administration.

3.4. Excretion

Renal excretion is the primary route of elimination depending on dosage and route of administration. 80% to 90% of the administered dose is excreted unchanged in urine within 24 hours when intravenously administrated, and a limited biliary excretion amounts to 10% or less. Enterohepatic recirculation of MTX also exists.

Renal excretion is through glomerular filtration and active tubular secretion. Duo to saturation of renal tubular reabsorption, nonlinear elimination is observed in psoriatic patients (dose of 7.5 - 30 mg). Renal disfunction, and concurrent use of medicine (e.g., weak organic acids) with tubular secretion, can significantly increase MTX levels in serum. Good correlation is reported between MTX clearance and endogenous creatinine clearance.

MTX clearance rates widely vary and are decreased at higher doses. Delayed drug clearance is identified as one of the major factors that are responsible for MTX toxicity. It is postulated that the toxicity of MTX for normal tissues is more dependent upon the duration of exposure to the drug rather than the peak level achieved. When a patient has delayed drug elimination due to compromised renal function, a third space effusion, or other causes, MTX serum concentrations may remain elevated for prolonged periods.

The most important transporters for MTX kidney or liver elimination are the organic anion transporters, organic anion transporting polypeptide, members of the multidrug resistance-associated protein subfamily and breast cancer resistance protein.

The potential for toxicity from high dose regimens or delayed excretion is reduced by the administration of leucovorin calcium during the final phase of MTX plasma elimination. Therapeutic monitoring of MTX serum concentrations may help identify those patients at high risk for MTX toxicity and aid in proper leucovorin dosage adjustment.

The terminal half-life of MTX approximately ranges from 3 to 10 hours during treatment for psoriasis, or RA or low dose antineoplastic therapy (less that 30 mg•m^{-2}), while it ranges from 8 to 15 hours with high doses of methotrexate in patients.

4. Clinical Applications

4.1. Rheumatoid Arthritis

For patients with rheumatoid arthritis, MTX starts to have a visible effect on articular swelling and tenderness as early as 3 to 6 weeks. Although MTX clearly ameliorates symptoms of inflammation (pain, swelling, stiffness), there is no evidence that it induces remission of RA nor has a beneficial effect been demonstrated on bone erosions and other radiologic changes which result in impaired joint use, functional disability, and deformity. Mostly, short term (3 - 6 m) studies of MTX were carried out in patients with RA . Lack of data from long-term studies indicates that an initial clinical improvement is maintained for at least two years with continued therapy.

4.2. Psoriasis

In psoriasis, the rate of production of epithelial cells in the skin is greatly increased over normal skin. This differential in proliferation rates is the basis for the use of MTXto control the psoriatic process. In a 6-month double-blind, placebo- controlled trial of 127 pediatric patients with juvenile RA (JRA) (mean age, 10.1 years; age range, 2.5 to 18 years; mean duration of disease, 5.1 years) on background non-steroidal anti-inflammatory drugs (NSAIDS) and/or prednisone, MTXgiven weekly at an oral dose of 10 mg•m-2 provided significant clinical improvement compared to placebo as measured by either the physician's global assessment, or by a patient composite (25% reduction in the articular-severity score plus improvement in parent and physician global assessments of disease activity). Over two-thirds of the patients in this trial had polyarticular-course JRA, and the numerically greatest response was seen in this subgroup treated with 10 mg•m^{-2}/wk methotrexate. The overwhelming majority of the remaining patients had systemic-course JRA. All patients were unresponsive to NSAIDS; approximately one-third were using low dose corticosteroids. Weekly MTX at a dose of 5 mg•m^{-2} was not significantly more effective than placebo in this trial.

5. Adverse Effects

During treatment with MTX, clinicians are supposed to evaluate contraindications and special precautions of MTX with great care. MTX has potential toxicity that may be related with administration frequency and severity. It is observed at all doses, and happens at any time during therapy, thus it is necessary to closely follow patients on MTX therapy.

Liver enzymes increases while using MTX with few clinic liver disease developed in patients. Hepatotoxicity is a common adverse effect. Liver damage may be immediately developed after MTX administration, especially with higher dose, and is characterized by a transient elevation of liver enzyme levels or hyperbilirubinaemia. MTX can induce acute increase of liver function tests (elevated serum transaminases in 15% of patients with RA on low-dose therapy) or chronic hepatotoxicity (fibrosis and cirrhosis). The average incidences of liver fibrosis and cirrhosis in patients with RA (low doses) are 3-7% and 0.1%, respectively. Meta-analysis revealed the incidence of progression of liver disease (worsening of 1 grade on the histological classification of Roenigk) in patients with RA or psoriatic arthritis averages 27%, or 7% per gram of MTX (total dose) given. Chronic hepatotoxicity typically that is developd only after chronic use of higher doses (2 years or more of total doses of 1.5 grams or more), is likely observed in patients who are aged or obese, or drink ethanol, or have chronic renal insufficiency or diabetes. MTX causes hepatotoxicity, fibrosis, and cirrhosis, but generally only after prolonged use. Acutely, liver enzyme elevations are frequently seen, but transient and asymptomatic without subsequent hepatic disease. Liver biopsy after sustained use often shows histological changes with fibrosis and cirrhosis reported, and these latter lesions may not be preceded by symptoms or abnormal liver function tests in the psoriasis population. For this reason, periodic liver biopsies are usually recommended for psoriatic patients who are under long-term treatment. Persistent abnormalities in liver function tests may precede appearance of fibrosis or cirrhosis in the RA population.

Most serious cytopenias are observed in patients with renal insufficiency to some degree or with significantly depleted folate storages without folic acid supplements applied. Hematologic side effects include myelosuppression that is one of the primary toxic effects of MTX. MTX suppressed hematopoiesis could caused anemia, aplastic anemia, pancytopenia, leukopenia, neutropenia, thrombocytopenia, lymphadenopathy, and lymphoproliferative disorders including reversible hypogamma globulinemia (which rarely reported).

Preexisting myelo suppression or small number of hematologic cell are contraindications of MTX application, particularly in patients with RA or psoriasis. Close monitoring of the CBC is mandatory. Profound count nadirs may require therapy discontinuation, at least temporarily. Folate therapy and/or leucovorin rescue may be preventive or palliative. Treated patients who become febrile should be assumed to have neutropenia until proven otherwise. Cytopenia occurs in 5% to 25% of patients with RA who receive long-term therapy. Risk factors include renal dysfunction, preexisting folate deficiency, increased mean corpuscular volume value, advanced age, concomitant use of other anti-folate medications (such as trimethoprim -sulfamethoxazole), and possibly hypoalbuminemia, concomitant infection, history of bone marrow injury, surgery, and concurrent use of NSAIDs or probenecid. Pancytopenia is rarely observed in patients with rheumatoid arthritis. Bone marrow recovery typically occurs within two weeks after the withdrawal of MTX.

Different from the toxicities in liver and blood that are reversible to some extent, that of the lung may be fatal. Lung injury secondary to MTX can occur almost at any time during its administration, even within few weeks of its initiation. MTX-induced lung disease is potentially dangerous, which may occur acutely at any time during therapy even at doses as low as 7.5 mg·week^{-1}. It is not always fully reversible. Pulmonary symptoms (especially a dry, nonproductive cough) may require interruption of treatment and careful investigation. MTX-induced lung toxicity was discussed about the recommendation on investigations required before MTXinitiation in patients with RA. Lower respiratory tract infections and immunoallergic pneumonitis are the main manifestations. These potentially life-threatening complications may occur at any time during treatment.

MTX is considered a co-carcinogenic that acts synergistically with other compounds to induce malignant changes. In addition to the manifestations discussed, patients receiving MTX may experience a number of other side effects such as carcinogenesis teratogenicity and direct potential mutagenic action. No controlled human data exist regarding the risk of neoplasia with MTX. MTX is evaluated in a number of animal studies for carcinogenic potential with inconclusive results. Although there is evidence that MTX causes chromosomal damage to animal somatic cells and human bone marrow cells, the clinical significance remains uncertain. Non-Hodgkin's lymphoma and other tumors are reported in patients receiving low-dose oral MTX. However, there are instances of malignant lymphoma arising during treatment with low-dose oral MTX, which have regressed completely following withdrawal of MTX, without requiring active anti-lymphoma treatment. Benefits should be weighed against the potential risks before using MTX alone or in combination with other drugs, especially in pediatric patients or young adults. MTX causes embryotoxicity, abortion, and fetal defects in humans. It is reported to cause impairment of fertility, oligospermia and menstrual dysfunction in humans, during and for a short period after cessation of therapy. These reported toxicities are numerous and involve almost any organ system.

6. Interactions

Concomitant administration of some NSAIDs and MTX with high dose is reported to increase and prolong MTX levels in serum, resulting in deaths from severe hematologic and gastrointestinal toxicity. Caution should be taken when NSAIDs and salicylates are administered concomitantly with MTX at lower dose, which could reduce the tubular secretion of MTX in animal model and may enhance its toxicity. However, there is no obvious problems observed in patients with RA who were treated with concurrent use of MTX and constant dosage regimens of NSAIDs. It may appreciated the lower doses doses used in RA (7.5 to 15 mg·week^{-1}) in comparison with that used in psoriasis.

MTX is partially bound to serum albumin. Toxicity may be increased if the binding sites are displaced by some medicines, such as salicylates, phenylbutazone, phenytoin, and sulfonamides. It need monitored with care for applications of MTX combined with probenecid that diminish renal tubular transport. Oral antibiotics such as tetracycline, chloramphenicol, and nonabsorbable broad spectrum antibiotics, may decrease intestinal absorption of MTX or interfere with the enterohepatic circulation by inhibiting bowel flora and suppressing metabolism of the drug by bacteria. Penicillins may reduce the renal clearance of MTX and increased MTX serum. Hematologic and gastrointestinal toxicity are observed during administration of Penicillins combined with MTX. Thus, Application of MTX combined with penicillins should be carefully monitored.

The potential hepatotoxicity of MTX is not evaluated yet while hepatotoxic agents are also applied, but some hepatotoxicity cases are reported. Therefore, patients receiving concomitant therapy with MTX and potential hepatotoxins, e.g., azathioprine, retinoids, sulfasalazine, should be closely monitored for possible increased risk of hepatotoxicity.

Therefore, theophylline levels should be monitored while being used concurrently with MTX, because MTX may decrease the clearance of theophylline. Vitamin containing folic acid or its derivatives may decrease responses to MTX systemically administered. Preliminary animal and human studies shows that small quantities of leucovorin (i.v.) is present in the cerebral spinal fluid primarily as 5-methyltetrahydrofolate and remain 1 - 3 orders of magnitude that is lower than the usual MTX concentrations following intrathecal administration. However, high doses of leucovorin may reduce the efficacy of MTX intrathecally administered.

Folate deficiency states may increase MTX toxicity. Trimethoprim -sulfamethoxazole rarely increases suppression of bone marrow in patients that receive MTX, which may be due to additive antifolate effects. Most adverse reactions are reversible if being detected early. When adverse reactions occur, dosage should be reduced, the medicine needs to be stopped, or appropriate corrective measures should be taken. If necessary, it also includes application of leucovorin calcium, and/or acute, intermittent hemodialysis with a high-flux dialyzer. If MTX therapy is reinstituted, great caution need to be taken during application to avoid possible recurrence of toxicity.

The clinical pharmacology of MTX is not well studied in older individuals. Due to diminished hepatic and renal function as well as decreased folate stores in this population, these patients should be given lower doses and closely monitored for early signs of toxicity. MTX is reported to cause fetal death and/or congenital anomalies. Therefore, it is not recommended for women of childbearing patients unless there is clear medical conformation that benefits can be expected to outweigh risks. Pregnant women with psoriasis or RA should not receive MTX. MTX elimination is reduced in patients with impaired renal function, ascites, or plural effusions. Such patients require especially careful monitoring for toxicity and dose reduction or, discontinuation of MTX administration in some cases.

Both the physician and pharmacist should emphasize that mistaken use of the recommended dose could lead to fatal toxicity to the patient with RA and psoriasis. Encourage patients to read the Patient Instructions attached. Prescriptions should not be written or refilled on a PRN basis. Patients should be informed of the potential benefit and risk of MTX. The risk of MTX effects on reproduction should be discussed with both male and female patients.

References

A. Lorico, G. Toffoli, M. Boiocchi, E. Erba, M. Broggini, G. Rappa, M. D'Incalci. Accumulation of DNA strand breaks in cells exposed to methotrexate or N10-propargyl-5, 8-dideazafolic acid, *Cancer Res.* 48 (1988) 2036–2041.

Allegra CJ, Chabner BA, Drake JC, Lutz R, Rodbard D, Jolivet J. Enhanced inhibition of thymidylate synthase by methotrexate polyglutamates. *J. Biol. Chem.* 1985; 260: 9720–6.

Allegra CJ, Drake CJ, Jolivet J, Chabner BA. Inhibition of phosphoribosyl aminoimidiazole carboxamide transformylase by methotrexate and dihydrofolic acid polyglutamates. *Proc. Natl. Acad. Sci. USA* 1985;82:4881–5.

Barry MA, Behnke CA, Eastman A. Activation of programmed cell death (apoptosis) by cisplatin, other anticancer drugs, toxins and hyperthermia. *Biochem. Pharmacol.* 1990;40:2353–62.

Caltayud S, Warner TD, Mitchell JA. Modulation of colony stimulating factor release and apoptosis in human colon cancer cells by anticancer drugs. *Br. J. Cancer* 2002;86:1316–21.

D.K. Hattangadi, G.A. DeMasters, T.D. Walker, K.R. Jones, X. Di, I.F. Newsham, D.A. Gewirtz. Influence of p53 and caspase 3 on cell death and senescence in response to methotrexate in the breast tumor cell, *Biochem. Pharmacol.* 68 (2004) 1699–1708.

de Silva CP, de Oliveira CR, de Conceicao PL. Apoptosis as a mechanism of cell death induced by different chemotherapeutic drugs in human leukemic T-lymphocytes. *Biochem. Pharmacol.* 1996;51: 1331–40.

Drake JC, Allegra CJ, Baram J, Kaufman BT, Chabner BA. Effects on dihydrofolate reductase of Methotrexate metabolites and intracellular folates formed following methotrexate exposure of human breast cancer cells. *Biochem. Pharmacol.* 1987;36: 2416–8.

el Alaoui S, Lawry J, Griffin M. The cell cycle and induction of apoptosis in a hamster fibrosarcoma cell line treated with anticancer drugs: its importance to solid tumor chemotherapy. *J. Neurooncol.* 1997;31:195–207.

Isaac N, Panzarella T, Lau A, Mayers C, Kirkbride P, Tannock IF, et al. Concurrent cyclophosphamide, methotrexate and 5-fluorouracil chemotherapy and radiotherapy for breast carcinoma: a well tolerated adjuvant regimen. *Cancer* 2002;95:696–703.

J.A. Houghton, Antimetabolites, in: D.A. Gewirtz, S.E. Holt, S. Grant (Eds.). Cancer Drug Discovery and Development, Apoptosis, Senescence and Cancer, Humana Press Inc., Totowa, NJ,2007, pp.361–382.

J.C. Li, E. Kaminskas, Accumulation of DNA strand breaks and methotrexate cytotoxicity. *Proc. Natl. Acad. Sci. USA* 81 (1984) 5694–5698.

J.H. Schornagel, J.G. McVie. The clinical pharmacology of methotrexate, *Cancer Treat. Rev.* 10 (1983) 53–75.

Kaufmann S. Induction of endonucleolytic DNA cleavage in human acute myelogenous leukemia cells by etoposide, camptothecin and other cytotoxic anticancer drugs: a cautionary note. *Cancer Res.* 1989;49:5870–8.

Lorico A, Toffoli G, Boiocchi M, Erba E, Broggini M, Rappa G, et al. Accumulation of DNA strand breaks in cells exposed to methotrexate or N10-Propargyl -5,8-dideazafolic acid. *Cancer Res.* 1998;48: 2036–41.

R.Singh, A.A.Fouladi-Nashta, N. Halliday, D.A. Barrett, K.D. Sinclair. Methotrexate induced differentiation in colon cancer cells is primarily due to purine deprivation, *J. Cell. Biochem.* 99 (2006) 146–155.

S. Hatse, E. De Clercq, E. Balzarini. Role of antimetabolites of purine and pyrimidine nucleotide metabolism in tumor cell differentiation, *Biochem. Pharmacol.* 58 (1999) 539–555.

Schilsky RL, Jolivet J, Bailey BD, Chabner B. Synthesis, binding and intracellular retention of methotrexate polyglutamates by cultured human breast cancer cells. *Adv. Exp. Med. Bio.* 1983;163: 247–57.

Tsurusawa M, Niwa M, Katano N, Fujimoto T. Flow cytometric analysis by bromodeoxyuridine/DNA assay of cell cycle perturbation of methotrexate-treated mouse L1210 leukemia cells. *Cancer Res.* 1988;48:4288–93.

Y.G. Assaraf, Molecular basis of antifolate resistance, *Cancer Metast. Rev.* 26 (2007) 153–181.

In: Methotrexate
Editors: V. S. Castillo and L. A. Moyano

ISBN: 978-1-62100-596-4
© 2012 Nova Science Publishers, Inc.

Chapter XII

Molecular Mechanisms of Methotrexate Resistance

Amit K. Tiwari[1], Dong-Hua Yang[2] and Zhe-Sheng Chen[1,*]
[1]Department of Pharmaceutical Sciences, College of Pharmacy and Allied Health
Professions, St. John's University, Queens, NY, US
[2]Biosample Repository Facility, Fox Chase Cancer Center, Philadelphia, PA, US

Abstract

Methotrexate (MTX) is a purine analog antimetabolite that is widely used in the treatment of neoplastic disease, rheumatoid arthritis, and severe psoriasis. Uptake of MTX into cells is dependent upon the reduced folate carriers (RFCs), while the cellular level of MTX is maintained by its polyglutamylation. The development of MTX resistance, which reduces MTX efficacy in a variety of disease treatments, has been discussed in many studies. Resistance factors include defective or slow uptake of MTX with RFCs or increased efflux via ATP-binding cassette (ABC) multidrug transporters, certain alterations in targeted enzymes, genetic polymorphisms, impaired MTX polyglutamylation, increased salvage and increased metabolism of MTX. However, the pharmacokinetic and cellular resistance mechanisms of MTX are still not completely understood. This chapter discusses current knowledge of the molecular basis of MTX resistance based on data obtained from both pre-clinical and clinical studies. In addition, emerging mechanisms for MTX treatment are also discussed. An in-depth understanding of the molecular mechanisms behind the MTX resistance could help facilitate the optimal use of antifolate therapy as well as new drug development.

* Corresponding author: Tel: 1-718-990-1432, Fax: 1-718-990-1877, Email: Chenz@stjohns.edu.

Introduction

Methotrexate (MTX), an antifolate and antimetabolite, was rationally synthesized by an Indian biochemist, Dr. Yellapragada Subbarao, to circumvent the toxic effect of its parent analog aminopterin, and thus replaced aminopterin in the treatment of childhood acute lymphocytic leukemia (ALL) in 1956 (Hertz et al., 1956; Bhargava, 2001). In almost 60 years, we have learned newer uses of MTX in severe psoriasis, adult rheumatoid arthritis (RA), autoimmune diseases, ectopic pregnancy, graft-versus-host diseases (Walling, 2006). The MTX is also used alone or in combination as an anti-neoplastic drug in a variety of tumors such as gestational choriocarcinoma, osteosarcoma, breast cancer, head and neck squamous cell carcinoma, small cell and squamous cell type lung cancer, and advanced stage non-Hodgkin's lymphomas (Walling, 2006). Optimizing the uses of MTX has been a challenge among the clinicians and scientists, as it has been fascinating to uncover cellular mechanism of action and resistance. In-depth knowledge about the drug resistance will not only facilitate effective use of this drug but also guide new drug developments. This chapter gives a brief overview on our current understanding of MTX resistance.

1. Cellular Mechanisms of MTX Action

MTX was rationally designed in 1948 on the basis of its homologue aminopterin, to inhibit key folate dependent enzyme dihydrofolate reductase (DHFR) (Farber and Diamond, 1948; Jackson et al., 1976; Bhargava, 2001). In the past 60 years or so, the interaction of MTX with several cellular molecules has been largely understood. MTX enters the cell either by reduced folate carriers (RFCs) or by endocytosis through folate receptors (FR) present on the plasma membrane (Figure 1). Next, MTX is metabolized by folypolyglutamate synthase (FPGS) to more active polyglutamated MTX-(Glu)n forms (n is from 2~7; It is MTX if n equals 1). Both MTX and MTX-(Glu)n bind tightly and inhibit dihydrofolate reductase (DHFR), a key enzyme in folate metabolism and thus cellular replication as well as DNA synthesis and repair (Figure 1). In addition, MTX-(Glu)n significantly inhibit other folate dependent enzymes such as thymidylate synthase (TS), 5-aminoimadazole-4-carboxamide riboneucleoside formyltransferase (AICARFT) and Glycinamide ribonucleotide formyltransferase (GARFT) which is involved in the *de novo* purine biosynthesis (Figure 1). However, clinical application of MTX is limited due to the development of resistance (Zhao and Goldman, 2003).

2. Resistance Mechanisms to MTX

Factors affecting the efficacy of MTX include its rate of cellular uptake, its expulsion from cells due to over-expression certain multidrug efflux transporters, its rate of polyglutamylation of MTX and the rate of hydrolysis of MTX-(Glu)n to MTX. In addition, the effect of MTX is also influenced by downstream target inhibition processes including changes in the microenviornment such as alterations in the level of glutathione or nucleotides (Wessels et al., 2008).

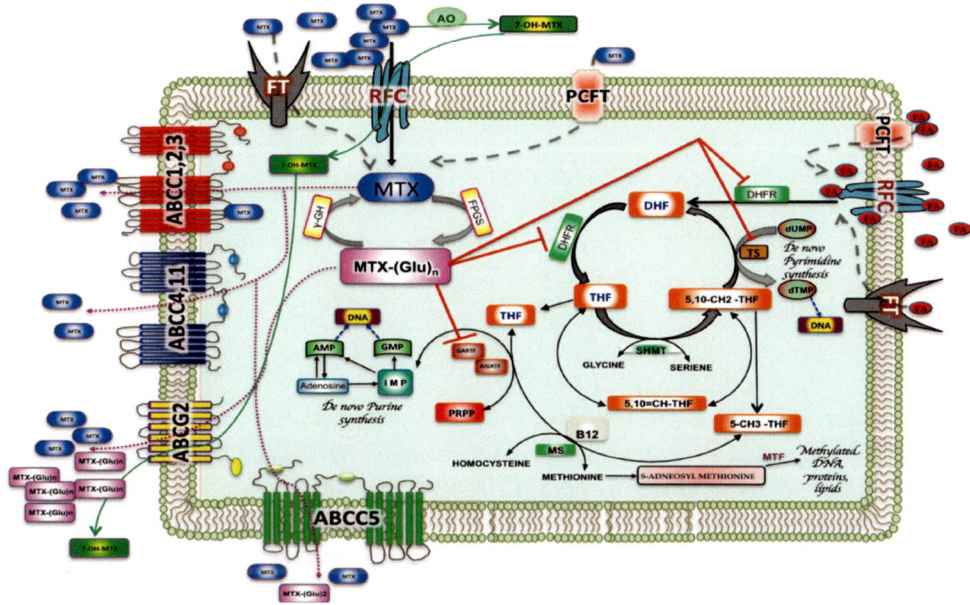

Tiwari *et al.*

MTX resistance could be due to (a) alterations in the expression and/or function of RFC and FR, resulting in poor intracellular import of MTX. (b) Impairment of FPGS activity resulting in decreased MTX-(Glu)n intracellular accumulation. (c) Increased activity of γ-GH will produce MTX (monoglutamate form). (d) The MTX(monoglutamated form) is effluxed by ABCCs 1-5, 11 and ABCG2 transporters, whereas MTX-(Glu)n (polyglutamated forms: n is up to 3) are only expelled by ABCG2 transporter, with an exception of MTX-Glu₂, which is also effluxed by ABCC5 transporter. (e) The effect of MTX is reduced with the increased expression or function of enzymes involved in *de novo* nucleotide synthesis pathway, such as DHFR, TS, AICARFT and GARFT. (f) Plasma concentration of MTX is reduced by metabolism of MTX in liver to its metabolite 7-OH-MTX, or (g) increased extracellular folate pool, which competes with MTX for cellular uptake via RFCs or FRs.

Abbreviations: ABC, ATP-binding cassette; AICARFT, 5-aminoimidazole-4-carboxamide ribonucleotide formyltransferase; DHF, dihydrofolate; DHFR, dihydrofolate reductase; dTMP, deoxythymidylate; dUMP, deoxyuridilate; FA, folic acid; FPGH, folylpolyglutamate hydrolase; FPGS, folylpolyglutamate synthetase; FR, folate receptor; GARTF, glycinamide ribonucleotide formyltransferase; ICCMTF, Isoprenylcysteine carboxyl methyltransferases; MTX, methotrexate; MTX-(Glu)n, MTX polyglutamate derivatives; PCFT, proton coupled folate transporter; RFCs, reduced folate carriers; SHMT, seriene hydroxymethyltransferase; THF, tetrahydrofolate; TS, thymidilate synthase; 5-CH3-THF, 5-methyltetrahydrofolate; 5,10-CH2-THF, 5,10-methylenetetrahydrofolate; 7-OH-MTX, 7-hydroxymethotrexate; γ-GH, γ-glutamyl hydrolase.

Figure 1. Model depicting bioconversions of folate, MTX mechanisms of action and development of MTX resistance. MTX, folic acid and reduced folates enter the cell via three different routes – facilitative carriers RFCs, FRs and PCFT. The RFCs mediate high affinity infflux of MTX, and also internalizes FA and reduced folates with comparatively less affinity. FRs endocytose MTX with low affinity compared with FA and reduced folates. PCFT on the other hand, mediates transport of both oxidized (FA) and reduced folates and MTX at low pH. Intracellularly, MTX is metabolized to highly active polyglutamated derivatives via FPGS. The MTX and MTX-(Glu)n (n is from 2~7; It is MTX if n equals 1) significantly block the activity of several key enzymes such as DHFR, TS, AICARFT and GARFT, which play a crucial role in folate metabolic pathway and thus *de novo synthesis of* purines and pyrimidines.

Reports have shown that the genetic polymorphism in any of the dynamic processes involved in MTX mechanism of action, or combination of any of the above factors could also lead to MTX resistance (van der Kooij et al., 2008).

2.1. Impaired Uptake of MTX

The optimum therapeutic concentration of MTX inside the cell is an important determinant of MTX's mechanism of action. However, resistance to MTX occurs because of defective transport of MTX by RFCs or reduced affinity of MTX by folate receptors (FRs) or overexpression of certain ATP-binding cassette (ABC) efflux transporters, leading to decreased accumulation of intracellular MTX (Figure 1).

2.1.1. Reduced Folate Carriers (RFCs)

The major member of RFCs also known as solute carrier family 19 member 1 (SLC19A1), is a predicted 12 transmembrane domain (TMD) facilitative transporter, devoid of ATP-binding site (Prasad et al., 1995). The RFCs are organic anion antiporters, which influx the reduced folates derivatives and various divalent hydrophilic antifolates (including MTX) into the cells, by binding with higher affinity and exchanging certain organic phosphates such as adenine nucleotides as well as thiamine mono- and pyro-phosphate (Yang et al., 1984; Zhao et al., 2001b). Decreased expression, transcriptional deregulation, and impaired mobility of the RFCs, either due to increased K_m (affinity for folates and antifolates), or decreased V_{max} (translocation activity), or both, was suggested to be the responsible factor for MTX resistance (Gorlick et al., 1997; Zhao and Goldman, 2003; Assaraf, 2007).

2.1.1a. Alteration in RFCs Expression and Translocation

Acquired MTX resistance is associated with decreased *RFCs* gene expression and/or downregulation of RFC transporters in a variety of tumors such as colorectal carcinoma, osteosarcoma, breast cancer, acute leukemias (lymphoblastic and lymphocytic), as well as primary CNS lymphoma (Gorlick et al., 1997; Moscow et al., 1997; Guo et al., 1999; Rots et al., 2000; Levy et al., 2003; Ferreri et al., 2004; Wettergren et al., 2005). The intrinsic resistance to high-dose MTX therapy in osteosarcoma patients was reported due to low levels of *RFCs* mRNA and low RFCs protein expression (Guo et al., 1999). The *RFC1* gene is localized at the end of the long arm of chromosome 21 (21q22.2-q22.3) (Moscow et al., 1997). It was reported that the reduction in *RFC1* gene copy numbers due to complete deletion of *RFC1* gene or allelic loss might be a responsible factor for MTX and other antifolate resistance (Ding et al., 2001b; Kaufman et al., 2006). Furthermore, it was reported that the loss of one or more *RFC1* alleles and the translocation of the remaining *RFC1* allele with the formation of chromosome 21/22 fusions disrupt *RFC1* gene expression (Ding et al., 2001b). Additionally, leukemia cells grown in a reduced folate environment produced chromosomal aberrations with frequent loss of a copy of chromosome 21, leading to amplification of *RFC1* gene fragments and translocation of these fragments to different chromosomal loci (Wong et al., 1998; Zhang et al., 1998). In children with hyperdiploid B-precursor ALL, the elevated *RFC1* gene expression is considered to be a prognostic factor for MTX uptake activity (Zhang et al., 1998).

2.1.1b. Functional Abberations in the RFC Transporters

One of the frequent causes of MTX resistance is the functional abberation of RFC transporters due to inactivating mutation, transcriptional silencing or allelic loss in *RFC* genes. Such change may disrupt substrate translocation activity ($\downarrow V_{max}$) or alter affinity of RFC for folates and antifolates i.e. ($\uparrow K_m$) (Jansen et al., 1998; Zhao et al., 1999; Drori et al., 2000; Kaufman et al., 2006). Following antifolate selection, Glu45Lys is the common mutations identified in the *RFC* genes (Jansen et al., 1998; Zhao et al., 1999; Drori et al., 2000). This mutation resulted in increased affinity for folates, while decreased the transport V_{max} for MTX. This is interesting because although the MTX and other antifolates were inhibited, the cellular uptake of folic acid and other natural folates were uninhibited, thus maintaining the cellular THF cofactor pool (discussed later). Another important mutation is Ser46Asn, which was seen in cell lines obtained from leukemia and osteosarcoma patients. These cell lines do not affect the transport of folates, lecovorin and 5-CH3-THF, but significantly reduce MTX transport V_{max} (Zhao et al., 1998; Flintoff et al., 2004). The Gly44Arg and Ser127Aspa mutations resulted in frameshift and early translational termination in *RFC* genes, and thus complete loss of RFC proteins (Wong et al., 1999). In addition, a SNP in *RFC* genes in leukemia cell line markedly decreased V_{max} for antifolates due to impaired mobility of these carriers (Brigle et al., 1995). Although, several missense and nonsense mutations completely disrupted the RFCs transport function, clinical studies on ALL patients failed to show any frequent mutations of *RFCs* (Gifford et al., 2002). In contrast, heterozygous *RFC* mutations were frequently seen in large clinical study done on osteosarcoma patients (Yang et al., 2003).

2.1.1c. Transcriptional Regulation and RFC Promoter Methylation

Another mechanism of MTX resistance may be due to alterations in transcriptional silencing of factors regulating for *RFC* genes under physiological conditions. The basal promoters of *RFC* genes are regulated by key transcription factors such as AP-1 like elements/c-AMP response element (CREB), AP-2,Sp1 families, USF, GATA families, p53 and Ikaros (Whetstine and Matherly, 2001; Payton et al., 2005; Liu et al., 2006). For example, the activation of tumor suppressor gene p53 in ALL was accompanied by significant decrease in *RFCs* transcription levels and MTX influx activity (Ding et al., 2001a).

2.1.2. Folate Receptors(FRs)

The transport of folates and antifolates is mediated by two membranous folate receptors (FRs) i.e. FR-α (adults) and FR-β (fetus) (Ratnam et al., 1989; Sadasivan and Rothenberg, 1989). These FRs mediate slow transport (1/100 of RFCs) with high affinity for folic acid (~1 nM) and relatively low affinity for MTX (~300 nM) (Westerhof et al., 1991; Sierra et al., 1995). An MTX selected leukemia cell line with defective RFCs function (Schuetz et al., 1989), when grown in folic acid depleted medium produced a subline, which expressed higher levels of FR-β with higher resistance to MTX (Brigle et al., 1994). However, even in the presence of RFCs, enhancing the uptake of folic acid, other reduced folates and THF cofactors with sufficient expression of FRs with activating mutations could increase the intracellular pool of folates (Jansen et al., 1989). Hence, if the folic acid is >2.3 µM in the medium, the MTX uptake by FRs is significantly reduced, whereas when folic acid is uptaken with 300 folds higher affinity, MTX resistance occurs (Kane et al., 1986; Chung et al., 1993). So far, the role of FRs in MTX resistance has not been determined clinically.

2.1.3. Proton Coupled Folate Transporter (PCFT)

The proton driven PCFT transporter, previously known as "low pH folate transporter", has an optimal activity in acidic condition (pH=5.5), and has a high affinity for folate transport (For 5-CH$_3$-THF, K$_m$ ~ 1-5 µM) and MTX (K$_m$ ~ 3.5 µM) (Assaraf et al., 1998; Sierra and Goldman, 1998; Zhao et al., 2004). However, polyglutamatable hydrophilic antifolates such as MTX-(Glu)n are not the substrate for PCFT (Qiu et al., 2007; Zhao et al., 2007). Recently, an inactivating mutation in the *PCFT* gene was identified to be the molecular basis of a rare recessive hereditary folate malabsorption (HFM) disorder (Qiu et al., 2006). At physiological pH, the PCFT is apically localized and expressed significantly in the small intestine, liver, kidney, spleen and to a lesser extent in testes, brain and colon (Qiu et al., 2006; Subramanian et al., 2008). In addition, significant levels of *PCFT* mRNA were detected in cervical and colon cancer cell lines (Qiu et al., 2006). This systematic localization of PCFT may be important in disposition of its transport substrates, such as MTX and other antifolates, into the acidic environment of malignant neoplasms, especially in tumors where RFCs are down regulated or inactivated. The role of PCFT in MTX resistance needs to be determined.

2.2. Augmented Efflux by ABC Transporters

2.2.1. ATP-Binding Cassette (ABC) Transporters

The ABC transporter family is one of the largest superfamily of transporters with 48 members, subdivided into seven distinct subfamilies, ABCA to ABCG, based on sequence homologies (Dean and Allikmets, 2001). These ABC transporters have a potential to extrude a wide range of drugs and thus cause multidrug resistance (Gottesman, 2002). Among these, seven members, ABCCs1-5, ABCC11 and ABCG2 have so far been reported, to actively efflux MTX from the cells, thus leading to MTX resistance (Hooijberg et al., 1999; Bakos et al., 2000; Zeng et al., 2001; Chen et al., 2002; Chen et al., 2005; Shafran et al., 2005; Wielinga et al., 2005). Although a higher expression of ABCB1 (P-gp) was seen in leukemia cell lines treated with antifolates, the role of ABCB1 could not be correlated as a resistance factor in these cells (Klohs et al., 1986).

2.2.1a. ABCC (MRP) Family

The ABCC subfamily contains thirteen members, and nine of these drug transporters are often referred to as the Multidrug Resistance Proteins (MRPs) (Dean and Allikmets, 2001; Chen and Tiwari, 2011). The MRP proteins are ubiquitously expressed, four of them, MRPs 4, 5, 8, 9 (ABCCs 4, 5, 11 and 12) are referred to as the "short" MRPs as they have a two membrane spanning domains (MSD1 and MSD2), each followed by a nucleotide binding domain (NBD1 and NBD2). MRPs 1, 2, 3, 6, 7 (ABCCs 1, 2, 3, 6 and 10), have an additional fifth domain, MSD0, at their NH2-terminus, hence they are called "long" MRPs. The MRP (ABCC) family members confer resistance to a variety of hydrophobic and hydrophilic chemotherapeutic agents and their conjugated metabolites such as nucleoside and nucleotide analogs, vinca alkaloids, anthracyclines, camptothecins, epipodophyllotoxins, tyrosine kinase inhibitors as well as antifolates (Kruh and Belinsky, 2003; Chen and Tiwari, 2011). MTX is transported by MRP1 to MRP5 and MRP8, as shown by transport assay in membrane vesicle overexpressing these transporters, with a Km value typically in millimolar range (Bakos et al., 2000; Zeng et al., 2001; Chen et al., 2002; Chen et al., 2005; Wielinga et al., 2005). MRPs have a high capacity for transporting MTX with a Vmax ~ 1 μmol/min/mg, despite having a low affinity for MTX. Nonetheless, the MRPs' capacity to transport MTX is approximately 100 times more than that of RFCs, which is likely to determine the disposition and bioavailability of MTX (Assaraf and Goldman, 1997). Cellular accumulation of MTX and cellular resistance to MTX are also dependent on the length of exposure of MTX in these MRPs 1-5 overexpressing cells i.e. with 1-4 h, MTX exposure showed significant resistance, that was not seen when exposed more than 24 h (Hooijberg et al., 1999; Wielinga et al., 2005). This phenomenon was later recognized to be due to folate polyglutamylation, suggesting that MRPs 1-4 cannot transport MTX-(Glu)n (Zeng et al., 2001; Chen et al., 2002). However, Wielinga et al. reported that MRP5 could transport MTX-di-glutamate (MTX-Glu2), but that function was lost by the addition of even a single glutamyl residue (Wielinga et al., 2005). Interestingly, MTX transport or resistance was not appreciably seen in MRP6 (Belinsky et al., 2002) and MRP7 transporters (Chen et al., 2003a). However, MRP8 overexpressing membrane vesicles showed robust transport of MTX, but not its polyglutamated forms (Chen et al., 2005). MRP9 transport activity in terms of MTX, MTX-(Glu)n or other antifolates has not been reported yet. Pharmacogenetic studies in relation to MTX efflux by highly polymorphic ABC transporters have not been studied in great detail. In pediatric ALL, higher MTX concentration was seen in SNP of ABCC2 24C>T form, whereas loss of function by another MRP2 variant lead to defective MTX excretion, altering MTX pharmacokinetics (Rau et al., 2006). However, in the case of rheumatoid arthritis, the effect of polymorphic ABC transporters on MTX resistance had inconsistent data (Ranganathan et al., 2008).

2.2.1b. ABCG2 (BCRP) Transporter

The human ABCG2/BCRP is a 72 kDa (655 amino acids) "half-transporter" encoded by *ABCG2* gene localized on chromosome 4q22 (Allikmets et al., 1998; Doyle et al., 1998). Normally, significant expression of ABCG2 is seen in a variety of tissues including the placenta, colon, breasts, apical membrane of the epithelium in the small and large intestine, pancreas, canalicular membrane of liver and bile duct, alveolar pneumocytes, adrenal gland, cortical tubules of the kidney, prostate epithelium, and brain tissues (Maliepaard et al., 2001; Mao and Unadkat, 2005). The ABCG2 transporter effluxes a variety of chemotherapeutic agents and at least in *in vitro* studies it has been shown to confer resistance to nucleoside analogues, organic anion conjugates, organic dyes, anthracyclines, camptothecin-derived indolocarbazole topoisomerase I inhibitors, flavopiridol, and a newer class of anticancer agents belonging to tyrosine kinase inhibitors (reviewed by (Mao and Unadkat, 2005; Tiwari et al., 2011).

Mitoxantrone-selected breast cancer cell line overexpressed ABCG2 and confered cross-resistance to MTX (Volk et al., 2002). In addition, the membrane vesicles prepared from ABCG2 transfected HEK293 cells showed that wild type ABCG2 with Arg at 482 position, but not R482T or R482G mutations, was responsible for efflux of folic acid, MTX and MTX-

(Glu)n, although transport gradually decreased as the polyglutamate chain length increased (Chen et al., 2003b; Volk and Schneider, 2003). Recently, overexpression of ABCG2 and ABCC1 on inflammatory cells in RA synovial tissue has been shown to contribute to reduced therapeutic efficacy of MTX and other disease modifying rheumatoid factors (DMARD) (van der Heijden et al., 2009). In Abcc2/Abcg2(-/-) mice, substantial accumulation of 7-OH-MTX (7-OH-MTX), a major toxic metabolite of MTX in the liver and kidney, and significantly decrease in biliary 7-OH-MTX excretion were seen, suggesting the role of Abcc1, Abcc2 and Abcg2 together in MTX and 7-OH-MTX disposition and pharmacokinetics (Vlaming et al., 2009a; Vlaming et al., 2009b). In fact, co-administration of MTX with proton pump inhibitors, another type of ABCG2 inhibitors, was shown to be a risk factor for delayed elimination of plasma MTX in high-dose MTX therapy for malignant diseases (Suzuki et al., 2009). A recent report suggests that changes in cellular folate concentration alter the expression of ABCG2 and MRP1 in a variety of cancer cells (Lemos et al., 2009). The SNPs in ABCG2 421C>A has not been found to produce any clinical response in children with ALL (Imanishi et al., 2007).

2.3. Impaired Polyglutamylation and Augmented Glutamylation Hydrolysis

The monoglutamate form 5-methyl-THF is the primary circulatory reduced folate derivative in the blood. The 5-methyl-THF, THF cofactors as well as MTX and other antifolates are uptaken via RFCs and are biochemically converted to polyglutamates [such as MTX-(Glu)n] by a unique transformation catalyzed by FPGS (Figure 1).

2.3.1. Folypolyglutamylation and Folylpolyglutamate Synthetase (FPGS)

Cellular uptake of CH_3-THF, other reduced folates, and various hydrophilic antifolates including MTX is catalyzed by the enzyme FPGS in both cytosol and mitochondria (Baugh et al., 1973; McGuire et al., 2000). Polyglutamylation of MTX by FPGS is catalyzed by sequential addition of glutamic acid, one at a time to γ-carboxyl group of antifolate and folate THF cofactors. Intracellular accumulation of polyglutamation enhances the antifolate drug action, because they are not substrates of MRPs (except MTX-Glu$_2$ which is exported by MRP5) (Figure 1). In addition, these polyglutamated derivatives are more potent inhibitors of enzymes involved in nucleotide biosynthesis. The polyglutamylation process could be altered by length of exposure of MTX, by changes in the MTX transport into the cells by RFCs and changes in FPGS levels and/or its activity. In addition, increased efflux of MTX by MRPs 1-5, 8 and ABCG2 transporters or impaired influx by RFCs may leave very little free monoglutamyl substrate available for FPGS exposure, decreasing the rate and extent of MTX-(Glu)n formation. Also, rapid recovery of TS activity, probably due to reduced polyglutamylation, was shown to be responsible for low FPGS activity (Lu et al., 1995). Decreased polyglutamylation leads to intrinsic and acquired resistance to MTX in a variety of cancer cells including those of leukemia, breast and colon cancer, soft tissue sarcoma and squamous carcinoma (Jackman et al., 1995; Lu et al., 1995; Barnes et al., 1999; Mauritz et al., 2002). Decreased FPGS activity due to decreased FPGS mRNA levels or posttranscriptional alterations in *FPGS* gene were shown to decrease FPGS at protein level in cancer cells (McGuire et al., 1995; Roy et al., 1997). In contrast, the FPGS activity increased in B- rather than T-lineage ALL after MTX treatment and is considered to be a prognostic factor for the level of MTX glutamates accumulation in ALL (Barredo et al., 1994).

Few inactivating mutations in the *FPGS* gene associated with decrease in FPGS-antifolate binding and/or decreased FPGS activities have also been reported (Zhao et al., 2000; Liani et al., 2003). Marked decrease in FPGS activity was seen due to heterozygous Cys346Phe mutations in antifolate selected leukemia cells (Sanghani et al., 1999). Leil et al. have reported many functionally relevant polymorphisms in FPGS encoding gene (Leil et al., 2007). However, these polymorphisms in *FPGS* seem to be neutral in altering toxicity, resistance, or even MTX action in clinical study on rheumatoid arthritis patients (van der Straaten et al., 2007). The pharmacogenetic studies on FPGS in ALL patients have not been reported.

2.3.2. Gamma-Glutamyl Hydrolase (γ-GH)

The γ-GH (previously known as folypolygammaglutamyl hydrolase) is a lysosomal glycoprotein, and in contrast to FPGS it mediates the hydrolysis of polyglutamated chains of folates and antifolates (Rhee et al., 1993; Galivan et al., 2000; Schneider and Ryan, 2006). Based on this property, it is possible that an increase in γ-GH activity would result in a decrease in polyglutamylation, and thus would be responsible for acquisition to antifolate resistance (Rhee et al., 1993; Schneider and Ryan, 2006). Increased γ-GH activity was seen in several sarcoma and hepatocellular carcinoma cells resistant to MTX (Li et al., 1993; Rhee et al., 1993). The lomotrexol (antifolate)-selected H35D rat hepatoma cells displayed a seven-fold increase in γ-GH activity and significant cross-resistance to MTX due to marked decrease (~90%) of MTX-(Glu)n (Yao et al., 1995). In a clinical study on childhood ALL patients, the γ-GH:FPGS ratio was shown to be the best predictor for MTX-(Glu)n (Longo et al., 1997). In addition, increased γ-GH plasma and tumor concentration were seen in metastatic breast cancer patients (Baggott et al., 1987), and later increased expression of γ-GH was found in breast and liver cancer (Galivan et al., 2000). Similarly, in acute myeloid leukemia patients, increased expression of γ-GH decreased MTX-(Glu)n formation, and this was associated with inherent MTX resistance (Rots et al., 1999). Certain epigenetic changes were also noted to regulate γ-GH activity in ALL patients, for example, reduced γ-GH activity and expression were seen when the CpG island methylation occurred in γ-GH promoter region (Cheng et al., 2006). Moreover, polymorphisms in the coding and promoter region of γ-GH gene were also shown to modulate γ-GH expression (Chave et al., 2003; Cheng et al., 2004). Whereas, most of these mutations lead to enhanced expression of γ-GH (Chave et al., 2003), one of the SNPs in the coding region, Thr127Ile, was linked to reduced expression and activity of γ-GH in both B- and T-lineage hyperdiploid lymphoblasts (Cheng et al., 2004).

It is also possible that overexpression of γ-GH may increase sensitivity towards antifolates due to increased hydrolysis of folate polyglutamates resulting in decreased folate pool intracellularly. Supporting this hypothesis, increased γ-GH activity was seen in γ-GH cDNA stably transfected into fibrosarcoma and breast cancer (Cole et al., 2001). Although there was no marked difference in MTX glutamate formation in fibrosarcoma cells, the breast cancer cells showed ~50% reduction in MTX-(Glu)n with no significant change in the sensitivity of either cells, probably due to compensation by comparable decrease of CH_3-THF levels (Cole et al., 2001). The role of γ-GH in MTX and other antifolates resistance needs further exploration, in order to modulate this important pathway to overcome antifolate resistance.

2.4. Alterations in Crucial Enzyme's

2.4.1. Dihydro Folate Reductase (DHFR)

The DHFR uses enzyme catalyses the regeneration of THF (and other 1-carbon donor cofactors) from DHF, using NADPH as a cofactor. Acquired resistance mechanism to MTX and other antifolates is frequently reported to be due to stable and unstable DHFR gene amplification resulting in DHFR enzyme overexpression (Alt et al., 1978; Dolnick et al., 1979; Mini et al., 1985). The *DHFR* gene is located at the chromosome 5q11.2-q13.3 (Smith SL, Patrick P, Stone D 1979). Gene amplification was associated with MTX-resistance in clinical samples obtained from MTX treated ALL, ovarian cancer and HD-MTX treated soft-tissue sarcoma (Horns et al., 1984; Trent et al., 1984; Li et al., 1992) The biochemical basis underlying this phenomenon is probably the polymorphisms in DHFR gene, leading to its enhanced gene expression and MTX sensitivity (Gorlick et al., 1997; Goto et al., 2001) In addition, the mutations in the DHFR gene were shown to have decreased affinity for MTX (Flintoff et al., 1976). After selection with MTX, several mutations in *DHFR* gene have been recorded in variety of cell lines obtained from different species (Simonsen and Levinson, 1983; Melera et al., 1988). Some mutations such as leu22Arg (murine) and Leu22Phe (hamster lung cancer cells) altered the binding affinity of MTX, antifolates and other DHF substrates with the DHFR enzyme (Simonsen and Levinson, 1983; Melera et al., 1988). Whereas, other mutations such as Gly15Trp (L1210 leukemia cells) decreased the affinity of 4-aminoantifolates for DHFR, less than the affinity for DHF, probably due to the influence of allelic variation at another site. However, so far no mutations in the coding region of *DHFR* gene have been reported (Gellekink et al., 2007). Also, these mutant forms of DHFR have not been reported in patients treated with MTX (Spencer et al., 1996).

Various studies have shown that transcriptional deregulations in *DHFR* gene may contribute to resistance phenotype in MTX treated samples (Albrecht et al., 1972; Flintoff and Essani, 1980; Goldie et al., 1980; Sowers et al., 2003). In osteosarcoma patient the E2F transcription factor was shown to regulate the tumor suppressor gene, retinoblastoma (Rb), which was pivotal in regulation of DHFR expression (Sowers et al., 2003). Antifolate treatment eventually leads to increased DHFR synthesis due to increase in DHFR message to enhance translation (Ercikan-Abali et al., 1997; Schmitz et al., 2001). Interestingly, this regulation process of DHFR is lost in malarial parasite, opening new avenues for therapeutic implications (Zhang and Rathod, 2002).

2.4.2. Thymidylate Synthase (TS)

The TS catalyzes the reductive methylation reaction between deoxyuridine monophosphate (dUMP) and 5,10-methylene tetrahydrofolate, leading to *de novo* formation of thymidine monophosphate (dTMP), which is subsequently phosphorylated to deoxythymidine triphosphate (dTTP) for use in DNA synthesis and repair, yielding DHF as a secondary product. Sustained levels of dTTPH also maintain increased DNA synthesis. At molecular level antifolate resistance is associated with high intrinsic levels of TS due to its overexpression, gene amplification or functional mutation leading to insufficient TS inhibition by antifolates, including MTX (Zhao and Goldman, 2003). Various human cell lines selected with TS inhibitors produced variable cross-resistance to different antifolates including MTX, due to the overexpression or gene amplification of TS enzyme (Tong et al., 1998a; Tong et al., 1998b; Bertino and Banerjee, 2004). This mechanism of resistance through TS was also seen in colorectal cancer patients treated with fluorinated compounds, such as 5-fluorouracil. Notably, 23% of 5-FU treated advanced colorectal cancer patients showed TS gene amplification, which was correlated with significantly shorter median survival rate (Wang et al., 2004).

Mutagenesis studies in TS showed different binding sites for different antifolates. For example, Gly52Ser, Lys47Glu, Asp49Gly, mutations in a highly conserved TS region were reported when HT1080 (human sarcoma cells) were selected with a non-polyglutamable, hydrophobic TS inhibitor, thymitaq in presence of ethyl methanesulfonate (mutagen) (Tong et al., 1998a; Tong et al., 1998b; Wang et al., 2004). The cells having Lys47Glu and Asp49Gly mutations were cross-resistant to 5-FU but not to other TS inhibitor such as GW1843U89 or ZD1694 (Tong et al., 1998a). Similarly, Ile108Ala mutation produced less resistance to GW1843U89 but significant resistance to AG337 and ZD1694 (Tong et al., 1998b). However, one should not forget other cellular factors such as cellular retention of MTX, polyglutamylation, uptake and efflux and THF cofactor pool expansion playing key role in variability of antifolate cytotoxicity (Bertino and Banerjee, 2004). Recently, SNPs in serine hydroxymethyltransferase (SHMT1), a key cytosolic enzyme in thymidine synthesis of the folate pathway, has been described with the lack of MTX toxicity in childhood ALL (Huang et al., 2008).

2.4.3. Glycinamide Ribonucleotide Formyltransferase (GARFT)

The GARFT enzyme is involved in *de novo* purine biosynthesis by its catalysis of the formation of N -formylglycinamide ribonucleotide from glycinamide ribonucleotide, and at the same time conversion of $10\text{-}CH_3\text{-}THF$ to THF. Hepatoma cells selected with lomotrel, a known inhibitor of GARFT, showed cross resistance to MTX, albeit through different pathways, including increased efflux of folic acid and MTX, impaired uptake of MTX, decreased FPGS, and increased γ-GH activity (Yao et al., 1995; Zhao and Goldman, 2003). So far, the role of GARFT in human MTX resistance has not yet been explored in great detail.

2.5. Alterations in Cellular Folate Pool

The accumulation of intracellular THF-cofactor pool largely affects the polyglutamylation process and thus modulates antifolate activity (van der Wilt et al., 2001; Zhao et al., 2001a). Antifolates requiring polyglutamylation show resistance due to increase in THF-cofactor pool intracellularly, either due to increased uptake by defective or mutated RFC carrier or decreased efflux by MRP1-5, 8 and ABCG2 transporter (Assaraf and Goldman, 1997; Jansen et al., 1999; Drori et al., 2000). The MTX and its polyglutamate derivatives potently inhibit DHFR activity, thus initiating the rapid oxidization of THF-cofactors to DHF. The DHF then competes with MTX and MTX-(Glu)n to bind with the target DHFR enzyme, thereby resulting in MTX and MTX-(Glu)n resistance (Tse and Moran, 1998; Jansen et al., 1999). The intracellular expansion of DHF and THF-cofactors strongly inhibits polyglutamylation process as they compete with MTX for FPGS at enzyme level. For example, when intracellular folate level was increased to significant levels antifolates, a potent TS inhibitor ZD9331, which does not undergo polyglutamylation, showed no resistance (Assaraf and Slotky, 1993; Jackman et al., 1995; Assaraf and Goldman, 1997). Another example is expansion of THF-cofactor pool in cells devoid of MRP1, which showed variable cross-resistance to polyglutamable antifolate such as AG2034, thymitaq and non-polyglutamylable antifolates such as trimetrexate and AG377. In addition, expansion of THF-cofactor levels also depends on the increased expression of RFCs and FPGS or decreased expression of γ-GH or efflux ABC transporters, as these natural folates are substrates of these enzymes/proteins. Expanded cellular folate pool was seen to cause significant resistance to lomotrexol and cross-resistance to ZD1694 and to MTX, when grown in mouse L1210 cells by two mechanisms. A mutation in the RFC gene was reported to increase the affinity and influx of folic acid levels, which then blocked the polyglutamylation of lomotrexol, however without affecting the binding affinity for FPGS (Tse et al., 1998; Tse and Moran, 1998).

2.6. Emerging Mechanisms of MTX Resistance

2.6.1. 7-Hydroxy Methotrexate (7-OH-MTX)

Extensive metabolism of MTX by aldehyde xidases in the liver to its primary metabolite 7-OH-MTX could lead to acquired resistance to MTX treatment. The 7-OH-MTX is a better substrate of FPGS, and thus the rate of 7-OH-MTX-(Glu)n formation exceeds that of MTX 3-fold, with a comparable transport Km for RFC for both drugs (Fabre et al., 1983). When a high dose MTX infusion was given to children with ALL, the plasma concentration of 7-OH-MTX was significantly higher than that of MTX. The leukemic cells MOLT-4 and CEM, when selected with 7-OH-MTX showed disparate mechanisms of antifolate resistance (Fotoohi et al., 2004). Molecular basis of resistance to 7-OH-MTX was due to 95% loss of FPGS activity, along with downregulation of transcriptional factors associated with RFC expression (Fotoohi et al., 2004). The 7-OH-MTX is readily effluxed by ABCG2 transporter at low pH (Breedveld et al., 2007). Overlapping roles of Abcg2 and Abcc2 in the elimination of the MTX and its toxic metabolite (7-OH-MTX) was seen in Abcc2/Abcg2(-/-) mice (Vlaming et al., 2009a). Recently, it was shown that the absence of Abcc2 and/or Abcg2 led to significantly increased levels of 7-OH-MTX in the liver and kidney. Moreover, overexpression of either ABCC2 or ABCG2 inhibition may result in decreased biovailability of MTX (Vlaming et al., 2011). Hence these findings suggest that 7-OH-MTX contributes to MTX resistance by competing with MTX for inward uptake by RFCs or polyglutamylation by FPGS.

2.6.2. High-Dose MTX (HDMTX) Treatment

Recently, rationale for the use of MTX treatment has been questioned for different indications. One such modality is the use of high-dose MTX (HDMTX) with leucovorin in the treatment of osteogenic sarcoma and ALL, which theoretically was thought to circumvent most mechanisms of MTX resistance (Holmboe et al., 2011). High extracellular MTX concentration allows it to diffuse passively even in the transport-defective resistant cells, and intracellular MTX levels are extremely high to produce action. In addition, it was recently shown that co-administration of proton pump inhibitors delays elimination of plasma MTX in high-dose MTX therapy (Suzuki et al., 2009). However, one can predict that increased intracellular MTX delivered by HDMTX therapy can saturate DHFR in cells whose resistance is a result of amplification of the DHFR gene or of lowered affinity of DHFR for MTX.

2.6.3. Isoprenylcysteine Carboxyl Methyltransferases (ICCMTF)

The MTX and its polyglutamated derivatives inhibit the folate metabolism and thus increase the level of S-adenosylhomocysteine (SAH) (Figure 1). Cellular hypomethylation of SAH leads to the formation of toxic homocysteine and inhibition of methyltransferases including that of ICCMTF (Rosenquist et al., 1996). The ICCMTF mediates carboxyl methylation and proper membrane targeting of Ras signaling (later being a substrate of this enzyme), which is a crucial pathway in cell differentiation and proliferation (Winter-Vann et al., 2003). Leukemic cells devoid of ICCMTF were significantly resistant to MTX. Downregulation and/or MTX-mediated inhibition of ICCMTF disrupted Ras-dependent signaling, accompanied by a decrease in AKT and p44 mitogen-activated protein kinase (MAPK), with this consequently abrogating DNA synthesis (Blum and Kloog, 2005). This is a novel pathway of MTX and antifolates resistance and it is possible that targeting this pathway may provide avenues for new therapies in the future.

Summary

The multiple mechanisms of MTX resistance can be summarized below –

1. Defective uptake of MTX due to alterations in the qualitative, quantitative and/or functional loss of facilitative reduced folate carriers (RFCs) or folate receptors (FRs).
2. Increased efflux of MTX by ABCCs 1-5 and ABCC11 while increased efflux of both MTX and MTX-(Glu)n by ABCG2.
3. Reduced intracellular MTX-polyglutamates concentration due to decreased expression and/or inactivating mutations of folypolyglutamate synthase (FPGS) or increased expression of γ-glutamyl hydrolase (γ-GH).
4. Increased expression or mutations in enzymes involved in folate metabolic pathway such as dihydrofolate folate reductase (DHFR), thymidylate synthase (TS), 5-aminoimidazole-4-carboxamide ribonucleotide formyltransferase (AICARFT), reduces the affinity for MTX and MTX-(Glu)n.
5. Increased accumulation of THF cofactor pool, leads to competition with MTX for enzymes involved in de novo purine biosynthesis, leading to MTX resistance.
6. Novel mechanisms in MTX treatment involve increased metabolism of MTX to 7-hydroxy-MTX, which competes with MTX to enter into the cells through RFCs. In addition, lack of key enzyme isoprenylcysteine carboxyl methyltransferases (ICCMTF) involved in mediating Ras-dependent signal pathway leads to MTX resistance.

Acknowledgments

We thank Miss Yanglu Chen (Montgomery High School, New Jersey, USA) for her critical reading and edition. This work was supported by funds from NIH R15 No. 1R15CA143701 (Z.S. Chen) and Ray Biotech. Co. (Z.S. Chen and A.K. Tiwari).

References

Albrecht AM, Biedler JL and Hutchison DJ (1972) Two different species of dihydrofolate reductase in mammalian cells differentially resistant to amethopterin and methasquin. *Cancer Res.* 32:1539-1546.

Allikmets R, Schriml LM, Hutchinson A, Romano-Spica V and Dean M (1998) A human placenta-specific ATP-binding cassette gene (ABCP) on chromosome 4q22 that is involved in multidrug resistance. *Cancer Res.* 58:5337-5339.

Alt FW, Kellems RE, Bertino JR and Schimke RT (1978) Selective multiplication of dihydrofolate reductase genes in methotrexate-resistant variants of cultured murine cells. *J. Biol. Chem.* 253:1357-1370.

Assaraf YG (2007) Molecular basis of antifolate resistance. *Cancer Metastasis Rev.* 26:153-181.

Assaraf YG, Babani S and Goldman ID (1998) Increased activity of a novel low pH folate transporter associated with lipophilic antifolate resistance in chinese hamster ovary cells. *J. Biol. Chem.* 273:8106-8111.

Assaraf YG and Goldman ID (1997) Loss of folic acid exporter function with markedly augmented folate accumulation in lipophilic antifolate-resistant mammalian cells. *J. Biol. Chem.* 272:17460-17466.

Assaraf YG and Slotky JI (1993) Characterization of a lipophilic antifolate resistance provoked by treatment of mammalian cells with the antiparasitic agent pyrimethamine. *J. Biol. Chem.* 268:4556-4566.

Baggott JE, Heimburger DC, Krumdieck CL and Butterworth CE, Jr. (1987) Folate conjugase activity in the plasma and tumors of breast-cancer patients. *Am. J. Clin. Nutr.* 46:295-301.

Bakos E, Evers R, Sinko E, Varadi A, Borst P and Sarkadi B (2000) Interactions of the human multidrug resistance proteins MRP1 and MRP2 with organic anions. *Mol. Pharmacol.* 57:760-768.

Barnes MJ, Estlin EJ, Taylor GA, Aherne GW, Hardcastle A, McGuire JJ, Calvete JA, Lunec J, Pearson AD and Newell DR (1999) Impact of polyglutamation on sensitivity to raltitrexed and methotrexate in relation to drug-induced inhibition of de novo thymidylate and purine biosynthesis in CCRF-CEM cell lines. *Clin. Cancer Res.* 5:2548-2558.

Barredo JC, Synold TW, Laver J, Relling MV, Pui CH, Priest DG and Evans WE (1994) Differences in constitutive and post-methotrexate folylpolyglutamate synthetase activity in B-lineage and T-lineage leukemia. *Blood* 84:564-569.

Baugh CM, Krumdieck CL and Nair MG (1973) Polygammaglutamyl metabolites of methotrexate. *Biochem. Biophys. Res. Commun.* 52:27-34.

Belinsky MG, Chen ZS, Shchaveleva I, Zeng H and Kruh GD (2002) Characterization of the drug resistance and transport properties of multidrug resistance protein 6 (MRP6, ABCC6). *Cancer Res.* 62:6172-6177.

Bertino JR and Banerjee D (2004) Thymidylate synthase as an oncogene? *Cancer Cell* 5:301-302.

Bhargava PM (2001) Dr. Yellapragada SubbaRow (1895-1948). He Transformed Science; Changed Lives. *Indian Academy of Clinical Medicine* 2:96-100.

Blum R and Kloog Y (2005) Tailoring Ras-pathway--inhibitor combinations for cancer therapy. *Drug Resist Updat.* 8:369-380.

Breedveld P, Pluim D, Cipriani G, Dahlhaus F, van Eijndhoven MA, de Wolf CJ, Kuil A, Beijnen JH, Scheffer GL, Jansen G, Borst P and Schellens JH (2007) The effect of low pH on breast cancer resistance protein (ABCG2)-mediated transport of methotrexate, 7-hydroxymethotrexate, methotrexate diglutamate, folic acid, mitoxantrone, topotecan, and resveratrol in in vitro drug transport models. *Mol. Pharmacol.* 71:240-249.

Brigle KE, Seither RL, Westin EH and Goldman ID (1994) Increased expression and genomic organization of a folate-binding protein homologous to the human placental isoform in L1210 murine leukemia cell lines with a defective reduced folate carrier. *J. Biol. Chem.* 269:4267-4272.

Brigle KE, Spinella MJ, Sierra EE and Goldman ID (1995) Characterization of a mutation in the reduced folate carrier in a transport defective L1210 murine leukemia cell line. *J. Biol. Chem.* 270:22974-22979.

Chave KJ, Ryan TJ, Chmura SE and Galivan J (2003) Identification of single nucleotide polymorphisms in the human gamma-glutamyl hydrolase gene and characterization of promoter polymorphisms. *Gene* 319:167-175.

Chen ZS, Guo Y, Belinsky MG, Kotova E and Kruh GD (2005) Transport of bile acids, sulfated steroids, estradiol 17-beta-D-glucuronide, and leukotriene C4 by human multidrug resistance protein 8 (ABCC11). *Mol. Pharmacol.* 67:545-557.

Chen ZS, Hopper-Borge E, Belinsky MG, Shchaveleva I, Kotova E and Kruh GD (2003a) Characterization of the transport properties of human multidrug resistance protein 7 (MRP7, ABCC10). *Mol. Pharmacol.* 63:351-358.

Chen ZS, Lee K, Walther S, Raftogianis RB, Kuwano M, Zeng H and Kruh GD (2002) Analysis of methotrexate and folate transport by multidrug resistance protein 4 (ABCC4): MRP4 is a component of the methotrexate efflux system. *Cancer Res.* 62:3144-3150.

Chen ZS, Robey RW, Belinsky MG, Shchaveleva I, Ren XQ, Sugimoto Y, Ross DD, Bates SE and Kruh GD (2003b) Transport of methotrexate, methotrexate polyglutamates, and 17beta-estradiol 17-(beta-D-glucuronide) by ABCG2: effects of acquired mutations at R482 on methotrexate transport. *Cancer Res.* 63:4048-4054.

Chen ZS and Tiwari AK (2011) Multidrug resistance proteins (MRPs/ABCCs) in cancer chemotherapy and genetic diseases. *FEBS J.*

Cheng Q, Cheng C, Crews KR, Ribeiro RC, Pui CH, Relling MV and Evans WE (2006) Epigenetic regulation of human gamma-glutamyl hydrolase activity in acute lymphoblastic leukemia cells. *Am. J. Hum. Genet.* 79:264-274.

Cheng Q, Wu B, Kager L, Panetta JC, Zheng J, Pui CH, Relling MV and Evans WE (2004) A substrate specific functional polymorphism of human gamma-glutamyl hydrolase alters catalytic activity and methotrexate polyglutamate accumulation in acute lymphoblastic leukaemia cells. *Pharmacogenetics* 14:557-567.

Chung KN, Saikawa Y, Paik TH, Dixon KH, Mulligan T, Cowan KH and Elwood PC (1993) Stable transfectants of human MCF-7 breast cancer cells with increased levels of the human folate receptor exhibit an increased sensitivity to antifolates. *J. Clin. Invest.* 91:1289-1294.

Cole PD, Kamen BA, Gorlick R, Banerjee D, Smith AK, Magill E and Bertino JR (2001) Effects of overexpression of gamma-Glutamyl hydrolase on methotrexate metabolism and resistance. *Cancer Res.* 61:4599-4604.

Dean M and Allikmets R (2001) Complete characterization of the human ABC gene family. *J. Bioenerg. Biomembr.* 33:475-479.

Ding BC, Whetstine JR, Witt TL, Schuetz JD and Matherly LH (2001a) Repression of human reduced folate carrier gene expression by wild type p53. *J. Biol. Chem.* 276:8713-8719.

Ding BC, Witt TL, Hukku B, Heng H, Zhang L and Matherly LH (2001b) Association of deletions and translocation of the reduced folate carrier gene with profound loss of gene expression in methotrexate-resistant K562 human erythroleukemia cells. *Biochem. Pharmacol.* 61:665-675.

Dolnick BJ, Berenson RJ, Bertino JR, Kaufman RJ, Nunberg JH and Schimke RT (1979) Correlation of dihydrofolate reductase elevation with gene amplification in a homogeneously staining chromosomal region in L5178Y cells. *J. Cell Biol.* 83:394-402.

Doyle LA, Yang W, Abruzzo LV, Krogmann T, Gao Y, Rishi AK and Ross DD (1998) A multidrug resistance transporter from human MCF-7 breast cancer cells. *Proc. Natl. Acad. Sci. USA* 95:15665-15670.

Drori S, Jansen G, Mauritz R, Peters GJ and Assaraf YG (2000) Clustering of mutations in the first transmembrane domain of the human reduced folate carrier in GW1843U89-resistant leukemia cells with impaired antifolate transport and augmented folate uptake. *J. Biol. Chem.* 275:30855-30863.

Ercikan-Abali EA, Banerjee D, Waltham MC, Skacel N, Scotto KW and Bertino JR (1997) Dihydrofolate reductase protein inhibits its own translation by binding to dihydrofolate reductase mRNA sequences within the coding region. *Biochemistry* 36:12317-12322.

Fabre G, Matherly LH, Favre R, Catalin J and Cano JP (1983) In vitro formation of polyglutamyl derivatives of methotrexate and 7-hydroxymethotrexate in human lymphoblastic leukemia cells. *Cancer Res.* 43:4648-4652.

Farber S and Diamond LK (1948) Temporary remissions in acute leukemia in children produced by folic acid antagonist, 4-aminopteroyl-glutamic acid. *N. Engl. J. Med.* 238: 787-793.

Ferreri AJ, Dell'Oro S, Capello D, Ponzoni M, Iuzzolino P, Rossi D, Pasini F, Ambrosetti A, Orvieto E, Ferrarese F, Arrigoni G, Foppoli M, Reni M and Gaidano G (2004) Aberrant methylation in the promoter region of the reduced folate carrier gene is a potential mechanism of resistance to methotrexate in primary central nervous system lymphomas. *Br. J. Haematol.* 126:657-664.

Flintoff WF, Davidson SV and Siminovitch L (1976) Isolation and partial characterization of three methotrexate-resistant phenotypes from Chinese hamster ovary cells. *Somatic Cell Genet.* 2:245-261.

Flintoff WF and Essani K (1980) Methotrexate-resistant Chinese hamster ovary cells contain a dihydrofolate reductase with an altered affinity for methotrexate. *Biochemistry* 19:4321-4327.

Flintoff WF, Sadlish H, Gorlick R, Yang R and Williams FM (2004) Functional analysis of altered reduced folate carrier sequence changes identified in osteosarcomas. *Biochim. Biophys. Acta* 1690:110-117.

Fotoohi K, Jansen G, Assaraf YG, Rothem L, Stark M, Kathmann I, Gregorczyk J, Peters GJ and Albertioni F (2004) Disparate mechanisms of antifolate resistance provoked by methotrexate and its metabolite 7-hydroxymethotrexate in leukemia cells: implications for efficacy of methotrexate therapy. *Blood* 104:4194-4201.

Galivan J, Ryan TJ, Chave K, Rhee M, Yao R and Yin D (2000) Glutamyl hydrolase. pharmacological role and enzymatic characterization. *Pharmacol. Ther.* 85:207-215.

Gellekink H, Blom HJ, van der Linden IJ and den Heijer M (2007) Molecular genetic analysis of the human dihydrofolate reductase gene: relation with plasma total homocysteine, serum and red blood cell folate levels. *Eur. J. Hum. Genet.* 15:103-109.

Gifford AJ, Haber M, Witt TL, Whetstine JR, Taub JW, Matherly LH and Norris MD (2002) Role of the E45K-reduced folate carrier gene mutation in methotrexate resistance in human leukemia cells. *Leukemia* 16:2379-2387.

Goldie JH, Krystal G, Hartley D, Gudauskas G and Dedhar S (1980) A methotrexate insensitive variant of folate reductase present in two lines of methotrexate-resistant L5178Y cells. *Eur. J. Cancer* 16:1539-1546.

Gorlick R, Goker E, Trippett T, Steinherz P, Elisseyeff Y, Mazumdar M, Flintoff WF and Bertino JR (1997) Defective transport is a common mechanism of acquired methotrexate resistance in acute lymphocytic leukemia and is associated with decreased reduced folate carrier expression. *Blood* 89:1013-1018.

Goto Y, Yue L, Yokoi A, Nishimura R, Uehara T, Koizumi S and Saikawa Y (2001) A novel single-nucleotide polymorphism in the 3'-untranslated region of the human dihydrofolate reductase gene with enhanced expression. *Clin. Cancer Res.* 7:1952-1956.

Gottesman MM (2002) Mechanisms of cancer drug resistance. *Annu Rev Med* 53:615-627.

Guo W, Healey JH, Meyers PA, Ladanyi M, Huvos AG, Bertino JR and Gorlick R (1999) Mechanisms of methotrexate resistance in osteosarcoma. *Clin. Cancer Res.* 5:621-627.

Hertz R, Li MC and Spencer DB (1956) Effect of methotrexate therapy upon choriocarcinoma and chorioadenoma. *Proc. Soc. Exp. Biol. Med.* 93:361-366.

Holmboe L, Andersen AM, Morkrid L, Slordal L and Hall KS (2011) High-dose Methotrexate Chemotherapy: Pharmacokinetics, Folate and Toxicity in Osteosarcoma Patients. *Br. J. Clin. Pharmacol.*

Hooijberg JH, Broxterman HJ, Kool M, Assaraf YG, Peters GJ, Noordhuis P, Scheper RJ, Borst P, Pinedo HM and Jansen G (1999) Antifolate resistance mediated by the multidrug resistance proteins MRP1 and MRP2. *Cancer Res* 59:2532-2535.

Horns RC, Jr., Dower WJ and Schimke RT (1984) Gene amplification in a leukemic patient treated with methotrexate. *J. Clin. Oncol.* 2:2-7.

Huang L, Tissing WJ, de Jonge R, van Zelst BD and Pieters R (2008) Polymorphisms in folate-related genes: association with side effects of high-dose methotrexate in childhood acute lymphoblastic leukemia. *Leukemia* 22:1798-1800.

Imanishi H, Okamura N, Yagi M, Noro Y, Moriya Y, Nakamura T, Hayakawa A, Takeshima Y, Sakaeda T, Matsuo M and Okumura K (2007) Genetic polymorphisms associated with adverse events and elimination of methotrexate in childhood acute lymphoblastic leukemia and malignant lymphoma. *J. Hum. Genet.* 52:166-171.

Jackman AL, Kelland LR, Kimbell R, Brown M, Gibson W, Aherne GW, Hardcastle A and Boyle FT (1995) Mechanisms of acquired resistance to the quinazoline thymidylate synthase inhibitor ZD1694 (Tomudex) in one mouse and three human cell lines. *Br. J. Cancer* 71:914-924.

Jackson RC, Hart LI and Harrap KR (1976) Intrinsic resistance to methotrexate of cultured mammalian cells in relation to the inhibition kinetics of their dihydrololate reductases. *Cancer Res.* 36:1991-1997.

Jansen G, Barr H, Kathmann I, Bunni MA, Priest DG, Noordhuis P, Peters GJ and Assaraf YG (1999) Multiple mechanisms of resistance to polyglutamatable and lipophilic antifolates in mammalian cells: role of increased folylpolyglutamylation, expanded folate pools, and intralysosomal drug sequestration. *Mol. Pharmacol.* 55:761-769.

Jansen G, Kathmann I, Rademaker BC, Braakhuis BJ, Westerhof GR, Rijksen G and Schornagel JH (1989) Expression of a folate binding protein in L1210 cells grown in low folate medium. *Cancer Res.* 49:1959-1963.

Jansen G, Mauritz R, Drori S, Sprecher H, Kathmann I, Bunni M, Priest DG, Noordhuis P, Schornagel JH, Pinedo HM, Peters GJ and Assaraf YG (1998) A structurally altered human reduced folate carrier with increased folic acid transport mediates a novel mechanism of antifolate resistance. *J. Biol. Chem.* 273:30189-30198.

Kane MA, Portillo RM, Elwood PC, Antony AC and Kolhouse JF (1986) The influence of extracellular folate concentration on methotrexate uptake by human KB cells. Partial characterization of a membrane-associated methotrexate binding protein. *J. Biol. Chem.* 261:44-49.

Kaufman Y, Ifergan I, Rothem L, Jansen G and Assaraf YG (2006) Coexistence of multiple mechanisms of PT523 resistance in human leukemia cells harboring 3 reduced folate carrier alleles: transcriptional silencing, inactivating mutations, and allele loss. *Blood* 107:3288-3294.

Klohs WD, Steinkampf RW, Besserer JA and Fry DW (1986) Cross resistance of pleiotropically drug resistant P338 leukemia cells to the lipophilic antifolates trimetrexate and BW 301U. *Cancer Lett.* 31:253-260.

Kruh GD and Belinsky MG (2003) The MRP family of drug efflux pumps. *Oncogene* 22: 537-7552.

Leil TA, Endo C, Adjei AA, Dy GK, Salavaggione OE, Reid JR and Ames MM (2007) Identification and characterization of genetic variation in the folylpolyglutamate synthase gene. *Cancer Res.* 67:8772-8782.

Lemos C, Kathmann I, Giovannetti E, Belien JA, Scheffer GL, Calhau C, Jansen G and Peters GJ (2009) Cellular folate status modulates the expression of BCRP and MRP multidrug transporters in cancer cell lines from different origins. *Mol. Cancer Ther.* 8:655-664.

Levy AS, Sather HN, Steinherz PG, Sowers R, La M, Moscow JA, Gaynon PS, Uckun FM, Bertino JR and Gorlick R (2003) Reduced folate carrier and dihydrofolate reductase expression in acute lymphocytic leukemia may predict outcome: a Children's Cancer Group Study. *J. Pediatr. Hematol. Oncol.* 25:688-695.

Li WW, Lin JT, Tong WP, Trippett TM, Brennan MF and Bertino JR (1992) Mechanisms of natural resistance to antifolates in human soft tissue sarcomas. *Cancer Res.* 52:1434-1438.

Li WW, Waltham M, Tong W, Schweitzer BI and Bertino JR (1993) Increased activity of gamma-glutamyl hydrolase in human sarcoma cell lines: a novel mechanism of intrinsic resistance to methotrexate (MTX). *Adv. Exp. Med. Biol.* 338:635-638.

Liani E, Rothem L, Bunni MA, Smith CA, Jansen G and Assaraf YG (2003) Loss of folylpoly-gamma-glutamate synthetase activity is a dominant mechanism of resistance to polyglutamylation-dependent novel antifolates in multiple human leukemia sublines. *Int. J. Cancer* 103:587-599.

Liu M, Ge Y, Payton SG, Aboukameel A, Buck S, Flatley RM, Haska C, Mohammad R, Taub JW and Matherly LH (2006) Transcriptional regulation of the human reduced folate carrier in childhood acute lymphoblastic leukemia cells. *Clin. Cancer Res.* 12:608-616.

Longo GS, Gorlick R, Tong WP, Lin S, Steinherz P and Bertino JR (1997) gamma-Glutamyl hydrolase and folylpolyglutamate synthetase activities predict polyglutamylation of methotrexate in acute leukemias. *Oncol. Res.* 9:259-263.

Lu K, Yin MB, McGuire JJ, Bonmassar E and Rustum YM (1995) Mechanisms of resistance to N-[5-[N-(3,4-dihydro-2-methyl-4-   oxoquinazolin-6-ylmethyl)-N-methylamino]-2-thenoyl]-L-glutamic acid (ZD1694), a folate-based thymidylate synthase inhibitor, in the HCT-8 human ileocecal adenocarcinoma cell line. *Biochem. Pharmacol.* 50:391-398.

Maliepaard M, Scheffer GL, Faneyte IF, van Gastelen MA, Pijnenborg AC, Schinkel AH, van De Vijver MJ, Scheper RJ and Schellens JH (2001) Subcellular localization and distribution of the breast cancer resistance protein transporter in normal human tissues. *Cancer Res.* 61:3458-3464.

Mao Q and Unadkat JD (2005) Role of the breast cancer resistance protein (ABCG2) in drug transport. *AAPS J.* 7:E118-133.

Mauritz R, Peters GJ, Priest DG, Assaraf YG, Drori S, Kathmann I, Noordhuis P, Bunni MA, Rosowsky A, Schornagel JH, Pinedo HM and Jansen G (2002) Multiple mechanisms of resistance to methotrexate and novel antifolates in human CCRF-CEM leukemia cells and their implications for folate homeostasis. *Biochem. Pharmacol.* 63:105-115.

McGuire JJ, Haile WH, Russell CA, Galvin JM and Shane B (1995) Evolution of drug resistance in CCRF-CEM human leukemia cells selected by intermittent methotrexate exposure. *Oncol. Res.* 7:535-543.

McGuire JJ, Russell CA and Balinska M (2000) Human cytosolic and mitochondrial folylpolyglutamate synthetase are electrophoretically distinct. Expression in antifolate-sensitive and -resistant human cell lines. *J. Biol. Chem.* 275:13012-13016.

Melera PW, Davide JP and Oen H (1988) Antifolate-resistant Chinese hamster cells. Molecular basis for the biochemical and structural heterogeneity among dihydrofolate reductases produced by drug-sensitive and drug-resistant cell lines. *J. Biol. Chem.* 263: 1978-1990.

Mini E, Srimatkandada S, Medina WD, Moroson BA, Carman MD and Bertino JR (1985) Molecular and karyological analysis of methotrexate-resistant and -sensitive human leukemic CCRF-CEM cells. *Cancer Res.* 45:317-324.

Moscow JA, Connolly T, Myers TG, Cheng CC, Paull K and Cowan KH (1997) Reduced folate carrier gene (RFC1) expression and anti-folate resistance in transfected and non-selected cell lines. *Int. J. Cancer* 72:184-190.

Payton SG, Whetstine JR, Ge Y and Matherly LH (2005) Transcriptional regulation of the human reduced folate carrier promoter C: synergistic transactivation by Sp1 and C/EBP beta and identification of a downstream repressor. *Biochim. Biophys. Acta* 1727:45-57.

Prasad PD, Ramamoorthy S, Leibach FH and Ganapathy V (1995) Molecular cloning of the human placental folate transporter. *Biochem. Biophys. Res. Commun.* 206:681-687.

Qiu A, Jansen M, Sakaris A, Min SH, Chattopadhyay S, Tsai E, Sandoval C, Zhao R, Akabas MH and Goldman ID (2006) Identification of an intestinal folate transporter and the molecular basis for hereditary folate malabsorption. *Cell* 127:917-928.

Qiu A, Min SH, Jansen M, Malhotra U, Tsai E, Cabelof DC, Matherly LH, Zhao R, Akabas MH and Goldman ID (2007) Rodent intestinal folate transporters (SLC46A1): secondary structure, functional properties, and response to dietary folate restriction. *Am. J. Physiol. Cell Physiol.* 293:C1669-1678.

Ranganathan P, Culverhouse R, Marsh S, Mody A, Scott-Horton TJ, Brasington R, Joseph A, Reddy V, Eisen S and McLeod HL (2008) Methotrexate (MTX) pathway gene polymorphisms and their effects on MTX toxicity in Caucasian and African American patients with rheumatoid arthritis. *J. Rheumatol.* 35:572-579.

Ratnam M, Marquardt H, Duhring JL and Freisheim JH (1989) Homologous membrane folate binding proteins in human placenta: cloning and sequence of a cDNA. *Biochemistry* 28:8249-8254.

Rau T, Erney B, Gores R, Eschenhagen T, Beck J and Langer T (2006) High-dose methotrexate in pediatric acute lymphoblastic leukemia: impact of ABCC2 polymorphisms on plasma concentrations. *Clin. Pharmacol. Ther.* 80:468-476.

Rhee MS, Wang Y, Nair MG and Galivan J (1993) Acquisition of resistance to antifolates caused by enhanced gamma-glutamyl hydrolase activity. *Cancer Res.* 53:2227-2230.

Rosenquist TH, Ratashak SA and Selhub J (1996) Homocysteine induces congenital defects of the heart and neural tube: effect of folic acid. *Proc. Natl. Acad. Sci. USA* 93:15227-15232.

Rots MG, Pieters R, Peters GJ, Noordhuis P, van Zantwijk CH, Kaspers GJ, Hahlen K, Creutzig U, Veerman AJ and Jansen G (1999) Role of folylpolyglutamate synthetase and folylpolyglutamate hydrolase in methotrexate accumulation and polyglutamylation in childhood leukemia. *Blood* 93:1677-1683.

Rots MG, Willey JC, Jansen G, Van Zantwijk CH, Noordhuis P, DeMuth JP, Kuiper E, Veerman AJ, Pieters R and Peters GJ (2000) mRNA expression levels of methotrexate resistance-related proteins in childhood leukemia as determined by a standardized competitive template-based RT-PCR method. *Leukemia* 14:2166-2175.

Roy K, Egan MG, Sirlin S and Sirotnak FM (1997) Posttranscriptionally mediated decreases in folylpolyglutamate synthetase gene expression in some folate analogue-resistant variants of the L1210 cell. Evidence for an altered cognate mRNA in the variants affecting the rate of de novo synthesis of the enzyme. *J. Biol. Chem.* 272:6903-6908.

Sadasivan E and Rothenberg SP (1989) The complete amino acid sequence of a human folate binding protein from KB cells determined from the cDNA. *J. Biol. Chem.* 264:5806-5811.

Sanghani SP, Sanghani PC and Moran RG (1999) Identification of three key active site residues in the C-terminal domain of human recombinant folylpoly-gamma-glutamate synthetase by site-directed mutagenesis. *J. Biol. Chem.* 274:27018-27027.

Schmitz JC, Liu J, Lin X, Chen TM, Yan W, Tai N, Gollerkeri A and Chu E (2001) Translational regulation as a novel mechanism for the development of cellular drug resistance. *Cancer Metastasis Rev.* 20:33-41.

Schneider E and Ryan TJ (2006) Gamma-glutamyl hydrolase and drug resistance. *Clin. Chim. Acta* 374:25-32.

Schuetz JD, Westin EH, Matherly LH, Pincus R, Swerdlow PS and Goldman ID (1989) Membrane protein changes in an L1210 leukemia cell line with a translocation defect in the methotrexate-tetrahydrofolate cofactor transport carrier. *J. Biol. Chem.* 264:16261-16267.

Shafran A, Ifergan I, Bram E, Jansen G, Kathmann I, Peters GJ, Robey RW, Bates SE and Assaraf YG (2005) ABCG2 harboring the Gly482 mutation confers high-level resistance to various hydrophilic antifolates. *Cancer Res.* 65:8414-8422.

Sierra EE, Brigle KE, Spinella MJ and Goldman ID (1995) Comparison of transport properties of the reduced folate carrier and folate receptor in murine L1210 leukemia cells. *Biochem. Pharmacol.* 50:1287-1294.

Sierra EE and Goldman ID (1998) Characterization of folate transport mediated by a low pH route in mouse L1210 leukemia cells with defective reduced folate carrier function. *Biochem. Pharmacol.* 55:1505-1512.

Simonsen CC and Levinson AD (1983) Isolation and expression of an altered mouse dihydrofolate reductase cDNA. *Proc. Natl. Acad. Sci. USA* 80:2495-2499.

Sowers R, Toguchida J, Qin J, Meyers PA, Healey JH, Huvos A, Banerjee D, Bertino JR and Gorlick R (2003) mRNA expression levels of E2F transcription factors correlate with dihydrofolate reductase, reduced folate carrier, and thymidylate synthase mRNA expression in osteosarcoma. *Mol. Cancer Ther.* 2:535-541.

Spencer HT, Sorrentino BP, Pui CH, Chunduru SK, Sleep SE and Blakley RL (1996) Mutations in the gene for human dihydrofolate reductase: an unlikely cause of clinical relapse in pediatric leukemia after therapy with methotrexate. *Leukemia* 10:439-446.

Subramanian VS, Reidling JC and Said HM (2008) Differentiation-dependent regulation of the intestinal folate uptake process: studies with Caco-2 cells and native mouse intestine. *Am. J. Physiol. Cell Physiol.* 295:C828-835.

Suzuki K, Doki K, Homma M, Tamaki H, Hori S, Ohtani H, Sawada Y and Kohda Y (2009) Co-administration of proton pump inhibitors delays elimination of plasma methotrexate in high-dose methotrexate therapy. *Br. J. Clin. Pharmacol.* 67:44-49.

Tiwari AK, Sodani K, Dai CL, Ashby CR, Jr. and Chen ZS (2011) Revisiting the ABCs of multidrug resistance in cancer chemotherapy. *Curr. Pharm. Biotechnol.* 12:570-594.

Tong Y, Liu-Chen X, Ercikan-Abali EA, Capiaux GM, Zhao SC, Banerjee D and Bertino JR (1998a) Isolation and characterization of thymitaq (AG337) and 5-fluoro-2-deoxyuridylate-resistant mutants of human thymidylate synthase from ethyl methanesulfonate-exposed human sarcoma HT1080 cells. *J. Biol. Chem.* 273:11611-11618.

Tong Y, Liu-Chen X, Ercikan-Abali EA, Zhao SC, Banerjee D, Maley F and Bertino JR (1998b) Probing the folate-binding site of human thymidylate synthase by site-directed mutagenesis. Generation of mutants that confer resistance to raltitrexed, Thymitaq, and BW1843U89. *J. Biol. Chem.* 273:31209-31214.

Trent JM, Buick RN, Olson S, Horns RC, Jr. and Schimke RT (1984) Cytologic evidence for gene amplification in methotrexate-resistant cells obtained from a patient with ovarian adenocarcinoma. *J. Clin. Oncol.* 2:8-15.

Tse A, Brigle K, Taylor SM and Moran RG (1998) Mutations in the reduced folate carrier gene which confer dominant resistance to 5,10-dideazatetrahydrofolate. *J. Biol. Chem.* 273:25953-25960.

Tse A and Moran RG (1998) Cellular folates prevent polyglutamation of 5, 10-dideazatetrahydrofolate. A novel mechanism of resistance to folate antimetabolites. *J. Biol. Chem.* 273:25944-25952.

van der Heijden JW, Oerlemans R, Tak PP, Assaraf YG, Kraan MC, Scheffer GL, van der Laken CJ, Lems WF, Scheper RJ, Dijkmans BA and Jansen G (2009) Involvement of breast cancer resistance protein expression on rheumatoid arthritis synovial tissue macrophages in resistance to methotrexate and leflunomide. *Arthritis Rheum.* 60:669-677.

van der Kooij SM, Wessels JA, Huizinga TW and Guchelaar HJ (2008) Comment on: The pharmacogenetics of methotrexate. *Rheumatology (Oxford)* 47:557; author reply 5557-5558.

van der Straaten RJ, Wessels JA, de Vries-Bouwstra JK, Goekoop-Ruiterman YP, Allaart CF, Bogaartz J, Tiller M, Huizinga TW and Guchelaar HJ (2007) Exploratory analysis of four polymorphisms in human GGH and FPGS genes and their effect in methotrexate-treated rheumatoid arthritis patients. *Pharmacogenomics* 8:141-150.

van der Wilt CL, Backus HH, Smid K, Comijn L, Veerman G, Wouters D, Voorn DA, Priest DG, Bunni MA, Mitchell F, Jackman AL, Jansen G and Peters GJ (2001) Modulation of both endogenous folates and thymidine enhance the therapeutic efficacy of thymidylate synthase inhibitors. *Cancer Res.* 61:3675-3681.

Vlaming ML, Pala Z, van Esch A, Wagenaar E, de Waart DR, van de Wetering K, van der Kruijssen CM, Oude Elferink RP, van Tellingen O and Schinkel AH (2009a) Functionally overlapping roles of Abcg2 (Bcrp1) and Abcc2 (Mrp2) in the elimination of methotrexate and its main toxic metabolite 7-hydroxymethotrexate in vivo. *Clin. Cancer Res.* 15:3084-3093.

Vlaming ML, van Esch A, Pala Z, Wagenaar E, van de Wetering K, van Tellingen O and Schinkel AH (2009b) Abcc2 (Mrp2), Abcc3 (Mrp3), and Abcg2 (Bcrp1) are the main determinants for rapid elimination of methotrexate and its toxic metabolite 7-hydroxymethotrexate in vivo. *Mol. Cancer Ther.* 8:3350-3359.

Vlaming ML, van Esch A, van de Steeg E, Pala Z, Wagenaar E, van Tellingen O and Schinkel AH (2011) Impact of abcc2 [multidrug resistance-associated protein (mrp) 2], abcc3 (mrp3), and abcg2 (breast cancer resistance protein) on the oral pharmacokinetics of methotrexate and its main metabolite 7-hydroxymethotrexate. *Drug Metab. Dispos.* 39:1338-1344.

Volk EL, Farley KM, Wu Y, Li F, Robey RW and Schneider E (2002) Overexpression of wild-type breast cancer resistance protein mediates methotrexate resistance. *Cancer Res.* 62:5035-5040.

Volk EL and Schneider E (2003) Wild-type breast cancer resistance protein (BCRP/ABCG2) is a methotrexate polyglutamate transporter. *Cancer Res.* 63:5538-5543.

Walling J (2006) From methotrexate to pemetrexed and beyond. A review of the pharmacodynamic and clinical properties of antifolates. *Invest. New Drugs* 24:37-77.

Wang TL, Diaz LA, Jr., Romans K, Bardelli A, Saha S, Galizia G, Choti M, Donehower R, Parmigiani G, Shih Ie M, Iacobuzio-Donahue C, Kinzler KW, Vogelstein B, Lengauer C and Velculescu VE (2004) Digital karyotyping identifies thymidylate synthase amplification as a mechanism of resistance to 5-fluorouracil in metastatic colorectal cancer patients. *Proc. Natl. Acad. Sci. USA* 101:3089-3094.

Wessels JA, Huizinga TW and Guchelaar HJ (2008) Recent insights in the pharmacological actions of methotrexate in the treatment of rheumatoid arthritis. *Rheumatology (Oxford)* 47:249-255.

Westerhof GR, Jansen G, van Emmerik N, Kathmann I, Rijksen G, Jackman AL and Schornagel JH (1991) Membrane transport of natural folates and antifolate compounds in murine L1210 leukemia cells: role of carrier- and receptor-mediated transport systems. *Cancer Res.* 51:5507-5513.

Wettergren Y, Odin E, Nilsson S, Willen R, Carlsson G and Gustavsson B (2005) Low expression of reduced folate carrier-1 and folylpolyglutamate synthase correlates with lack of a deleted in colorectal carcinoma mRNA splice variant in normal-appearing mucosa of colorectal carcinoma patients. *Cancer Detect. Prev.* 29:348-355.

Whetstine JR and Matherly LH (2001) The basal promoters for the human reduced folate carrier gene are regulated by a GC-box and a cAMP-response element/AP-1-like element. Basis for tissue-specific gene expression. *J. Biol. Chem.* 276:6350-6358.

Wielinga P, Hooijberg JH, Gunnarsdottir S, Kathmann I, Reid G, Zelcer N, van der Born K, de Haas M, van der Heijden I, Kaspers G, Wijnholds J, Jansen G, Peters G and Borst P (2005) The human multidrug resistance protein MRP5 transports folates and can mediate cellular resistance against antifolates. *Cancer Res.* 65:4425-4430.

Winter-Vann AM, Kamen BA, Bergo MO, Young SG, Melnyk S, James SJ and Casey PJ (2003) Targeting Ras signaling through inhibition of carboxyl methylation: an unexpected property of methotrexate. *Proc. Natl. Acad. Sci. USA* 100:6529-6534.

Wong SC, Zhang L, Proefke SA, Hukku B and Matherly LH (1998) Gene amplification and increased expression of the reduced folate carrier in transport elevated K562 cells. *Biochem. Pharmacol.* 55:1135-1138.

Wong SC, Zhang L, Witt TL, Proefke SA, Bhushan A and Matherly LH (1999) Impaired membrane transport in methotrexate-resistant CCRF-CEM cells involves early translation termination and increased turnover of a mutant reduced folate carrier. *J. Biol. Chem.* 274:10388-10394.

Yang CH, Sirotnak FM and Dembo M (1984) Interaction between anions and the reduced folate/methotrexate transport system in L1210 cell plasma membrane vesicles: directional symmetry and anion specificity for differential mobility of loaded and unloaded carrier. *J. Membr. Biol.* 79:285-292.

Yang R, Sowers R, Mazza B, Healey JH, Huvos A, Grier H, Bernstein M, Beardsley GP, Krailo MD, Devidas M, Bertino JR, Meyers PA and Gorlick R (2003) Sequence alterations in the reduced folate carrier are observed in osteosarcoma tumor samples. *Clin. Cancer Res* 9:837-844.

Yao R, Rhee MS and Galivan J (1995) Effects of gamma-glutamyl hydrolase on folyl and antifolylpolyglutamates in cultured H35 hepatoma cells. *Mol. Pharmacol.* 48:505-511.

Zeng H, Chen ZS, Belinsky MG, Rea PA and Kruh GD (2001) Transport of methotrexate (MTX) and folates by multidrug resistance protein (MRP) 3 and MRP1: effect of polyglutamylation on MTX transport. *Cancer Res.* 61:7225-7232.

Zhang K and Rathod PK (2002) Divergent regulation of dihydrofolate reductase between malaria parasite and human host. *Science* 296:545-547.

Zhang L, Taub JW, Williamson M, Wong SC, Hukku B, Pullen J, Ravindranath Y and Matherly LH (1998) Reduced folate carrier gene expression in childhood acute lymphoblastic leukemia: relationship to immunophenotype and ploidy. *Clin. Cancer Res.* 4:2169-2177.

Zhao R, Assaraf YG and Goldman ID (1998) A reduced folate carrier mutation produces substrate-dependent alterations in carrier mobility in murine leukemia cells and methotrexate resistance with conservation of growth in 5-formyltetrahydrofolate. *J. Biol. Chem.* 273:7873-7879.

Zhao R, Gao F and Goldman ID (2001a) Marked suppression of the activity of some, but not all, antifolate compounds by augmentation of folate cofactor pools within tumor cells. *Biochem. Pharmacol.* 61:857-865.

Zhao R, Gao F and Goldman ID (2001b) Molecular cloning of human thiamin pyrophosphokinase. *Biochim. Biophys. Acta* 1517:320-322.

Zhao R, Gao F, Hanscom M and Goldman ID (2004) A prominent low-pH methotrexate transport activity in human solid tumors: contribution to the preservation of methotrexate pharmacologic activity in HeLa cells lacking the reduced folate carrier. *Clin. Cancer Res.* 10:718-727.

Zhao R and Goldman ID (2003) Resistance to antifolates. *Oncogene* 22:7431-7457.

Zhao R, Min SH, Qiu A, Sakaris A, Goldberg GL, Sandoval C, Malatack JJ, Rosenblatt DS and Goldman ID (2007) The spectrum of mutations in the PCFT gene, coding for an intestinal folate transporter, that are the basis for hereditary folate malabsorption. *Blood* 110:1147-1152.

Zhao R, Sharina IG and Goldman ID (1999) Pattern of mutations that results in loss of reduced folate carrier function under antifolate selective pressure augmented by chemical mutagenesis. *Mol. Pharmacol.* 56:68-76.

Zhao R, Titus S, Gao F, Moran RG and Goldman ID (2000) Molecular analysis of murine leukemia cell lines resistant to 5, 10-dideazatetrahydrofolate identifies several amino acids critical to the function of folylpolyglutamate synthetase. *J. Biol. Chem.* 275:26599-26606.

Index

B

D

E

H

N

Q

R

S

W

Y